Patient
AND
Person

Patient
AND
Person

EMPOWERING INTERPERSONAL
RELATIONSHIPS IN NURSING

Chris Stevenson
Reader in Nursing
School of Health and Social Care, University of Teesside
Middlesbrough, UK

Marion Grieves
Principal Lecturer
School of Health and Social Care, University of Teesside
Middlesbrough, UK

Jane Stein-Parbury
Professor of Mental Health Nursing
South Eastern Sydney Area Health Service and
Faculty of Nursing, Midwifery and Health, University of Technology
Sydney, Australia

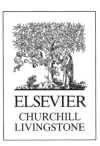

ELSEVIER
CHURCHILL
LIVINGSTONE

ELSEVIER
CHURCHILL
LIVINGSTONE

PATIENT AND PERSON   ISBN 0 443 07475 5
© 2004 Chris Stevenson, Marion Grieves and Jane Stein-Parbury. Published by Elsevier Ltd.
All rights reserved

First published 2004

British Library Cataloguing in Publication Data

A catalogue record for this book is available from the British Library.

Library of Congress Cataloging in Publication Data

A catalog record for this book is available from the Library of Congress.

Commissioning Editor: *Susan Young*
Development Editor: *Catherine Jackson/Kim Benson*
Production Manager: *Yolanta Motylinska*
Design: *Steven Gardiner Ltd, Cambridge*

The
Publisher's
Policy is to use
Paper manufactured
from sustainable forests

Printed in China

CONTENTS

PREFACE

Patient and Person: Developing Interpersonal Skills in Nursing was first published in Australia in 1993. Jane Stein-Parbury offered the text as an aid to nurses who want to learn about establishing interpersonal contact with patients, not as patients but as people. The book encourages readers to practise the use of interpersonal skills in order to have the wherewithal to understand patients' experiences not simply on a theoretical level, important though that is, but on a personal level. The starting point of the book is that nurses need to know that interactions with patients are central to their care, and know how to make those interactions meaningful. Thus, the important skills are isolated and discussed in context later in the book. Stein-Parbury incorporated experiential learning activities and the use of real-life case scenarios to focus on the development of skills in a practical, workable manner, including guidance about what skill to use and when. This new adaptation *Patient and Person: Enacting Empowering Interpersonal Relationships in Nursing* builds on this foundation.

Stein-Parbury recognizes that one of the major changes in the second edition of *Patient and Person* (2000; Australia) is the addition of relevant research findings that serve to reinforce the practice wisdom and expert opinion that filled the pages of the first edition. As she points out, discussion and analysis of relevant research material challenge readers to expand their theoretical understanding of the practical skills of relating to patients. For Stein-Parbury, selecting appropriate research findings from the variety of available published studies proved both challenging and rewarding. We were similarly challenged in producing the new adaptation. It is absolutely necessary to focus and limit the amount of information to keep the book from being unduly long or losing its ease of reading. The task is compounded because the text is generic. It would be impossible to include up-to-date literature that is highly specific, say to risk assessment in Mental Health nursing, because the same would have to be done for all other nursing specialities. With this in mind, although we have added more up-to-date literature, we have tried to do so to support the general principles set out in the text.

Stein-Parbury was aware in producing the 2000 edition that the type of evidence that is available on the topic of patient–nurse relationships is descriptive and theoretical in nature, perhaps not the 'strongest' evidence possible in the sense that cause–effect relationships between health-care interventions and patient outcomes are not established. But as Stein-Parbury points out, the evidence is appropriate because the material in this book is not concerned with clinical interventions as such. It is not a book about psychotherapy, that is, intervening through particular ways of talking to patients in order to alter their thoughts, feelings or behaviours. Rather, it is a book with information about how nurses can be therapeutic in their everyday interactions with patients.

Thus, in Part III of the new adaptation, we merge descriptive and theoretical evidence to explore how empowering interpersonal relationships (between nurses and people/patients and other disciplines) can help to underpin therapeutic encounters. These ideas are presented as two new chapters, 'Empowering interpersonal relationships' and 'Interprofessional working', and in a revision of the existing chapter 'Themes in health and illness', now Chapter 9, 'Health, illness and crisis'. This major change in Part III was made possible because we took previous material on age and cultural differences produced by Sue Nagy and Jackie Crisp and threaded it through the text in order to create space for what we believe to be important concerns for nursing in the early 21st century.

Stein-Parbury recognized that in writing a book about interpersonal aspects of nursing there is a tension between the need to capture the complexity of interpersonal connections and the need to present concrete guidelines and general rules for beginning nurses. She addressed this by emphasizing the need to consider every clinical encounter as a unique, intricate interaction, as well as suggesting guidelines and rules that might support the beginning nurse. In this new adaptation, we have adopted Stein-Parbury's idea and presented Part II as a 'how to' develop and use skills section, although we have chosen to discuss self-awareness in Part I. The material in Part II, therefore, bears a strong resemblance to that in the 2000 edition.

At its inception, *Patient and Person* was intended primarily for use as a textbook for undergraduate nursing courses. The material was prepared in a manner to assist educators planning a programme of interpersonal skill development in these courses. The second edition was academically more rigorous, with the inclusion of a stronger evidence base and probably met the needs of a slightly wider audience. The new adaptation still offers itself to these audiences. However, we have contextualized Part II (on skills development) with a theoretical framework, symbolic interactionism, outlined in Part I. In the new Chapter 1, we argue that symbolic interactionism offers a means for nurses to understand the process of interpersonal interactions and a tool for analysing what happens when interpersonal relationships break down. This meets a general aim of the text (old and new), which is to encourage the reader to consider her/his own reactions and position in relation to the person/patient. The explicit use of the theoretical framework in the revised version of Chapter 2 makes the aim more achievable through providing an exemplar. In Chapter 3 we re-focus on 'Why interpersonal skills?' from a symbolic interactionist perspective. In Chapter 4 we look at the importance of self and self-awareness (in the symbolic interactionist tradition) in establishing how the nurse works out how to present her/himself win the therapeutic encounter. The development of the theoretical framework in Part I and the exploration in Part III of the philosophy of empowerment underpinning care make the text useful for nurses progressing to Master's level.

In the 1993 and 2000 editions, Stein-Parbury chose to use the word 'patient', believing that it is the most commonly used in nursing. She felt that the central point of the book, that patients should be treated as persons, spoke for itself about the humanistic basis of her philosophical beliefs. We have taken a different stance and used the terms 'person/patient' and 'people/patients' where referring to our own ideas, while using 'patient' when reporting more impersonal theory and research. We think that it is worth reflecting the book title through the text as a means of reinforcing the inseparability of the person and their position within health care. As Nyatanga and Dann (2002)[1] point out, the continued use of the term 'patient' militates against empowerment as it reinforces the sick role. In common with previous editions, the term 'nurse' is used in the generic sense to refer to any level of nurse, from students of nursing to experienced registered nurses. However, we would point out that the text would have great relevance for other health disciplines and that the term 'nurse' could have been substituted with the descriptor 'health-care professional'.

Stein-Parbury concluded the Preface to the 1993 edition by stressing that skills are not learnt simply by reading about them in a book. We are in full agreement with her when she points out that the book offers guidelines and suggestions for the development of interpersonal skills in nursing, and that the best way to learn them is through interacting with patients. In listening to and understanding patients' experiences of health and illness, nurses will come to appreciate that their real teachers are the persons who happen to be patients.

Chris Stevenson and Marion Grieves
Teesside 2004

---

[1] Nyatanga, L. and Dann K. L. (2002) 'Empowerment in nursing: the role of philosophical and psychological factors'. *Nursing Philosophy* 3: 234–9.

ACKNOWLEDGEMENTS

The new adaptation of this book was based on the previous work of Jane Stein-Parbury and her contribution cannot be over-stated. It is fitting, therefore, to adopt part of her (2000 edition) acknowledgements: 'A special note of appreciation is extended to all of the students of nursing whom I have had the pleasure of teaching over the years. Your questions, although often challenging, expanded my thinking, sharpened my focus and enriched my insights into the struggles of learning interpersonal skills. The many experiences that you shared in class helped in the development of the stories in this book. Also, your comments on the activities used in this book assisted in their development and refinement'.

We appreciate the assistance provided by Elsevier, especially Susan Young and Catherine Jackson.

We would also like to acknowledge the support received from our colleagues in the Mental Health, Learning Disabilities and Child teams who shared their experiences to enable us to ensure that the accounts in this book reflect interpersonal issues for students entering their chosen pathway of care.

We would like to acknowledge our families' continuing support and patience over the past year, with a special mention from Marion to David, Anne and Alan for being excellent sounding boards, and Paul and Sue for their valued discussions on the interpersonal skill requirements for care providers in the mental health environment.

Chris Stevenson
Marion Grieves

LIST OF ACTIVITIES

In the text, activities are differentiated by symbols in the left margin:

indicates that the activity is to be completed in solitude.

indicates that the activity requires group interaction and discussion.

indicates that the activity can be completed in solitude, although learning is enhanced through group interaction.

Part I

THE INTERPERSONAL RELATIONSHIP: THEORY AND SKILLS

In Part I of the book we make clear our position that all nursing care takes place in the context of interpersonal relations (Peplau 1952). To date, theorizing about interpersonal relationships in nursing has been based in psychodynamic theory, often implying pathology. Nurses need a theoretical tool that will help them to make sense of their interactions with people who are patients in a more constructive way. We think that symbolic interactionism is an appropriate theoretical approach. Its main features are set out in Chapter 1. 'Symbolic interactionism as a theoretical tool for understanding interpersonal relationships in nursing'. In the chapter, symbolic interactionist principles are applied to nursing examples. In Chapter 2. 'The drama of the interpersonal relationship', symbolic interactionism is used to make sense of how the interpersonal relationship and care are negotiated. In Chapter 3. 'Why interpersonal skills?', we illustrate how interpersonal skills are central to the process of negotiation that occurs to establish and maintain the interpersonal relationship and the care that is offered within it. In Chapter 4. 'Self-awareness', we use the symbolic interactionist perspective on self as outlined in Chapter 1 and look at why awareness and assessment of self are important and the routes to achieving them.

Nurses provide the majority of day-to-day care, for people who are patients, although we think that our ideas are relevant to all health disciplines. For this reason in Part I, and throughout the book, we use 'nurse' as a summary term for all levels of nurse and professionals. The book is entitled 'Patient and Person', and the book is oriented towards foregrounding the personal aspects of care. For this reason, we have taken the decision to use the terms 'person/patient' and 'people/ patients' as the most apt descriptors where we are referring to our own position and ideas, but to use 'patient' where more impersonal theories ideas or are being described.

CHAPTER 1

SYMBOLIC INTERACTIONISM AS A THEORETICAL TOOL FOR UNDERSTANDING INTERPERSONAL RELATIONSHIPS IN NURSING

RATIONALE FOR SYMBOLIC INTERACTIONISM AS A THEORETICAL PERSPECTIVE

Nurses need to know how to relate effectively to and interact with people in their care. As such, nursing is a social activity. In addition to being technically proficient, nurses need to be socially competent. Peplau (1952) goes so far as to say that the interpersonal relationship is the crux of nursing. The quality of the relationship therefore, by definition, has a huge impact on the whole of the care process.

In our experience, it is easy to teach nurses to use certain 'core' skills in relation to interacting with others. They can rehearse and become competent in these skills. In Part II of this book we devote some space to helping nurses do just this. However, the reality of nursing practice is that it is a context in which the unexpected often happens, because nursing involves people who have different needs and expectations and preferences. Dealing with the unusual demands a special kind of nurse, using a special kind of nursing. In particular, we think that a nurse prepared with theoretical as well as practical abilities can operate in a more responsive way. Having recourse to 'practical theory' can help the nurse to understand what has happened, work with what is happening and predict what might happen next.

Much of nursing involves 'performance', by which we mean acting together with the person/patient and professional colleagues in order to produce 'health outcomes'. Performances may be scripted or improvised. A study by Haney *et al.* (1973) demonstrates the power of scripted performance via an experiment with a simulated prison. The researchers randomly allocated male college students to role-play either prison guards or prisoners for eight hours a day. The students stayed in role for nearly one full week. Neither of the groups was trained or otherwise prepared to take on the roles. Using multiple measures, Haney *et al.* found that the '. . . simulated prison developed into a psychologically compelling prison environment'. It elicited strong and often pathological responses from many of the participants.

> The prisoners experienced a loss of personal identity and the arbitrary control of their behaviours which resulted in a syndrome of passivity, dependency, depression and helplessness. In contrast, the guards (with rare exceptions) experienced a marked gain in social power, status and group identification which made the role playing rewarding. (Haney *et al.* 1973: 69)

The study demonstrates the power of context and language (in this case, labelling) in constructing who we are and how we act and interact. For the nurse, using the knowledge, skills and competencies that are attached to specific care situations amounts to a scripted performance.

However, in nursing, the nurse often has no well-defined script to follow, as the unpredictable occurs. In this circumstance, the nurse has to have a means to reflect on the process of what is occurring, second by second, minute by minute and hour by hour in order to make her/himself up as s/he goes along (Peplau 1952). In other words s/he must engage in reflection 'in and on practice' Schön (1987) describes. Some nursing theorists, for example Peplau (1952) and Menzies (1961), have used psychodynamic theory to make sense of interpersonal relations, either proactively or retrospectively. Menzies (op. cit.) argued that nurses use ego defence mechanisms, e.g. denial, in order to prevent anxiety provoked by emotionally tense situations. In particular, Menzies noted that nurses tended to avoid contact with dying patients in general medical wards. She believed that anxiety arises because the nurse has her own internal fantasy world, constructed during infancy, in which the child, and people who the child ties with emotionally, play out different relationships. Because of the aggressive forces within the child (id drives), many of the fantasies are negative or destructive. 'Unconsciously, the nurse associates the patient's and relatives' distress with that experienced by the people in her fantasy world, which increases her anxiety and difficulty in handling it' (Menzies Lyth 1988: 48). Thus, Altschul's (1972) finding that nurses spend only 10 per cent of their time with people/ patients and the remainder in the office or completing non-person/patient centred tasks fits with Menzies' analysis.

However, we think that symbolic interactionism can be used as the basis of a practice framework that puts the interpersonal relationship with the person/ patient at the centre. Its advantage over psychodynamic explanations is that there is less tendency to pathologize the individuals involved in the interpersonal encounter. Symbolic interactionism is a theory of human communication that can account for the process by which everyday nursing situations become defined and re-defined. In being together, people act into the actions of the other and so create a sense of who they are, their social abilities and their social world. For example, in dealing with potentially violent episodes, it is common for psychiatric nurses to congregate at 'the scene', in numbers and fast. The action of rushing and the show of strength in numbers is read as 'forceful' by the person who wants to act out her/his dissatisfaction or distress. In response to the reading, s/he begins to create a story about being personally dangerous, which may become a story lived as the person acts into that possibility and lashes out at the nearest nurse. The nurse (and colleagues) may then confirm the 'reading' by restraining the person.

That action creates action is well illustrated by the following two contrasting approaches to surveillance of psychiatric people/patients who are seen as at high risk of harm to self or others. In some acute psychiatric in-person/patient facilities there is a practice of appointing a sentry, someone who watches the door of an open psychiatric ward to alert staff if someone tries to leave the ward while under observation. People/patients are being watched and so behave as if being watched, for example, 'teasing' staff by standing with one foot on either side of the threshold or finding a way to cross over without being noticed and triggering the 'absent without leave' (AWOL) procedure. In contrast, staff at Oakburn Unit, Bradford have abolished sentry and 'special' observations. Instead, they respectfully request that people/patients complete a whereabouts book left at the door of the ward before going out. They have reported a significant drop in the number of people going AWOL, and most of those who do have recorded where they are going (Dodds and Bowles 2001).

CHAPTER OVERVIEW

The chapter aims to help the student understand the basics of symbolic interactionism, how it accounts for the social production of meaning, and the contribution of language and thought. We look at how 'self' is conceptualized within symbolic interactionism, as 'self' is often seen as a nursing tool. In the final section, an exploration of nursing as performance is presented based in symbolic interactionism and using real clinical examples.

SYMBOLIC INTERACTIONISM

Although the roots of symbolic interactionism can be traced back to the eighteenth century (Benzies and Allen 2001), these roots were synthesized into a theory of human 'meaning-making' and action by George Hebert Mead in the early part of the twentieth century. However, Mead never published his work, but passed it on by word of mouth. It was left to his main disciple, Herbert Blumer, to publish Mead's teaching and further develop the theory that Blumer named symbolic interactionism. Put simply, the theory describes the humanizing effect of communication. It is a theory that respects the inseparability of the person from her/his environment. For Blumer, there were three important parts to the theory: meaning, language and thought. We will deal with each in turn, using illustrations from the world of nursing practice.

(i) Meaning and the construction of social reality

Humans are meaning making, in that they constantly seek to ascribe meaning to their social worlds. People act towards people or things on the basis of the meanings they give to those people or things. A good example can be found in the hospital space where people who have deliberately self-harmed meet the nursing face of generalist medicine. The nurses have a shared social meaning for people who overdose as taking up time and resources needed by the 'really ill, poorly people' (Hopkins 2002: 147). In these circumstances, Pembroke (1998) reports feeling alienated when seeking help and a sense of hostility from the potential carers. Thus, the nurses' definition of the self-harm 'situation' has negative outcomes for the person/patient. In other words, the definition of the social reality has real consequences.

As argued above, making meaning is not an end in itself. Rather, the shared social reality is the basis from which to act. Within symbolic interactionism, the accuracy of the definition is not what counts. Rather, it is the agreement that the definition is real. Take another nursing example: the nursing team is gathered in the office for 'report' at the shift change over. They have been looking after Mrs Green, who is described as a 'sweet old lady who never complains and who never makes demands on the nursing staff'. There has been a call from Mrs Green's daughter, who lives abroad and who cannot, therefore, come to visit. Implicitly, Mrs Green is seen as 'worthy' and 'lonely' and in 'need of company'. It is no surprise that through the afternoon nurses are seen on several occasions sitting with Mrs Green and looking at her family photographs.

Meaning-making is a community activity. The construction of meaning does not occur within people's heads. They need cognitive processes to deal with the symbols required for negotiating meaning, for example, in recognizing words, retrieving concepts from memory and having 'inner' conversations referred to below. However, it is through the interaction with others that meaning arises. A negative case might help to make the idea clearer. Community nurses (irrespective of speciality) have a peculiar sphere of practice because they are not in the immediate proximity of other team members. One of the aspects of the role that they often point out is that they have to work autonomously and make decisions immediately in the person's home. This makes their job more demanding. A symbolic interactionist analysis would connect the challenge of working autonomously with the lack of facility for shared 'meaning making' because the practitioner is detached from her/his community. In the ward context, there is the opportunity to try out different ideas in relation to a person's care before reaching a consensus and enacting it. Similarly, interprofessional working discussed in Chapter 11 offers support for re-constructing meaning where it is un-negotiated in the care episode.

(ii) Language is the source of meaning

Within symbolic interactionism, meaning is not deliberately forced. Neither does it necessarily directly reflect some external reality. For example, the words that we use do not of themselves convey an impression about the world. They are symbols that have learned meaning and value for people. We teach children to use a particular word 'cat' to refer to a furry, four-legged, purring animal. However, we could just as easily use the word 'wood' (or any other word) to refer to the same animal if we agreed to do so socially. Of course, our ability to name things is the basis for society. We freight the words with meanings through the use of the words in a social context. For example, if we take the word 'section' the common meaning would be 'a part (noun)' or 'to divide (verb)'. However, in a maternity ward, the word will be freighted with the meaning 'a way of delivering a baby (as in Caesarean section)'; in psychiatry, section refers to compulsory detention (Stevenson and Beech 2001). When we agree certain meanings for a word, we begin to build up a discourse. Discourses are patterns of meaning that organize the systems that people live within, and without which it would be difficult to understand one another. For example, in Western cultures, we have an 'illness discourse' that describes relationships as lay versus professional, nurse versus person/patient, etc. Phrases that are incongruent with the illness discourse, like 'a lay nurse', hold no meaning. We behave as if the illness discourse is simply a natural and universal structure. However, the language is not a way to capture the external reality of a situation. It constructs something that is beyond, though related to, the physical world. Because of this, it is possible for the meaning of a situation to arise from the use of language within that situation. For example, as the word 'section' is used in the context of a particular woman's labour, the situation may come to be understood as not natural or dangerous. Alternatively it may be construed as a positive choice in the case of a woman electing to give birth by that means.

(iii) Thought as a way to take the role of other people

Having the capacity for abstract thought means that people can modify the interpretation of symbols. They do this through having 'inner' conversations – taking a kind of reflective pause – in order to sort out meaning. For example, they may compare past, present and future potential meanings that have been attached to a symbol. They also use symbols in order to take the (theoretical) role of the other. For example, a nurse who encounters a parent who has lost a full-term baby, even if childless herself, has the capacity to read the symbols of grief and put her/himself in the place of the parent. This kind of accomplishment is similar to being able to play a part in a play, a point we develop in Chapter 2.

First, however, we look at the concept of 'self' from a symbolic interactionist perspective. It is important to think about 'self' as nurses often talk about the therapeutic use of self (Travelbee 1971) in relation to their encounters with people/patients. However, whether this is a use of a pre-existing self or a self that is responsive to the situation is not thoroughly discussed in nursing texts. Symbolic interactionism has a well-defined set of ideas in relation to the self that we believe to be helpful in understanding the fluid, reflexive practice of nursing.

THE SELF AND OTHERS

For many people, the self is either something that is given at birth or that develops in response to genetic and environmental factors during the formative years. Once developed, there is an assumption that the self is more or less stable and so it is possible to distinguish the 'real' self. On the other hand, symbolic interactionism describes the self as the product of interconnections of meaning, language and thought. The self is not discovered through introspection, looking inwards, as

Descartes argued. Rather, the self is constructed in two ways: (a) through the person's ability to take the role of the other, for example, the nurse who has her/himself experienced being in hospital for treatment can imagine what the new person/patient is thinking of, or the emotions that are present; or (b) by being able to 'read' the response of the other person to the particular self that we are presenting. For example, if the nurse, as her/his professional self, tries to offer therapy to the person/patient, the person/patient may try to engage the nurse in more ordinary conversation. The nurse reads this as a cue to alter her/his presentation (self) and s/he may tell the person/patient something more personal. The process allows the person to explore the possibilities for self in relation to the reflection offered by the other. Cooley (1902) first described this process, which he named 'the looking-glass self'. Because the processes require the symbolic use of language, self is a function of language. Self is fluid, as it always has the opportunity to adapt according to the reflections that are current.

Of course, we have a sense of self that seems to endure. Harré (1998) has a schema for accounting for the continuous experience of self that is coherent with symbolic interactionism. Harré argues against a 'singular self' (as in one given or developed early in life) in favour of a self that is derived from three factors. First, there is individuality. By this Harré means that we are distinct as people in time and space (rather than genetically). Therefore, our experience of situations is, inevitably, unique. For example, the nurse who is at the bedside of the person necessarily has a different perspective on the person/patient than the nurse who is managing the clinical area. Second, Harré notes that the cluster of attributes, the repertoire, that we have at any one time defines the sense of self. Thus, we can be jealous, open-minded, generous, mean, sad, happy, etc. sequentially and at the same time. For example, a nurse working in a busy emergency care setting may be feeling very organized and competent. However, when a new piece of technology is introduced s/he might feel deskilled and unable to cope – and feel inadequate as a person. Finally, Harré notes that a sense of self is defined through the contact with the community of others who ascribe to us attributes, dispositions and skills. For example, the student nurse who encounters a nursing team who identifies her/his strengths is likely to have a different sense of self than a learner who is consistently evaluated in terms of deficits.

Why is this relevant for nurses? If nurses are to use the interpersonal interaction as the foundation for caring, then it is critical to have an understanding of people, a theory of human nature. Theories that suggest the rigidity of self underpin a view that the person (as person/patient or as nurse) is not going to present her/himself in different ways on different occasions. It allows people to state, 'S/he is just a dependent personality' or 'I am the kind of person who likes to concentrate on nursing tasks'. Yet, common sense tells us that we are different people on different occasions and in different contexts. If we think that people are constantly making themselves up as they go along (Peplau 1952), then each encounter is an opportunity for change.

In this book, the emphasis is on the person/patient as a person, and on how interpersonal skills are the foundation of nursing practice. Interpersonal skills are important for without the skills to 'read', understand and interpret the symbols of communication, 'senses of self' and shared meaning cannot be built. When we talk about interpersonal skills in the remainder of this book, we are helping the reader to rehearse the use of these skills in order that s/he can function in the interpersonal encounter with a presentation that is helpful. It is to this perform-ative function that we turn next.

NURSE/PERSON/PATIENT PERFORMANCE: KNOWING YOU, KNOWING ME

When we take a symbolic interactionist perspective on nursing as everyday activity, we can understand better how nurses can present a professional persona while, simultaneously, being responsive to the situations that they encounter. It can also help us to make sense of how some problems arise in working with people who are patients.

As a person/patient comes to the encounter with the nurse, s/he expects a high level of professionalism. To some extent, this is judged with reference to how consistent and coherent the nurse's actions are. In other words, how far nurses have a shared social identity – a front – that is demonstrated in 'manner', 'appear-ance' and 'behaviour'. As Goffman puts it, the front is 'that part of an individual's performance which regularly functions in a general and fixed fashion to define the situation for those who observe the performance' (Goffman 1959: 22). Taking some nursing examples, it is customary for nurses in many clinical settings to wear a uniform and to adhere to certain standards of personal hygiene and appearance. Another example is the practice of offering people/patients an explanation of the procedure that they are about to be involved in. At a more macro level, there are behaviours that are prescribed and proscribed by the Nursing and Midwifery Council that govern nursing performance in practice. In relation to Harré's description of the sense of self, this represents the ascription of attributes, disposition and skills by the community of significant others. In order to perform professionally from the 'other's' point of view, one important attribute the nurse is meant to embody is knowledge in relation to people/patients and their needs.

In synthesizing results of field studies in a variety of nursing settings, Liaschenko and Fisher (1999) have differentiated three different types of knowl-edge that nurses use in their work. The first of these knowledge types is referred to by Liaschenko and Fisher (1999) as *case knowledge*. This is knowledge generalized and objective, and includes areas such as the knowledge of anatomy and physiology, physical disease processes and pharmacology. The knowledge is based on statistics and probabilities of the clinical situation. Nurses need not interact with people/patients in order to use this knowledge. They can understand the mechanics of a myocardial infarction without ever seeing a person/patient who has experienced one. In symbolic interactionist terms, this is the kind of 'background knowledge' that may be used within an encounter with the person, according to how the nurse reads the individual person/patient's need for factual information.

The second type of knowledge in Liaschenko and Fisher's (1999) schema is referred to as *patient knowledge*. It is the knowledge of how individual people/patients are responding to their clinical situations. This knowledge allows nurses to negotiate the care of people/patients within a health care system The type of knowing is based on an understanding of what individual people/patients are experiencing and so it requires interaction between the nurse and person/ patient.

A third type of knowledge involves an understanding of the unique individuality of the person/patient, knowing the person/patient's personal and private biography and understanding how that person's actions make sense for them. It is *person knowledge*. Patient knowledge and person knowledge encompass what is currently identified in the nursing literature as 'knowing the person/patient' (Henderson 1997; Liaschenko 1997; Radwin 1995a) – 'knowing you' – and associated with expert clinical nursing practice (Benner *et al.* 1992). Knowing the person/patient aids clinical decision-making (Radwin 1995a; Tanner *et al.* 1993; Jenks 1993; Jenny and Logan 1992).

In symbolic interactionist terms, these kinds of knowledge are important because they are readings of the situation of the person/patient and of their presentation. Reading the symbols within the situation, and being able to take the role of the other, in turn defines the presentation of the nurse (her/his nursing self – 'knowing me'). 'Knowing you–knowing me–knowing you' implies a joint performance from which a tailored package of care can emerge. What constitutes care is socially agreed. Thus, clinical decision-making is not based simply in case knowledge or patient knowledge or person knowledge, although all three are important. For example, nurses in Jenny and Logan's (1992) study used individual responses in determining how to wean the person/patient from mechanical ventilation. The physiology of respiratory functioning and the mechanics of artificial ventilation provide nurses with 'case knowledge' (Liaschenko and Fisher 1999) based on standardized, statistical evidence, generalizable to a majority of people/patients. Case knowledge of this kind is part of the professional front. But the professional front, while expected, might be experienced as over-rigid if maintained without reference to the evolving interpersonal relationship where patient and person knowledge becomes available. Nurses in Jenny and Logan's study also used knowledge of how an individual person/patient was responding to the gradual discontinuation of mechanical ventilation. The nurses took 'readings' of the people/patients' responses to their nursing actions, and adapted care accordingly, even though the people/patients were unable to communicate verbally.

NURSING PERFORMANCE

Working with people who are patients is not straightforward, and this is where symbolic interactionism as a tool to reflect in and on practice is invaluable. Barnhart (1994) rightly points out that symbolic interactionism as applied to everyday activities provides a detailed description and analysis of process. Jackson and Stevenson (2000) studied what people need psychiatric and mental health nurses for. They found that people/patients wanted nurses to be able to anticipate when a friendly, ordinary approach was called for and when they wanted an expert therapeutic encounter. Jackson and Stevenson (op. cit.) concluded that a symbolic interactionist analysis might help to unpick how these different meanings of the situation emerge. Here we offer two examples of just what such an analysis might lead us to.

(i)   *The 'good and bad person/patient'*   Sometimes nurses describe people/
        patients in evaluative terms, as good or bad. The judgement is often based
        on an assessment of how demanding (physically or emotionally) the person
        is, and reference to case knowledge may be made to establish if the
        person/patient is over-reacting to the illness. However, once the description
        arises it becomes a self-fulfilling prophecy. The expectation that the good
        or bad person/patient will behave in certain ways evokes responses that
        confirm what was originally expected. Indeed, as each of us affects how
        others view themselves, the person/patient her/himself may adhere to the
        good/bad descriptor.

(ii)   *Diagnosis as 'naming'*   In health care, we often try to assign a diagnosis
        based on symptoms and signs, on case knowledge. The diagnosis becomes
        a symbol of disease. We justify this as a means to ensure that a proper
        treatment regime is established. However, when the person is described as a
        diagnosis, they become only the diagnosis and this forces the person/patient
        to view her/himself through the lens of that diagnosis. Of course, this is
        an inaccurate reflection in that it represses the individuality of the person/
        patient. For example, Aldridge and Stevenson (2001) describe their
        encounter with Beth, a person who had been described as schizophrenic.
        Initially, Beth had wanted a diagnosis in order to help her account for some
        of the altered states of reality that she was experiencing. However, she
        quickly learnt that the diagnosis invaded other parts of her life, so that
        she was treated differently, either with artificial 'niceness' or with obstacles
        if she wanted to do things that would be available to ordinary people. Beth's
        own words illustrate:

> [T]here's a bad press of mental illness. . . . If I applied for a normal job
> I doubt I would get some work. . . . Recently, I sent off for a charity
> parachute jump . . . and it had a lot, one of these things, and if you had
> any of these . . . one of them was a mental illness . . . they wouldn't let
> you jump . . . maybe they think you're not going to pull the cord! At the
> optician's they ask you what medications you're on and what they are
> . . . so I said antipsychotic and ever since then the receptionist says, 'HI
> YA BETH, HI YA!' . . . it feels they're being jolly *in case*. (Aldridge and
> Stevenson 2001, 25–6)

These examples demonstrate how the interpretation of language and symbols
and expectations of others within interpersonal relationships can serve to create
shared meaning. But they serve also as a warning that we need to pay attention to
these factors in our encounters with people/patients. Meanings can become one-
sided or out of date and need to be re-worked. For, to paraphrase Blumer (1986),
when people define a situation as real, it is real in its consequences.

CHAPTER SUMMARY

In this chapter we have established that interpersonal relationships are an integral
part of nursing. We have set out our rationale for why nurses need to have
a theoretical framework for understanding the processes and outcomes of

interpersonal relationships. Symbolic interactionism is an approach that can help in understanding the everyday realities of practice. It is a way to analyse how social reality is constructed through language and interpretation. It helps us to see nursing as performance, based in the ways that nurse and person/patient call and respond to one another.

In Chapter 2. 'The drama of the interpersonal relationship', we build on the symbolic interactionist approach to interpersonal relationships by looking in more detail at how the interpersonal relationship is defined, and how a shared meaning of caring arises. In Chapter 3. 'Why interpersonal skills?' we develop the argument that nurses need interpersonal skills in order to present a professional persona and to be proficient in reading and responding to the symbols of communication in their encounters with people/patients.

REFERENCES

Aldridge, D. and Stevenson, C. (2001). Social poetics as research and practice: living in and learning from the process of research. *Nursing Inquiry*, 8, 19–27.

Altschul, A. (1972). *Patient–Nurse Interactions*. Edinburgh: Churchill Livingstone.

Barnhart, A. (1994). *Erving Goffman: The Presentation of Self in Everyday Life.* www.cfmc.com/adamb/writings/goffman.htm (Accessed 30 June 2003).

Benner, P., Tanner, C. and Chesla, C. (1992). From beginner to expert: gaining a differentiated clinical world in critical care nursing. *Advances in Nursing Science*, 14(3), 13–28.

Benzies, K. M. and Allen, N. N. (2001). Symbolic interactionism as a theoretical perspective for multiple method research. *Journal of Advanced Nursing*, 33(4), 541–7.

Blumer, H. (1986). *Symbolic Interactionism*. California: University of California Press.

Cooley, C. H. (1902). Human Nature and Social Order. New York: Scribners.

Dodds, P. and Bowles, N. (2001). Commentary. Dismantling formal observation and refocusing nursing activity in acute inpatient psychiatry: a case study. [Journal article case study]. *Journal of Psychiatric & Mental Health Nursing*, 8(2), 183–8.

Goffman, E. (1959). *The Presentation of Self in Everyday Life*. New York: Doubleday.

Haney, C., Banks, C. and Zimbardo, P. (1973). Interpersonal dynamics in a simulated prison. *International Journal of Criminology and Penology*, 1: 69–97.

Harré, R. (1998). *The Singular Self*. London: Sage.

Henderson, S. (1997). Knowing the patient and the impact on patient participation: a grounded theory study. *International Journal of Nursing Practice*, 3, 111–18.

Hopkins, C. (2002). 'But what about the really ill, poorly people?' (An ethnographic study into what it means to nurses on medical admissions units to have people who have harmed themselves as their patients). *Journal of Psychiatric and Mental Health Nursing*, 9(2), 147–54.

Jackson, S. and Stevenson, C. (2000). What do people need psychiatric and mental health nurses for? *Journal of Advanced Nursing*, 31, 378–88.

Jenks, J. M. (1993). The pattern of personal knowing in nurses' clinical decision making. *Journal of Nursing Education*, 32(9), 399–415.

Jenny, J. and Logan, J. (1992). Knowing the patient: one aspect of clinical knowledge. *Image: Journal of Nursing Scholarship*, 24(4), 254–8.

Liaschenko, J. and Fisher, A. (1999). Theorizing the knowledge that nurses use in the conduct of their work. *Scholarly Inquiry for Nursing Practice: An International Journal*, 13(1), 29–41.

Liaschenko, J. (1997). Knowing the patient? In S. E. Thorne and V. E. Hayes (eds), *Nursing Praxis: Knowledge and Action* (pp. 23–38). Thousand Oaks, CA: Sage.

Menzies, I. (1961). A case study of the functioning of social systems as a defence against anxiety. *Human Relations*, 13(2), 95–123.

Menzies Lyth, I. (1988). *Containing Anxiety in Institutions*. London: Free Association Press.

Pembroke, L. (1998). Self-harm – a personal story. *Mental Health Practice*, 2(3): 22–4.

Peplau, H. (1952). *Interpersonal Relations in Nursing*. New York: Putnam.

Radwin, L. E. (1995a). Knowing the patient: a process model for individualized interventions. *Nursing Research*, 44(6), 364–70.

Schön, D. (1987). *Educating the Reflective Practitioner*. San Francisco: Jossey-Bass.

Stevenson, C. and Beech, I. (2001). Paradigms lost, paradigms regained: defending nursing against a single reading of postmodernism. *Nursing Philosophy*, 2, 143–50.

Tanner, C., Benner, P., Chesla, C. and Gordon, D. R. (1993). The phenomenology of knowing the patient. *Image: Journal of Nursing Scholarship*, 25(4), 273–80.

Travelbee, J. (1971). *Interpersonal Aspects of Nursing*. Philadelphia, PA: F. A. Davis.

CHAPTER 2

THE DRAMA OF THE INTERPERSONAL RELATIONSHIP

INTRODUCTION: INTERPERSONAL RELATIONSHIPS IN NURSING HISTORY

Interpersonal relationships between people/patients and nurses humanize nursing care because the relationships are the vehicles through which nurses are responsive to people/patients' subjective experiences. The relationship meshes the nurse's compassion and knowledge with the person/patient's experience. Through their relationships with people/patients, nurses express concern, care and commitment. In the absence of interpersonal relationships with nurses, patients can be viewed as objects, clinical conditions or a set of problems to be solved. Nursing care that is offered without a human connection is impoverished. Peplau (1952) believed that the nurse needs to be sensitive to the person/patient's need at different times and adopt a role of 'friend' or 'teacher' or 'parental figure', and so on, accordingly. Almost 50 years later, Jackson and Stevenson (2000) have supported Peplau's findings in a study that researched 'What do people need psychiatric and mental health nurses for?' They found that people wanted nurses to 'toggle' along a continuum of friend to professional. People expected nurses to be able to divine, or somehow read, what particular nursing response was required at a given time.

A connection is created by the way nurses and people/patients interact, and every interaction between person/patient and nurse takes place within the overall context of an interpersonal relationship. For example, listening without judging and responding with understanding symbolically represent the will to create a relationship based on acceptance and respect. Thus, each interaction helps to develop and define the relationship, but each interaction is merely a snapshot of the entire moving picture that is the relationship.

The act of aligning oneself alongside another person, in an attempt to help or be of assistance, serves to distinguish that interpersonal relationship from other social relationships. How nurses relate to and are with people/patients creates their own sense of self as a nurse. In this sense, understanding the nature of the relationship between nurse and person/patient is akin to understanding the nature of nursing itself. For these reasons, it is not surprising that the exploration of interpersonal relations in nursing has a long history. For example, Nightingale's (1859) *Notes on Nursing* contains numerous references to the need to understand the idiosyncrasies of individual people/patients and how to relate to them.

From the standpoint of symbolic interactionism, each individual person/patient's point of view and expectations is a communication that affects the response of the nurse, which, in turn, affects the views of the person/patient. Thus, the basis of the relationship between nurses and people/patients is mutual understanding – alignment that enables them to engage in mutual endeavours. Through the process of alignment, nurses are able to work out with people/patients what might be of most benefit in terms of care.

Despite the lengthy history, there are claims that centralizing the interpersonal relationship between person/patient and nurse is a new concern (see, for example, Barthow 1997; Porter 1994; May 1992b; Ramos 1992; Salvage 1990). Making explicit the beneficial aspects of interpersonal interventions (helping people/patients by talking and relating to them) is an attempt to move away from care that is predominantly physical and task oriented. An orientation toward the completion of tasks is associated with the nurse's functional role in a health care organization, that is, a job. Under such an impersonal system, nurses are discouraged from relating to individual people/patients because doing so has the potential to distract them from their allocated tasks (May 1993). Likewise, work is organized in such a way to protect nurses from involvement. People/patients are regarded as sets of tasks and nurses are regarded as sets of skills to accomplish the tasks. Unfortunately, the political agenda reinforces this state of affairs. For example, DoH (2003a) promotes combining tasks in a different way to develop new roles; DoH (2003b) acknowledges that knowledge and skills are intermixed but the descriptors within the package suggest that sets of tasks are more important.

The meaning arising from such briefing is that nurses practise on patients, that collaborative care is not valued and that the patient is not a person but a collection of problems that need to be solved. Encouraging people/patients and nurses to relate as subjective beings alters such arrangements, and has further implications for how nurses organize themselves. For example, primary nursing, a system for allocating nursing care of individual people/patients to individual nurses for an entire episode of care (for example a hospital stay), is based on the notion that a relationship between the primary nurse and the person/patient will develop. Relating to people/patients as individual people also helps to humanize the health care environment in which increasing technology threatens to dehumanize people/patients. Finally, ideas about holistic care are contingent on knowing more about the person/patient than a diagnostic category or an anticipated clinical pathway.

The 'move to relate' has not been without its critics. There are suggestions that requiring nurses to relate to patients more personally is a questionable form of control and surveillance (May 1992b; Armstrong 1983). May (1992a) cautions nurses that transforming patients from objects (of physical care) to subjects (with psychological needs) carries with it the risk of 'inventing' living and coping problems for patients when such problems are matters of daily living. Solving problems such as these through the development of therapeutic relationships becomes the vehicle for nurses to legitimate their interpersonal work. However, from a symbolic interactionist viewpoint, these issues disappear. As nurses and people/patients encounter each other, it is inevitable that they read meaning into each other's presentation, that certain expectations lead to reciprocal responses. From this a definition of the situation arises which may, or may not, include a description of psychosocial needs. The definition is an achievement by *agents*, implying that all parties contribute. In other words, it is not simply the nurse as agent who constructs the person/patient's need, or the way to meet it.

CHAPTER OVERVIEW

It is clear that there is no template for the perfect interpersonal relationship in nursing. As every nurse and person/patient is different, and clinical environments vary, there can be no simple description or definition or model for nurses to aspire to. In Chapter 1 we looked at how symbolic interactionism, with its ideas about performance, could aid an analysis of relationships between nurses and people who are patients. This is because symbolic interactionism allows us to assume that the meaning of a relationship arises from the symbolic communication between participants. In the remainder of this chapter, we look at the process in detail. We adopt the metaphor of a play to help explore in more depth the dimensions of the encounter between the nurse and the person who is a patient. Entrances and exits, acts, scenes and intervals, players, roles, scripts, cues, improvisation, performance, prologue and epilogue, prompts and stage management all have a place in the interpersonal relationship.

THE INTERPERSONAL RELATIONSHIP AS A DRAMATIC ENCOUNTER

Rather than imagine that a 'correct' interpersonal relationship within nursing can be defined, we have taken the view that the participants construct the meaning of the relationship, with reference to the context in which they are operating. For example, the nurse and patient discussing the pros and cons of palliative surgery might choose to interact as counsellor and counselled, or as patient and therapist. In other words, the role of the nurse can be defined in different ways: as carer, supporter, advocate, counsellor, therapist, and so on. A more inclusive description is that of being a helper or helping. 'Helping another human being is basically a process of enabling that person to grow in directions that the person chooses, to solve problems and face crises' (Brammer 1988: 5). Thus, helping seems to describe negotiating different roles and possibilities of care. As Benner recounts, 'helping encompasses transformative changes in meanings, and sometimes simply the courage to be with the patient, offering whatever comfort the situation allows' (Benner 1984: 48).

Of course, the interpersonal relationship entails roles that are freighted with expectations. For example, people have expectations that nurses will offer care and comfort. People/patients are expected to present with descriptions of symptoms or complaints. Yet, there is still scope for negotiation, as implied in the definition of helping. Establishing the right level and kind of involvement is not simply a matter for the nurse, because relationships are mutual endeavours between nurses and people/patients. Each participant influences the level of involvement. Mutuality implies that the care situation has been defined to the satisfaction of the participants. Although it is more common for nurses to initiate the care relationship, either participant, nurse or person/patient, may make the initial overtures. The other person must respond in some way to this initiative. For example, the nurse solicits the person/patient's participation in the relationship by exploring the person/patient's experience, and the person/patient responds by disclosing information; or, the person/patient solicits the nurse's help and the nurse responds by offering assistance, perhaps involving some self-disclosure (Marck 1990). This call-and-response can be called reciprocity, or, in symbolic interactionist terms, the process of meaning-making, of defining the situation. Through the reciprocal exchange of thoughts and feelings a care relationship is defined. Thus, the care relationship will vary. The patient who perceives her/his situation as minor or routine will call out for routine, technical nursing care (Morse 1991). For example, a person/patient visiting the GP surgery for a routine cervical smear might not expect any more than a nurse who listened, explained the procedure in understandable language, and provided privacy and comfort through the procedure. People/patients do not seek connection and involvement under these circumstances, just instrumental care (Ramos 1992). Conversely, nurses describe patients who touch or appeal to them on a personal or emotional level and these are the patients they choose to become involved with (Morse 1991). Here, the nurse is likely to be responding to expectations from the person/patient of the need for some special care and concern, perhaps because of the acute or critical nature of their illness, for example, by connecting with a person/patient who is dying to help them face death with dignity, peace and comfort. The nurse's ability to reach out in these circumstances may also be due to her/his capacity to take the role of the other (see discussion in Chapter 1 and the section on symbolic exchanges later in this chapter). There may be occasions when mutuality is not possible or desirable. When the patient's condition warrants a quick response, nurses engage in unilateral decision-making, not taking person/patient understandings into account (Ramos 1992: 502). However, overall, mutuality gives a firm basis from which to enact care.

In order to explore further how people/patients and nurses mutually construct the meaning of their relationship and care, we use a case scenario based on the structure and process of a drama. Relationships have beginnings, middles and ends, as do plays. In other words, relationships progress. The keepers of the relationship will give themselves different roles and responses at different times. For example, without trust – a major issue in beginning relationships – challenging (see Chapter 8) may alienate people/patients and reflecting feelings (see Chapter 7) could be perceived as intrusive. Tracking the progress of the relationship is like following the plot of a play:

- *Prior to interacting* The prologue describes the context of the person's journey in seeking help.
- *Establishing the relationship* The cast is chosen and makes an entrance to the care stage. The cast has scripts (nurse, patient and so on) but it has room for improvisation.

■ *Building the relationship* Cues are offered by the players that call out responses from others (for example, signs of loneliness leads to the nurse chatting). Action occurs within various care scenes. Roles are defined (friendly nurse, co-operative patient and so on).

■ *Helping is enacted* A performance is given (for example, a new dressing is applied). Prompts come from within and without the performance (for example, feedback from the audience of colleagues).

■ *Ending the relationship* Intervals (going off duty, going on leave and so on) and exits (for example, discharge).

■ *Reflection on care occurs* The epilogue (in clinical supervision, with friends/family and so on).

Not all relationships pass through each phase. Careful 'stage management' uses the stages as a guide and does not dogmatically treat them as rigid. Relationships between people/patients and nurses are fluid, flexible and dynamic.

Having proposed a structure for the progress of the interpersonal relationship (albeit one that allows variation), we pause to apply a symbolic interactionist perspective that helps us to enquire about the content by looking at three areas:

(i)   The processes that can be uncovered within a dramatic encounter
(ii) Expectations of role; the repertoires that people bring to the encounter
(iii) The symbolic exchanges that occur.

(i) Processes within the interpersonal encounter

There are three important processes that occur within the interpersonal encounter. If they are enacted to the satisfaction of the participants they facilitate the definition of the interpersonal relationship and of the situation. They are: (a) Negotiating distance: interpersonal distance versus involvement; (b) Negotiating the degree of intimacy; (c) Establishing trust.

(a) Negotiating distance: interpersonal distance versus involvement

The very fact that a relationship exists between person/patient and nurse implies a degree of interpersonal involvement, although the depth of relationship is varied. Superficial relationships tend to be seen as non-threatening, but nurses are often warned of the dangers of being 'involved' with people/patients. Two main reasons are often presented as the basis for warning about over-involvement. First, there is a perceived danger that involvement will bring with it emotions that will interfere with cognitive processes and impair clear thinking. Second, nurses are advised against over-involvement because it may be emotionally draining, leaving nurses unable to cope with the, sometimes harsh, reality of nursing. Nurses may believe that they can protect themselves from hurt, from the emotional aspects of illness, from depletion of their own internal resources through distancing strategies that remove them from the situation emotionally and numb them from the reality of pain and suffering (Jourard 1964; Menzies 1961). From a symbolic interactionist standpoint, nurses who become over-involved are losing their professional front (see Chapter 1), something that people/patients expect. Over-involvement might be experienced by the person/patient as the nurse being too personal, or not being able to distinguish between the nurse and personal friends. The nurse may find her/himself dreading the end of the relationship. The following is an example of an over-involved relationship, told in the first person by the nurse:

> When I heard Pat's account of how she received a gunshot wound to her spine at close range, from her husband during a domestic argument, I felt anger towards her husband and a deep sense of sympathy for Pat. There was virtually no hope that she would walk again as the bullet had severed her spine. We instantly 'hit it off' and over the next three weeks of her hospitalization became quite close. The fact that I often thought about her when off duty did not seem remarkable to me. But there was something different about our relationship. We came to know each other on a deeply personal basis, and I no longer thought of her as a patient. My anger towards Pat's husband grew as I held him responsible for putting her in a wheelchair. But Pat never demonstrated any anger. She accepted her situation, the complex physical problems that accompany a spinal injury and her altered future with equanimity and remarkable resilience. I admired her strength and supported it and I began to feel I was the only one who could care for her properly. If I had been on my days off and found that she had a 'set back' during that time, I would accuse my colleagues of not caring for her adequately. When she was discharged from hospital to the rehabilitation centre, I visited as often as I could even though it was a long drive away. When my own personal circum-stances meant that I had to move away, Pat and I lost touch, even though we wrote to each other for a while. To this day, I feel pangs of guilt because it seemed I had abandoned Pat when I moved away. The rational part of me tries to assuage my guilt, but in my heart I cannot reconcile the fact that it is my fault that I am no longer part of Pat's life. For all I did for Pat, it felt as if I had failed her.

Could or should this nurse have avoided the over-involvement? In all likelihood the answer is no. It happens, and when it does, most nurses learn from the experience. Benner (1984: 209) found that expert nurses coped with regulating distance by reminding themselves 'of their "otherness" whenever their identi-fication with the person/patient distorted their caring'. These nurses had come to terms with what has been described as the 'paradox of helping' (Brammer 1988: 47). They were involved enough to participate emotionally, spiritually and intellectually in their relationships with people/patients, yet remained distant enough to use their involvement to help people/patients.

Of course, it does happen that people/patients and nurses develop into lifelong friends even though their initial meeting was not of a social nature. However, if this becomes an everyday occurrence in the nurse's life, it does signal the need for self-reflection. It could indicate that the nurse is unable to focus energy on people/patients, or that she/he is putting her/his own needs for friendship and companionship before the person/patient's needs. She/he may be misinterpreting the cues given by people/patients as requests for friend*ship*, when what is requested is friend*liness*.

(b) Negotiating the degree of intimacy

All relationships between person/patient and nurse begin at a level of super-ficiality as the person and nurse begin to work out how to position themselves in relation to the other. Relationships at this level are characterized by minimal self-disclosure and focus primarily on 'safe', non-personal content areas. At this time, there is minimal knowledge and understanding of the other, and trust has yet to be established (Coad-Chapman 1986). The participants are operating on rough expectations in relation to how people/patients and professionals behave. Social exchanges and 'chit-chat' are common at this level. Some nurses fail to recognize the value of such interactions, believing that they are not really benefiting people/patients during these superficial interchanges. Yet, these inter-actions serve in the development of the relationship – there is relational benefit. Being friendly and informal helps to break down authoritarian barriers sometimes associated with professional roles. Loosening expectations can lead to the offering of different relational cues.

An awareness that different levels of relationship exist between themselves and people/patients enables nurses to feel confident in maintaining a relationship at a superficial level, and, at times, in choosing to engage in a relationship that progresses to a more intimate level. From a symbolic interactionist framework, therapeutic intimacy is not something to be expected; rather, the level of the relationship is the emergent property of the exchanges that occur between nurse and person/patient. People/patients and nurses engage in the exchange and interpretation of symbols in order to decide mutually whether to be together at the superficial level (with little being known beyond the formal roles of person/patient and nurse) or an intimate level (where formalized roles fade and person/patient and nurse become known to each other as unique beings).

(c) Establishing trust

The formation of trust is essential if the relationship is to progress beyond a superficial level, because trust enables the person/patient and nurse to place confidence in each other. Interpersonal trust means that one person in the relationship believes that the other person can be relied and depended upon. They are secure in the knowledge that acceptance, support and regard will be forth-coming. Without trust, there is little self-disclosure and little chance that people/patients will share their experiences with nurses or that nurse will come to understand people/patients. Building trust is not a one way street. It is a mutual process; it must be reciprocated. Nurses must trust people/patients' inherent capabilities and resources, as well as their judgements about what is best for them. Nurses demonstrate their trust in people/patients by treating them with respect and regard (see Chapter 10) and accepting and supporting them as capable human beings.

From the person/patient's perspective, nurses must be perceived as trustworthy. Nurses are fortunate because their professional role is viewed as trustworthy by most people/patients. This is because nurses are seen to have a repertoire of skills and qualities that underpin a 'professional front'. People/patients expect that nurses will care for them, meet their physical needs and provide comfort. In fact, when nurses 'don't seem to care' people/patients will often express shock and dismay, feeling betrayed by an apparent failure of the nurses to fulfil their role. Nurses can rely on people/patients' inherent trust in their role only to a limited extent. They must live up to people/patients' expectations that they are trustworthy through consistent actions, behaviours and attitudes. Self-disclosure must be met with feedback from nurses; otherwise people/patients who are sharing information may feel naked and vulnerable. 'Understanding responses' (see Chapter 6) are the most trust enhancing. Moralizing, evaluative and judgemental responses early in the relationship lead to people/patients feeling rejected. The call and response function of symbols of trust is discussed further in the section on symbolic exchanges later in this chapter.

(ii) **Expectations of role/repertoires**

(a) Caring

Caring is often considered as an essential ingredient to nursing. It is seen by nurses themselves and by people/patients as part of the nursing role or repertoire. Quite simply, caring means 'it matters' (Benner and Wrubel 1989). Some nursing leaders (Leininger 1994; Watson 1985) have asserted that caring is the most central concept to good nursing. As such, understanding the theoretical construct of caring is akin to understanding nursing itself. Caring and nursing are intrinsically linked (Cheung 1998).

In the 1980s, research on caring in nursing became more prominent. Researchers were trying to explicate the unique meaning of nursing. However, the concept remained poorly defined, with ongoing disagreements about its meaning (Morse *et al.* 1990; Kyle 1995; Sourial 1997). In their analysis of the nursing literature, Morse *et al.* (1990) identify five aspects of caring: caring as a human trait; caring as a moral imperative or ideal; caring as an affect; caring as the nurse–person/patient relationship; and caring as a therapeutic intervention. Although there are different conceptualizations, the predominant construction of caring in nursing encompasses an emotive, intimate, interpersonal relationship (Van Hooft 1987; Macdonald 1993). This is reinforced by a number of studies in which nurses refer to and describe caring through expressive behaviours that promote involved and intimate interaction with people/patients (Larson 1986; Wolf 1986; Forrest 1989; Morrison 1991; Astrom *et al.* 1993; Cheung 1998). Likewise, philosophical analyses of caring in nursing have stressed a moral commitment to and respect for a person/patient's unique humanness (Griffin 1983; Gaut 1986; Kitson 1987; Gadow 1988). Thus, the prevalent view of caring puts interpersonal engagement with the person/patient central.

However, caring tends to be defined by nurses themselves because that is how studies have been directed (Benner 1984; Larson 1986; Wolf 1986; Benner and Wrubel 1989; Forrest 1989; Morrison 1991; Astrom *et al.* 1993; Cheung 1998). Morse (1992) contends that focusing on caring directs nurses to consider their intentions. Alternatively, she suggests comfort as the aim and outcome of caring. What the person/patient experiences then becomes central.

When nurse-driven conceptualizations of caring are compared with people/patients' ideas, there is a disjuncture found in many studies across populations and geographic locations (Larson, 1984, 1986; Keane *et al.* 1987; Mayer 1987; Cronin and Harrison 1988; Koromita *et al.* 1991; von Essen and Sjorden 1995). Nurses in these studies reveal that they perceive the most important caring behaviours to be expressive (that is, feeling-oriented), for example, listening to the person/patient. The caring behaviours that the people/patients most value are instrumental (action-oriented), for example being given medications on time, notifying medical staff when necessary and explaining what is physically wrong with the person/patient. In other words, nurses were pre-occupied with social competence and people/patients with technical competence. Dunlop (1986) points out that caring cannot be understood as compassion and concern while ignoring physical aspects of nursing. However, these differences may be an artefact of the measures used to access ideas about caring. First, McKenna (1993) notes that the studies reported what nurses thought was important and did not assess actual behaviour. Second, McKenna (1993) points out that nurses who placed expressive items in a questionnaire as a priority may have been assuming the technical aspects of caring would be in place automatically. This is borne out by a study by Astrom *et al.* (1993) who found that skilled nurses' narratives about caring were built around both technical and social competence. The nurses reported that they based their caring actions on a conscious judgement of what would be best for the person/patient. Those judgements included both emotional distancing in order to intervene in a technical manner, and deliberately interacting on a deeper emotional level in order to intervene in a social manner. Recent studies that have explored people/patients' perceptions of nursing care (Appleton 1993; Fosbinder 1994; Webb and Hope 1995; Hegedus 1999) demonstrate that people/patients do value nurses' interpersonal skills. In one study (Webb and Hope 1995), 'listening to people/patients' worries' was top of the list of important nursing activities, followed by more instrumental nursing activities: 'relieving pain' and 'teaching people/patients'. Fosbinder (1994) confirms that people/patients value the interactive style of nurses who cared for them.

Astrom *et al.*'s (1993) study is consistent with a symbolic interactionist perspective on caring as it describes how the meaning of caring was constructed through exchange of symbols. Other work has tended to look at either the nurse's or person/patient's point of view, without considering how the meaning of caring is constructed in the interpersonal space between nurse and person/patient. Attempts to find the essence of caring that transcends all clinical encounters are flawed. Concept analysis is problematic when it is oblivious to the subtleties of context and interpersonal nuances that can influence whether a shared meaning arises (Ellis *et al.* 2004). No single definition could possibly capture the rich, complex and distinctive caring relationships between nurses and people/patients. Each participant brings particular experiences to the relationship. The meaning of caring arises from this mêlée.

(b) The professional nurse–person/patient relationship

'Beginning nurses' are told that they are to 'be professional' in their relationships with people/patients, but their experience to date has been in the comfortable arena of social relationships. A common distinction made between the social relationships of friendship and professional relationships is that the professional relationship is goal directed. To be professional is sometimes seen as being distant, detached and aloof. However, the nature of the relationship is constructed through the process of interaction. Thus the nurse can be friendly, sociable, personable, helpful, caring, therapeutic, and so on, with people/patients, according to the shared social agreement between nurse and person/patient. However, because the nurse–person/patient relationship often takes place within a defined time/space, there are some constraints on how the professional–person/patient relationship can be defined. Gadow (1980) offers a useful analysis in differentiating personal and professional relationships by describing the differences in terms of focus, intensity and perspective. In professional relationships, the nurse's focus of concern is away from her/himself and towards the other, the person/patient. There is no expectation that the person/patient is mutually concerned about the nurse, as would be the case if the nurse and person/patient were friends (Gadow 1980). In addition, the intensity of the situation is experienced differently in personal and professional relationships. In professional relationships, nurses may become emotionally aroused, and feel the person/patient's concern, distress, or sense of urgency. Therefore, nurses may experience emotional intensity along with the person/patient in a given situation, but in a reflective manner, rather than in the immediate way that people/patients do (Gadow 1980). Nurses are meant to be more skilled in the thoughtful manipulation of symbols, for example, the signs of pain that people/patients offer. This is a part of the nurse's professional repertoire. The reflective nature of nurses' experience of the intense emotional situation means that nurses use their experience of people/patients' distress as a way of considering what would be of help to people/patients. Nurses integrate this experience with their knowledge of how to be of help. In personal relationships, more value is placed upon sharing experiences than helping (Gadow 1980). The final difference in Gadow's (1980) analysis is that of perspective. The professional maintains an objectivity that is impossible for friends to sustain. Nurses try to maintain some objectivity while considering how their own subjective experiences create a context for the relationship with the person/patient. Gadow's analysis indicates that it is not the level of personal involvement that differentiates friendship from professional relationships, but the form and direction of the involvement.

(iii) Symbolic exchanges

Within the processes described above, symbolic exchanges occur. They are part of the call–response pattern of the interpersonal relationship. We have chosen two examples to illustrate the place and function of symbols in interpersonal relationships.

In the first example, Benner (1984) looked at how expert nurses managed involvement with people/patients. The experts in this study involved themselves with people/patients by identifying symbolically with them, that is, by imagining that they, or someone they loved, were in a similar predicament (Benner 1984: 209). From a symbolic interactionist point of view, this makes sense. In order to contribute to the definition of the situation (in this case, caring), the nurses in Benner's study were using significant symbols of attachment (their own loved ones) in order to interpret what people/patients needed. Of course, the nurses still made reference to the symbols derived from their own professional repertoires, for example, nursing knowledge and skills. However, in caring, they saw the other's reality as a possibility for themselves (Noddings 1984). Identification invokes involvement in the situation, not as a passive observer but as an active participant. Through identifying with people/patients, nurses involve themselves in a personal way in people/patients' experiences. This involvement, being close to the heart of a situation, enables nurses to notice what is significant and to notice subtle changes in people/patients. Rather than hampering nurses' clinical judgement, involvement has the potential to enhance it. Additionally, not only did Benner's (1984) expert nurses not become drained or depleted by their involvement with people/patients, but they also had the experience of being affirmed and stronger for it.

In the second example, in promoting mutual trust, nurses sometimes share something of themselves with people/patients (see Chapter 8). This amounts to the symbolic offering of self. Self-disclosure that is reciprocated builds trust. People/patients often ask nurses personal questions in an attempt to establish the nurse's trustworthiness. These questions, although personal in nature, are not intimate questions, but rather ones that request factual information about the nurse, for example, 'Do you have any children?' The question is freighted with a call to the nurse to respond with a symbol of trust, in this case, the personal information. Thus, honest, non-defensive responses to such questions help people/patients to sense that the nurse trusts them. This is not to say that nurses should immediately share deeply personal information about themselves in an effort to promote trust. Symbols of trust have to be offered and received that are at an acceptable level. The nurse and person/patient will look for cues to make sure that what they are offering is acceptable. The following section illustrates this.

THE DRAMA OF THE INTERPERSONAL RELATIONSHIP AND CARING

We have demonstrated how processes, expectations and symbolic exchanges work together to define a situation, in this case the nurse–person/patient relationship and the meaning of caring. We now set these processes, expectations and symbolic exchanges in a fictional, generic case study – a care drama – to illustrate further how the interpersonal relationship (and care) becomes defined.

Prologue

The drama begins in a hospital setting. Sally has been looked after in the community but now her nurse feels that she needs more intensive, structured care. Sally has never been in hospital before.

Casting and entrances

Sally arrives at the ward and is greeted by the person designated as her primary nurse, John. He introduces himself and explains carefully what he can offer, and who else may be involved in Sally's care if he is away. He checks what Sally's expectations are in relation to the admission, and the involvement of the nursing team generally and himself in particular. John explains it is his role to make a nursing assessment. Sally is anxious and worried because she does not know her way around the ward and she has never been in hospital before. She is a little nervous about being allocated a male nurse and says, 'I didn't think there was such a thing as a male nurse on this kind of ward'. John decides not to follow his agenda of making an assessment but to improvise and spend some time 'walking' Sally around the ward and explaining the daily routine.

Cues and roles

Sally has recently looked after her mother who died of breast cancer. She was very impressed by the way in which the (female) nurses were attentive to her mother's needs and wishes and seemed to 'really care' about her comfort. John notices that Sally invites him to ask her about her life outside her own illness, by making statements like, 'My mum had to have this done'. He expresses interest in hearing about Sally's recent experience and tells her that he too has recently been caring for a family member with cancer. He speaks enthusiastically about his experiences of nursing on the ward as he shows her around. Sally interprets this as John being likeable, kind, empathic and a 'good nurse', who transcends common gender boundaries.

The performance – Act I

John and Sally get together so that John can make a fuller assessment. John has a formal nursing history/assessment format to prompt him in his task, and that will form the basis of care planning. John has thought through carefully why person/patient assessment information of this kind is needed. So, rather than performing 'automatically', he is able to give Sally a thorough explanation of why the assessment is needed and he is prepared to answer fully any questions that Sally raises. John does not stick rigidly to the assessment format, but ensures that he is covering points that Sally thinks it is useful to talk about. Mindful of Sally's anxieties, he asks questions carefully, giving Sally time to respond rather than using a rapid succession of questions that might leave Sally feeling 'interrogated'. He explores what she says and listens to (and hears) her responses. He is sensitive to cues that Sally gives in relation to her preferred boundaries around a topic. John does not expect Sally to be an 'obedient' interviewee, but to ask him questions in return. He is trying to hear the person and not just the patient. John explains what will be done with the information Sally shares. He describes how other nurses and health care professionals will be able to access information that relates directly to her care, but that not every detail of her 'illness story' has to be heard by everyone. John is carefully setting the boundaries of confidentiality by stating that information that has no direct bearing on the nursing or other health care of the person/patient should be considered as confidential and treated as such. Sally feels invited to ask how information is stored and how she might be able to access it herself. John begins the assessment process with 'safe' topics that allow some rapport to be established, before moving on to more sensitive areas. He knows that delving into deeply subjective experiences is inappropriate as a beginning focus, when the relationship is new and possibly fragile. Once they have established a trusting relationship, more highly personal information (from both sides) may be requested or offered, if appropriate. John knows that Sally is the expert on how her health situation is affecting her life, although he has plenty of knowledge about similar 'cases'.

Sally is keen to engage with John as her primary nurse. She has already read some signs that he is a good nurse and she tries to determine whether he is also a 'good person'. She asks him more personal questions, aimed at having him self-disclose (see the discussion of symbolic exchanges above). Sally tests John's ability to keep a confidence by sharing a minor secret. He passes the test and Sally makes friendly overtures to him, by asking him what time his shift finishes and if he is going out for the evening. Although Sally has not been able to influence which nurse was allocated to her care, she has made a definite decision to become involved with John. John recognizes this and mutually shows interest in Sally's life outside the care arena.

Intervals and exits

Sally's treatment has gone well and she is ready for discharge. John is aware that, unlike social relationships, professional relationships between people/patients and nurses are usually time-limited. Sally knows this too, but has a sense of sadness in relation to ending the relationship with John. Both need to find a way to bring the relationship to an end, to gain a sense of closure. They take an opportunity when John is talking about Sally's follow-up treatment to say how much it has meant for both of them to be able to laugh together and how they both have a sense of something lost, as well as the gain of discharge. John says that he will miss Sally and feels that she has not been 'just a patient'. They revisit several scenes that have featured during Sally's stay.

Epilogue

John reflects on his care relationship with Sally through a case presentation. Sally goes home and tells people how marvellous 'her' nurse was and that she would not hesitate to recommend the hospital to anyone with a similar problem to her own.

WHEN SYMBOLS ARE MISINTERPRETED OR IGNORED: THE MIS-DEFINED SITUATION

The above drama describes a positive experience of caring for the participants. However, there are occasions when symbols are misinterpreted, or the presentation of the other is misread. In these circumstances, the definition of the situation is not agreed. There is confusion and conflict and unhelpful consequences arise. While technical care is provided, the relationship falters. One example of a mis-defined situation is that of a nurse expressing dislike for a person/patient. Nurses who feel such dislike first need to admit the feeling to themselves.

Through taking a symbolic interactionist perspective, nurses may be able to unravel their reasons for feeling negative about a person/patient. For example, the nurse may interpret a person/patient's anxiety about coming into hospital as hostility towards her/himself and respond by disliking the person/patient. Often, the nurse feels an accompanying sense of guilt, which may be enacted in over-compensation, for example, being over-protective towards a person/patient.

Admitting negative feelings about a particular person/patient to colleagues serves a useful purpose. Usually there are other nurses working in the same area who do not react negatively to the particular person/patient. This indicates that it is the interpretation of the person/patient (and the reciprocal interpretation of the nurse by the person/patient) rather than any real characteristic of the person/patient that generates the feeling of dislike. Often an agreement can be reached whereby those nurses who do not feel dislike towards a certain person/patient can offer the care.

CHAPTER SUMMARY

The skills described in detail in the next chapters offer nurses a range of alternatives when interacting with people/patients. The skills of listening, understanding, exploring and intervening are not ends in themselves, but are related to the roles that nurses and people/patients adopt with each other within the interpersonal relationship. Using such skills effectively increases the possibility that people/patients and nurses will connect and negotiate their relationship and the care that is delivered from within it. These skills enable nurses to establish with people/patients the meanings of the situations or episodes for both the nurse and person/patient. Operating from within shared meanings enhances the possibility that nursing care will be individualized and context specific, as opposed to mechanical, procedural or task-oriented. General guidelines for the appropriate utilization of each skill are presented in Chapters 5, 6, 7, and 8, but these guidelines may not determine which skill is most fitting to use under a given set of circumstances. This is because the 'best' approach can be determined only within the context of the relationship between person/patient and nurse. No single response is ever correct in itself; no magical formula can be applied out of this context. Taking a symbolic interactionist viewpoint, the context of the relationship and the broader environmental context contribute to the making of meaning. Thus, nurses' professional repertoires; the personal experiences of nurses and people/patients; and the person/patient's immediate situation and their perceptions of it are but a few of the contextual variables that interplay in the determination of the care episode.

REFERENCES

Appleton, C. (1993). The art of nursing: the experience of patients and nurses. *Journal of Advanced Nursing*, 18, 892–9.

Armstrong, D. (1983). The fabrication of the nurse–patient relationship. *Social Science and Medicine*, 17, 457–60.

Astrom, G., Norberg, A., Hallberg, I. R. and Jansson, L. (1993). Experienced and skilled nurses' narratives of situations where caring action made a difference to the patient. *Scholarly Inquiry for Nursing Practice: An International Journal*, 7(3), 183–93.

Barthow, C. (1997). Negotiating realistic and mutually sustaining nurse–patient relationships in palliative care. *International Journal of Nursing Practice*, 3, 206–10.

Benner, P. and Wrubel, J. (1989). *The Primacy of Caring: Stress and Coping in Health and Illness*. Menlo Park, CA: Addison-Wesley.

Benner, P. (1984). *From Novice to Expert: Excellence and Power in Clinical Nursing Practice*. Menlo Park, CA: Addison-Wesley.

Brammer, L. M. (1988). *The Helping Relationship: Process and Skills*, fourth edition. Englewood Cliffs, NJ: Prentice-Hall.

Cheung, J. (1998). Caring as the ontological and epistemological foundations of nursing: a view of caring from the perspectives of Australian nurses. *International Journal of Nursing Practice*, 4, 225–33.

Coad-Chapman, A. (1986). Therapeutic superficiality and intimacy. In D. C. Longo and R. A. Williams (eds), *Clinical Practice in Psychosocial Nursing: Assessment and Intervention*. East Norwaek, CT: Appleton-Century Crofts.

Cronin, S. N. and Harrison, B. (1988). Importance of nurse caring behaviours as perceived by patients after myocardial infarction. *Heart & Lung*, 17(4), 374–80.

Department of Health (2003a). Changing Workforce Programme *NHS Modernisation Agency*, Manchester, Crown copyright. www.modern.nhs.uk/cwp

Department of Health (2003b). *The NHS Knowledge and Skills Framework (NHS KSF) and Development Review Guidance – Working Draft – Version 6*, Department of Health, Crown copyright.

Dunlop, M. (1986). Is a science of caring possible? *Journal of Advanced Nursing*, 11, 661–70.

Ellis, D., Jackson, S. and Stevenson, C. (2004). A concept analysis of support. In J. Cutcliffe and H. McKenna (eds), *The Essential Concepts of Nursing: A Critical Review*. Oxford: Elsevier.

Forrest, D. (1989). The experience of caring. *Journal of Advanced Nursing*, 14, 815–23.

Fosbinder, D. (1994). Patient perceptions of nursing care: an emerging theory of interpersonal competence. *Journal of Advanced Nursing*, 20, 1085–93.

Gadow, S. (1980). Existential advocacy: philosophical foundation of nursing. In S. F. Spiker and S. Gadow (eds), *Nursing: Images and Ideals* (pp. 79–101). New York: Springer.

Gadow, S. (1988). Covenant with cure: letting and holding on in chronic illness. In J. Watson and M. Ray (eds), *The Ethics of Care and the Ethics of Cure: Synthesis in Chronicity* (pp. 5–14). New York: National League for Nursing.

Gaut, D. A. (1986). Evaluating caring competencies in nursing practice. *Topics in Clinical Nursing*, 8(2), 77–83.

Griffin. A. P. (1983). A philosophical analysis of caring in nursing. *Journal of Advanced Nursing*, 8, 289–95.

Hegedus, K. S. (1999). Providers' and consumers' perspectives of nurses' caring behaviours. *Journal of Advanced Nursing*, 30, 1090–6.

Henderson, S. (1997). Knowing the patient and the impact on patient participation: a grounded theory study. *International Journal of Nursing Practice*, 3, 111–18.

Jackson, S. and Stevenson, C. (2000) What do people need psychiatric and mental health nurses for? *Journal of Advanced Nursing*, 31, 378–88.

Jourard, S. M. (1964). *The Transparent Self*. Princeton, NJ: Van Nostrand.

Keane, S. M., Chastain, B. and Rudisill, K. (1987). Caring: nurse–patient perceptions. *Rehabilitation Nursing*, 12(4), 182–4.

Kitson, A. L. (1987). A comparative analysis of lay-caring and professional (nursing) caring relationships. *International Journal of Nursing Studies*, 24(2), 155–65.

Koromita, N. I., Doehring, K. M. and Hirchert, K. (1991). Perceptions of caring by nurse educators. *Journal of Nursing Education*, 30(1), 23–9.

Kyle, T. V. (1995). The concept of caring: a review of the literature. *Journal of Advanced Nursing* 21, 506–14.

Larson, P. J. (1984). Important nurse caring behaviours perceived by patients with cancer. *Oncology Nursing Forum*, 11(6), 46–50.

Larson, P. J. (1986). Cancer nurses' perceptions of caring. *Cancer Nursing*, 9(2), 86–91.

Leininger, M. (ed.) (1994). *Care: The Essence of Nursing and Health*. Thorofare, NJ: Charles B. Slack.

Macdonald, J. (1993). The caring imperative: a must? *Australian Journal of Advanced Nursing*, 11(1), 26–30.

McKenna, G. (1993). Caring is the essence of nursing practice. *British Journal of Nursing*, 2(1), 72–6.

Marck, P. (1990). Therapeutic reciprocity: a caring phenomenon. *Advances in Nursing Science*, 13(1), 49–59.

May, C. (1992a). Individual care? Power and subjectivity in therapeutic relationships. *Sociology*, 26(4), 589–602.

May, C. (1992b). Nursing work, nurses' knowledge, and the subjectification of the patient. *Sociology of Health and Illness*, 14(4), 472–87.

May, C. (1993). Subjectivity and culpability in the constitution of nurse–patient relationships. *International Journal of Nursing Studies*, 30(2), 181–92.

Mayer, D. K. (1987). Oncology nurses' versus cancer patients' perceptions of nurse caring behaviors: a replication study. *Oncology Nursing Forum*, 14(3), 49–52.

Menzies, I. (1961). A case study of the functioning of social systems as a defence against anxiety. *Human Relations*, 13(2), 95–123.

Morrison, P. (1991). The caring attitude in nursing practice: a repertory grid study of trained nurses' perceptions. *Nurse Education Today*, 11(1), 3–12.

Morse, J. M. (1991). Negotiating commitment and involvement in the nurse–patient relationship. *Journal of Advanced Nursing*, 16, 455–68.

Morse, J. M. (1992). Comfort: the refocusing of nursing care. *Clinical Nursing Research*, 1(1), 91–106.

Morse, J. M., Solberg, S. M., Neaner, W. L., Bottoroff, J. L. and Johnson J. L. (1990). Concepts of caring and caring as a concept. *Advances in Nursing Science*, 13, 1–14.

Nightingale, F. (1859). *Notes on Nursing: What it Is and What it Is Not*. Reprinted 1992, Lippincott, Philadelphia PA, originally published by Harrison & Son, London.

Noddings, N. (1984). *Caring: A Feminine Approach to Ethics and Moral Education*. Berkeley CA: University of California Press.

Peplau, H. (1952) *Interpersonal Relations in Nursing*. New York: Putnam.

Porter, S. (1994). New nursing: the road to freedom? *Journal of Advanced Nursing*, 20, 269–74.

Radwin, L. E. (1995a). Knowing the patient: a process model for individualized interventions. *Nursing Research*, 44(6), 364–70.

Radwin, L. E. (1995b). 'Knowing the patient': a review of research on an emerging concept. *Journal of Advanced Nursing*, 23, 1142–6.

Ramos, M. C. (1992). The nurse–patient relationship: theme and variations. *Journal of Advanced Nursing*, 17, 496–506.

Salvage, J. (1990). The theory and practice of the 'new nursing'. *Nursing Times*, 86(4), 42–5.

Sourial, S. (1997). An analysis of caring. *Journal of Advanced Nursing*, 26, 1189–92.

Van Hooft, S. (1987). Caring and professional commitment. *Australian Journal of Advanced Nursing*, 4(4), 29–38.

von Essen, L. and Sjorden, P. (1995). Perceived occurrence and importance of caring behaviours among patients and staff in psychiatric, medical and surgical care. *Journal of Advanced Nursing*, 21, 266–76.

Watson, J. (1985). *Nursing, Human Science and Human Care: A Theory of Nursing*. East Norwaek CT: Appleton-Century-Crofts.

Webb, C. and Hope, K. (1995). What kind of nurses do patients want? *Journal of Clinical Nursing*, 4(2), 101–8.

Wolf, Z. R. (1986). The caring concept and nurse identified caring behaviours. *Topics in Clinical Nursing*, 8(2), 84–93.

CHAPTER 3

WHY INTERPERSONAL SKILLS?

INTRODUCTION

The basis of good care is effective interpersonal contact and relationship building. To develop effective relationships professionals need to know how to relate to and interact with people in their care. As such caring is a social activity. In addition to being technically proficient, nurses need to be socially competent. Every person as they join the health care profession brings with them previously developed interpersonal skills, their own personal behaviours that they have acquired influenced by their social, environmental and cultural backgrounds. The professional needs to reflect on these skills and develop them further to enhance the caring role they undertake. 'Interpersonal skills refer to those interpersonal aspects of communication and social skills that people [need to] use in direct person to person contact' (Kagan, Evans and Kay, 1986, p. 1). As professional carers, nurses need to know what to do for people/patients, know how to do it, and know how to be while they are doing it. That is, caring involves knowing, doing and being: knowing how and doing that is accompanied by being with people/patients in ways that are helpful and healthful. This book explores the 'being with' part of caring, the social aspects of caring that are therapeutic to people/patients. It looks at how nurses and people/patients join together to construct the definition of the care situation. According to the definition that arises, the care encounter may be perceived as more or less therapeutic by the participants.

Throughout the course of their professional lives nurses are with a variety of people, in a variety of contexts and for a variety of reasons. The nurse may be working with people/patients, families, colleagues, students, and other nurses on a one-to-one basis or as a group. They may be, for example, taking a person/patient's history, facilitating a group discussion, breaking bad news, and supervising others, all of which require different interactions with the people/patients and a broad range of skills. The interpersonal skills utilized during these interactions need to be adapted by the professional to enable them to relate to the individual thus ensuring the actions meet the person/patient's needs. The ability to demonstrate this flexibility and adaptation to the situation is what makes them 'professional interpersonal skills' (Kagan and Evans 2001).

Numerous other professions outwith the caring environment also require the ability to interact with and relate to people. In fact, good interpersonal skills are needed for successful employment across a range of disciplines. In this respect the health care profession is not unique. What differs in the health care context is what qualifies as 'effective' in interaction with people/patients. 'Effective' in the health care context refers to interpersonal interactions between nurses and people/patients that are helpful to the people/patients. In effective person/patient–nurse interactions there is an orientation on the part of the nurse *to be* of benefit to the person/patient, and, more importantly, the person/patient feels assisted in some way by the interaction.

Persons in need of health care are often in vulnerable positions and look to the nurse to provide them with the support to reduce or remove this vulnerability. Nurses interacting with people/patients need to demonstrate sensitivity to their vulnerability. In reducing the person/patient's vulnerability, nurses need to be able to occupy the 'position of the other', symbolically imagining what it is like to be the person/patient. The nurses can then operate from a position of 'being for' the person/patient, that is, they can function as a useful resource. For example, the restful state of feeling reassured by knowing what to expect, through preparation for a procedure, is of benefit to people/patients. Fear, anxiety and worry are not part of an environment most conducive to healing. Decreasing a person/patient's fear of the unknown through explanations requires interpersonal skills to effectively communicate and relate.

Kagan, Evans and Kay (1986) identified four levels at which interpersonal skills in nursing should be considered: level one, *insight* into self and others; level two, *development* of specialist interpersonal skill; level three, *strategic use* of particular interpersonal strategies; and level four, *overcome constraints* on the effective use of interpersonal skill. They suggest that nurses should develop an insight into their own interpersonal skills so they can consider the effectiveness of these. From a symbolic interactionist standpoint, the nurse must read the response of people/patients, and take their position, when s/he is exercising skills in order to refine and develop what s/he is doing to a more specialist level. In being more flexible and adaptable to differing situations Kagan *et al.* (1986) suggest that nurses need to become more strategic in their use of interpersonal skills. From a symbolic interactionist viewpoint, they must respond to patient expectations, for example detecting when a patient wants to be listened to rather than advised. Finally, according to Kagan *et al.* (1986), nurses need to be able to identify and overcome internal and external constraints on the effective use of interpersonal skills. For example, from a symbolic interactionist perspective, the nurse may compare past, present and possible future interpretations of her/his own caring, how caring has been described professionally, in order to act out 'caring'. To work through the above levels assumes that the nurse has skills in self-awareness, listening, responding, and understanding: this chapter covers these fundamental elements of interpersonal skill development to provide a basis for the nurse with insight.

CHAPTER OVERVIEW

This chapter provides a series of accounts from nurses, people/patients and their carers that illustrate the importance of interpersonal aspects of care provision. All possible concepts of the interpersonal aspects of caring are not covered in this chapter. Rather, a selection has been made in an attempt to highlight the value of the use of interpersonal skills by examining the positive and the negative experiences of nurses and people/patients. The accounts provide examples of understanding and not understanding, responding and not responding, listening and not listening, from both a person/patient and nursing perspectives. They show how the use, or absence, of skills can contribute to, or obstruct, the construction of shared meaning in relation to care. One obstacle to interpersonal care is task orientation, and we give an example before turning to the importance of self-awareness.

UNDERSTANDING MARGARET

From a symbolic interactionist perspective, one person can take the (theoretical) role of the other. Taking the time and expending the effort to understand the world as the person/patient experiences it results in provision of care that integrates the person/patient's experiences. Consider the following, told by a nurse:

> I met Margaret during my clinical placement at a large rehabilitation unit that was established to provide services for people who were disabled and/or chronically ill. On my first day in the placement we were taken on a tour of the unit and told that the average age of the residents was 72. There were a few people/patients in their thirties and forties who were suffering from progressive conditions such as multiple sclerosis. The place looked like an enormous nursing home. Margaret caught my attention on that first day I was on the ward. She was a frail-looking lady who sat in a wheelchair the entire day, being transported from bed to dining table and back to bed at various times during the day. Margaret captured my attention because she kept repeating the same phrase over and over again. 'Why am I being chastised?', she kept saying. The word 'chastise' struck me as quaint and curious, as if it was a relic from a bygone era. I had to look in a dictionary to find its meaning. Once I discovered the meaning of the word, I became intrigued by Margaret's thought that she was being punished. 'Punished for what?', I thought. What is making Margaret feel she is being punished? I thought that being a permanent resident of this unit could be perceived as punishment, but there was more than this in Margaret's experience.
>
> I set out to learn more about Margaret. It did not take long for me to get to know her. The fact that I was willing to sit with her and listen to her was sufficient to establish a rapport. During the two days a week that I spent on the ward I sat next to her and listened, mostly to her comments about being punished. For what, I still did not know. I accepted her comments but wondered why she felt his way.
>
> Whenever we talked, I could not get past her expression of the feeling that she was being chastised, so I went to the case notes to learn more about Margaret. There I saw the words 'legally blind' and 'nearly deaf'. I began to wonder how much sensory input Margaret was receiving and how much this was contributing to her feelings. I explored the available literature that

described the possible effects of reduced sensory input. I learnt that one of these effects is suspicious feelings.

I also discussed Margaret with the regular staff working in this ward. They told me that Margaret was a 'bit crazy' and definitely 'paranoid'. Because I thought there was more to Margaret than her suspicion, labelling her as paranoid did not satisfy me. I could see how easily such a label could dismiss Margaret's behaviour. I still wanted to learn more about Margaret and only she could help me to do so. Week after week I came to Margaret, sat next to her, encouraged her to talk to me and then just listened.

Eventually Margaret began to trust me and talk to me about more than just her feelings of being punished. We talked about her family and discussed other things. Eventually I learnt more about Margaret, beyond her paranoia. I think that just being there, showing an interest in her and listening to her, gave her the opportunity to open up and share her thoughts and feelings with me. As I listened to Margaret's account I began to piece together bits of what she said.

She mentioned that when she entered the unit her handbag had been taken away and put into a room somewhere. She frequently questioned where the handbag was being kept. I began to realize that the handbag was very significant to Margaret. I asked, 'What's in the handbag?' She told me it contained a card that had her nephew's address written on it. Her nephew, who lived in the next county, was her only living relative. Margaret's husband had died and so had all of her brothers and sisters. She had no children. Her nephew was her only link with her family and she didn't have his address! Margaret wanted desperately to write to her nephew but could not.

With the aid of my practice assessor, I found the room that held Margaret's possessions that had been taken from her when she was admitted and placed in a locked cupboard for 'safe keeping'. I was able to retrieve the handbag and find her nephew's card. Margaret was relieved and happy with the return of her handbag. With it came the possibility of re-establishing contact with her family. On Margaret's request I wrote her dictated letter to her nephew and ensured that it was posted to him. Margaret seemed to settle after this, although she continued to complain about being punished and I continued to wonder why this feeling persisted.

While the contact with her nephew had helped to calm Margaret, she remained quite anxious about being in the unit. So I kept listening. One day she mentioned that sitting near the window hurt her eyes. Her diminishing eyesight was the result of cataracts and the bright summer sun through the window created discomfort for her. Each day after lunch she was wheeled to the window to 'enjoy the sunshine'. But instead of enjoying this afternoon ritual Margaret found the experience quite uncomfortable. Could this be perceived by Margaret as punishment? I explored these thoughts with Margaret, directing my questions toward the subject of her daily seating near the window. She confirmed my fears. In Margaret's mind, the afternoon ritual of being placed in the sun was equivalent to a daily punishment. Punishment for what, she did not know. But in her mind she thought it was because she had done something wrong and this was punishment for the transgression. This new information increased my understanding of Margaret's feelings of punishment. These now made more sense.

My next plan of action was to try to get the other staff on the ward to appreciate Margaret's experience. I spoke with the nursing staff when I realized what was happening to Margaret. They agreed that placing her in direct contact with the sunshine was counterproductive to what they planned. Even placing her near the sun but not in its direct flow would help her. Care was planned to ensure that Margaret would no longer be placed in the direct sunlight.

When it came close to the end of the placement experience I could hardly contain my feelings of sadness. Saying goodbye to Margaret was going to be difficult for me. When the time finally came to do so, Margaret reached into her 'newly found' handbag, pulled out an embroidered handkerchief and placed it in my hand. 'Here,' she said, 'this is for you.' In the back of my mind I recalled the warnings I had heard about accepting gifts from people/ patients. I ignored the warnings, placed the handkerchief in the pocket of my uniform and thanked Margaret. We had shared a special understanding and the handkerchief became a symbol of this understanding. I cherished this gift because it served as a reminder of the importance of being interested in the individual, listening to and accepting their beliefs, not labelling or accepting other people's pre-conceived ideas and, most importantly, understanding their experiences.

This account illustrates the essence of this book: the significance and value of taking the time to understand patients as people, to stand in their shoes, of taking the time to notice, of being concerned enough to explore and understand their world as they experience it, to interpret their symbolic offerings and respond accordingly. It highlights that nurses using their interpersonal skills effectively can provide positive outcomes to person/patient care and reduce the negative effects that can happen when inappropriate labels are given or no time is taken to listen to or understand the patient's personal needs. Interpersonal skills enable nurses to make almost a unique contact with the private, subjective experiences of people/patients in a vulnerable situation.

UNDERSTANDING STEPHEN

Sometimes nurses become so accustomed to the routine of health care that they treat people/patients in a routine manner, asking the same questions and failing to demonstrate an appreciation that, to people/patients, illness and health are not merely routine – they are personal and significant. When nurses demonstrate awareness of the highly personal and unique experiences of people/patients, they are connecting on an interpersonal level. Consider the following account, told by a person/patient:

As I awaited my coronary bypass surgery I was filled with mixed emotions. I was pleased that technological advances in health care enabled such surgery to be performed, but at the same time I was worried about the outcome. When the surgeons explained the surgical procedure, they did so with a detail that I appreciated. Everything I wanted to know had been covered and they answered each of my questions with patience and complete explanations. But

I could still see that to them the procedure was routine. They had successfully completed hundreds, even thousands, of these procedures and approached the explanations with a matter-of-fact manner that would be expected with such familiarity. But to me, the surgery could never be routine.

After they left my hospital room the nurse who was caring for me that day, Jan, came in to see me. I had come to know and trust Jan during my stay in hospital. She had been present as the surgical team explained what was to happen during the bypass procedure. Jan also had many years of experience in caring for people/patients who were undergoing coronary bypass surgery.

I did have a few more questions that Jan answered with knowledge and detail. She then sat down next to my bed and explained that sometimes people/patients need more than factual details. Sometimes they also have fears related to the surgery that cannot be allayed through information alone. She asked me if I had any fears.

Because I knew and trusted Jan, I told her that my greatest fear was that of becoming a cripple, unable to care for myself and function as an independent person. Some of the possible complications that the surgeons reviewed led me to believe that this was a possibility. I was surprised at how freely the words came out, as I am not a person who discusses feelings easily, especially when these feelings are related to my fears. Obviously I had some fears and Jan's concern and interest helped me to express them. I told her that I was not afraid of dying, only afraid of living half a life following the surgery.

She understood what I was telling her. She didn't try to alleviate my fears by offering me statistics about the probability of my becoming a cripple. The surgeons had already presented the statistics. There is not much consolation in knowing that there is a 10 per cent chance of this complication or a 5 per cent chance of that complication. Although I was somewhat reassured on hearing these facts, how was I to know whether I'd be the 90 per cent or the 10 per cent?

Instead of focusing on further details, Jan just listened to me. And she showed me that she understood. When my daughter came to visit me that evening I relayed my conversation with Jan to her. I told my daughter how impressed I was with the fact that Jan initiated this discussion with me. Talking about my conversation with Jan provided an opportunity for me to discuss my fears with my daughter, who also listened and understood. Without the trigger from Jan, I'm not sure I would have discussed my feelings with my daughter. Jan demonstrated that she knew my impending surgery was more than just another statistic or a routine event. I was facing a major event in my life and she was there to understand what this event might mean to me. She was concerned about me as a person.

Nurses sometimes shy away from discussing people/patients' feelings because they fear that they may 'upset people/patients' through such discussions. People/patients' feelings are part of their experiences. Bringing them out into the open demonstrates acknowledgement of the fears, it does not *create* them.

Like any interaction with people/patients, nurses need to approach discussion of feelings with people/patients with sensitivity. The person/patient in this account demonstrated that he was comfortable discussing his feelings. He also indicated that he trusted Jan, an essential prerequisite for the discussion of feelings. Had he responded to Jan's exploration with reluctance it would have been insensitive of her to continue. From a symbolic interactionist viewpoint, the meaning of the care relationship between Stephen and Jan was successfully negotiated.

RESPONDING TO TONY'S FATHER

'How can you be a nurse and witness suffering and pain?' is a question often asked of nurses. It reflects feelings of distress at the thought of human pain and implies that such pain is often hard to bear. But the fact that nurses do encounter situations of human suffering means that they cannot avoid it. Not only must nurses face such realities but, on a personal and professional level, they need to learn how to make contact with people who are experiencing human pain and suffering.

The situations that nurses encounter often create feelings of helplessness within them when the person/patient's circumstances cannot be changed. Nurses may fear that because they cannot change the situation there is nothing else that can be done. They have developed an account, or definition of the situation, that means that they are unable to act. When this happens, nurses may avoid interaction and interpersonal contact, or limit contact with people/patients to those times when physical aspects of care require attention.

At other times, nurses recognize the comfort and solace that comes as a result of establishing interpersonal contact. Consider the following, told by a nurse:

> Tony, age five, was hospitalized as a result of serious injuries he sustained in a motor vehicle accident. He was a passenger in the vehicle driven by his mother, who also sustained injuries and required hospitalization in a different ward to Tony. Although Tony's mother was in hospital, her injuries were minor. Because Tony's injuries were to his head and spine, he was initially admitted to the intensive care unit of the hospital, but eventually was transferred to a general medical ward. This is when we first met.
>
> Tony's father remained by his son's side day and night throughout the entire hospitalization. He did not say much and most of our interactions were either nonverbal or limited to brief and factual information about Tony's condition. I noticed that Tony's father looked increasingly tired and drained as the days went by.
>
> After five days on the ward Tony's condition deteriorated, necessitating a transfer back to the intensive care unit. This setback was overwhelming for Tony's father. I could see it in his face. Initially I concerned myself with the details of getting the transfer under way. After the transfer was complete Tony's father returned to the ward area to collect his son's belongings. He didn't look at me and seemed quite distant. I wanted to say something to him in an effort to offer some degree of comfort but knew better than to deliver a trite cliché such as 'It will be all right'. After all, how was I to know it would be? Instead I approached him in the hallway as he was about to leave the ward area and told him how sorry I was that his son had to be transferred back to intensive care. I expressed my genuine sympathy for the turn of events that led to the transfer. He didn't respond but rather looked at me with a vacant stare, as if he was looking through and past me. I wanted to say more. I could not leave it at just that. So I said: 'I can only imagine one-hundredth of what you must be feeling. It seems like Tony has taken two steps forward and three steps back.'

Tears welled in his eyes and he said, 'I keep hoping . . . but something always happens.' He began to cry and talk about how much he loved his son and how helpless he felt in this situation. I placed my hand on his shoulder and guided him to a private area of the ward. He expressed his thoughts and feelings about what was happening to his son, describing his condition in detail and expressing feelings of despair. Although I too felt extremely sad for Tony and his father, I controlled my emotions at the time because I wanted to focus on him, not me (although I did cry later). I said nothing but simply placed my hand on his hand and squeezed it. It seemed enough. After a few minutes he composed himself, told me how much he appreciated my concern, thanked me and left the ward. I recall how helpless I felt about Tony's situation. It was likely that he would not walk again.

Although I felt helpless I focused my energy on making contact with Tony's father. I *had* to make contact and was glad I found the courage to do so. In some small way I knew my concern for him and his son helped Tony's father. I could not change the situation but I was there for him. I demonstrated that I cared and that I wanted to understand how he felt, no matter how helpless this made me feel.

This account illustrates how conveying concern and understanding enables nurses to connect with people/patients and their families. Tony's clinical situation was not altered, but the emotional pain that Tony's father was experiencing was shared by this nurse. The nurse demonstrated the use of a number of positive strategies to enable Tony's dad to express his feelings of loss. The nurse chose a quiet private place, used techniques such as comforting touch and appropriate silence, and demonstrated confidence and honesty, all features that Hacking (1981) suggests are features of good interpersonal skill practice when discussing fears and anxieties.

This account also demonstrates that the helpless feelings nurses sometimes experience, as a result of clinical situations that are devastating and sad, does not mean that they *are* helpless. It does not mean that nothing more can be done. Rather, the nurse can engage with people to construct an alternative definition of the situation that is more liberating for the participants.

RESPONDING TO ANGER

As the previous account illustrates, patients themselves are not the only people with whom nurses need to establish interpersonal contact. Connecting with the friends and relatives of patients is often part of connecting with patients. When anger and frustration are being experienced by people/patients or their family and friends, the challenge of establishing contact with them is especially daunting for nurses. Consider the following told by a nurse:

As I came on duty to begin my night shift in the paediatric ward, I noticed two distraught women in the nursery. They were engaged in what appeared to be a heated discussion. One of the women was Eve, the nurse who was finishing her evening shift. The other woman was Tracey, the mother of one of the babies in the nursery. Tracey's child was hospitalized for respiratory problems. I caught only the tail end of their conversation and although I could not understand the content, I sensed hostility and anger in both of them. Tracey was walking away from Eve as I entered the nursery. I sat down to receive the handover report from Eve and she began to tell me of her frustration with Tracey. 'It seems that I cannot do anything to make her happy', Eve said. She then went on to tell of the numerous complaints made by Tracey. I listened to Eve, knowing in the back of my mind that I would have to listen to Tracey as well. I told Eve I would try to sort out the situation and would see her the next day. She seemed relieved.

After the report I went to find Tracey. She was packing her baby's belongings and informed me that she was taking her baby home. I knew from the report that Tracey's baby had not taken any fluids by mouth during the previous shift and was at risk of dehydration. I was quite concerned about Tracey's plan to leave. Slowly I said, 'I know you are upset –' but was cut off mid-sentence by Tracey.

'That person is typical of everything here, just typical. You bet I'm upset.' She continued to pack her belongings. 'And I don't want to discuss it. I'm going home with my baby.'

At this point I felt at a loss, but also knew I had to try and make contact with Tracey, even though she was shutting me out.

'Look,' I said in an almost pleading manner, 'I want to help but I don't know what is going on. I don't know what is wrong.'

Tracey picked up her belongings and her baby and said, 'Well, it's too late to start worrying now.'

I protested, 'I *am* worried, even if it is too late. I am concerned for you and your baby.'

'Don't give me that, nobody cares around here, not you or any of the others,' she said.

I blurted out, 'Oh, is that what's wrong?'

She looked straight at me for the first time, 'Yes, that's exactly what's wrong.'

I knew I had to think fast. The contact that I had made with her seemed tenuous and I wanted to strengthen it. I did not want this mother to leave. 'Please, let's talk', I said, 'I was just about to have a cup of coffee. Come with me and I'll get you one too.' To my relief she agreed. I added, 'And I'll get a bottle for your baby.'

We went together into the kitchen area, where I prepared coffee for us and a bottle for Tracey's baby, who had been crying the entire time we had been talking. I didn't want to take over but thought it essential to get the baby settled. Her distressed baby could have been half of Tracey's problem. When the bottle was ready I asked Tracey if she would like to feed her baby.

She replied, 'Look, that's what I've been trying to do all evening. He just won't take anything. I can't do it, and he'll end up needing a drip.'

I sensed her anger and frustration which was now starting to escalate again. 'OK', I said, 'I'll feed the baby and you drink your coffee.' I noticed how directive I'd become, but decided that Tracey needed some concrete assistance in settling her baby. Besides, it was becoming increasingly difficult to carry on a conversation in the presence of the crying baby.

'Nobody has been able to feed him today and they said he may need a drip. They expect me to feed him but what can I do when he keeps fussing and refusing to suck', she explained. She felt useless and helpless, while at the same time responsible. She was trapped by the circumstances. I decided to take over a bit more. In proceeding to feed her baby, I explained how his respiratory problems were interfering with his ability to suck. Thankfully, Tracey's baby began to feed and settle. At this point I turned to Tracey and said, 'You must be so frustrated and angry. I know I would be if I were you.' I held my breath, hoping that this statement would connect with Tracey. She nodded and looked at me, some of her anger was dissipating. I continued, 'Sometimes it's hard for us to know exactly when to take over and when to let mothers care for their own babies.'

I really didn't expect her to have much sympathy for the plight of the nurses, but fortunately I had struck a chord with Tracey. She responded by saying, 'Right now, I do need you to take over and care for my baby. I can't bear the thought that he would get a drip because I am unable to feed him.' With this statement I began to understand what this mother was going through.

Eventually Tracey's baby settled and I managed to put him to bed and get him off to sleep. Tracey also prepared to settle for the night. She was lying down in the bed next to her baby's cot as I prepared to leave the nursery. As I began to exit, she called me over and whispered, 'Thank you.' Even though I now had what seemed like a hundred other chores to complete, I knew I had spent my time wisely. I looked at my watch. Twenty minutes was all that it had taken to turn these events around. I had taken the time to become involved in what might have been a most unfortunate situation. I had taken the time to understand. I felt satisfied.

Situations like this are demanding of nurses. They must contain their natural instincts to defend themselves, their colleagues and their care provision. Tracey was distressed because she felt unable to care for her baby. She felt responsible for her baby's deteriorating condition and blamed the staff for not carrying out what she thought was *their* responsibility.

When this other member of staff arrived on the scene, the situation was almost out of control. By involving herself in a non-defensive, concerned manner she was able to make contact with Tracey and begin to see the situation through her eyes, to take the role of the other. This took effort, energy and time, all of which she knew were well spent in the end. The nurse used her interpersonal skills effectively to defuse the situation. Maddux (1988) identified five different styles of conflict resolution that nurses can adopt to resolve conflict: avoidance, accommodation, win/lose, compromise and problem-solving. As the professional becomes more experienced in dealing with these situations they tend to use a mix of styles as the situation demands.

Dealing with conflict requires time to listen, to understand and to respond in an appropriate manner. Often nurses believe that no time exists to listen to and understand what people/patients are experiencing. While this is sometimes the case, lack of time can become an easy excuse for not becoming involved in difficult and emotionally draining interactions. What might have happened if the nurse in this situation had not taken the time to understand?

LISTENING TO PITA

Interactions with people/patients occur in a particular environment. Often this environment means caring for people/patients in ways that are not exclusively interpersonal. That is, nurses often find that they engage in meaningful interaction with people/patients as they are going about what seems to be routine nursing care. Consider the following told by a nurse working within an insurance-driven health care system:

> When I answered her call light I did not know much about Pita, other than the fact that she had undergone a surgical procedure, an abdominal hysterectomy, two days ago. I had not cared for her during her hospitalization but was aware of her physical condition and knew her post-operative care was progressing as expected, although she was experiencing a great deal of post-operative pain. The named carer assigned to her care was at morning tea and I was covering for him during his break. As I entered her room Pita was moaning and clearly in some sort of distress. When I asked how I could help her, she requested medication for the pain. She was clutching her lower abdominal area and complaining of pain at her wound site. I assessed Pita's pain whilst I tried to help her become more comfortable by repositioning her in bed. I checked her documentation and medication kardex for the time of her last medication dosage and knowing that enough time had elapsed I offered her an injection for pain. She said that this is what she wanted. I explained that I would get her injection and left the room to prepare it.
>
> When I returned to her room Pita was moaning more loudly than before and rolling from side to side in her bed. After administering the medication I again tried to help Pita to become more comfortable in bed. She began moaning more loudly and I noticed tears in her eyes. Although I thought I had done what I could, I felt I needed to stay with Pita a bit longer. 'What is it?' I said softly but directly into her ear. 'Tell me, please.'
>
> She began to cry and I began to become more concerned. I placed my hand on her shoulder and looked at her. She looked at me and said, through her tears, 'It's the pain. It is so awful.'
>
> 'I know,' I said, 'sometimes the pain can be awful.'
>
> I was going to explain that the injection she had just received should alleviate some of the pain but she interrupted me. 'I just got off the phone to my husband', she blurted out. 'He told me that the hospital wants payment of my bill right away. There has been some mix up with our health insurance or something like that. I don't know what we are going to do.' With this she began to cry almost uncontrollably.
>
> I stood there feeling more than just a bit useless. What could I do about her financial difficulties? 'Oh, I'm sorry', I said. 'This must be so distressing for you, first the surgery, then the pain and now money worries.' My comment sounded a bit pathetic to me, but to my surprise she began to calm down and cry less.
>
> She looked at me and said, 'You have no idea how worried I am. We do not have much money. My husband is out of work at the moment.' With this statement she stopped crying, wiped the tears from her eyes and looked at me.
>
> 'I cannot do anything about your money situation personally but I will find someone who can help you with it. Maybe it can be sorted out', I told her. I could see Pita begin to relax. I thought to myself that the medication was beginning to take effect, but I realized it was not simply the medication. I knew that my being there to listen and understand was helping Pita. I told her I would get the social worker to come and discuss the financial situation with her. She looked relieved. I asked if she would like her husband to be present when the social worker came to visit.

'Yes', she said.

'I will go and try to contact the social worker now', I told her.

'Thank you,' she said, 'thank you so very much.' As I left her room I thought to myself, now this is holistic care provision. Although I knew I could not directly assist with Pita's financial worries, these worries were part of her overall care needs. And to think that all I initially did was answer her call light. Her physical pain was compounded by her emotional worry. I was glad that I had looked beyond the obvious.

Looking beyond the obvious enables nurses to see the complexity of the entire person who is the patient. The nurse sees symbols, for example tears, and does not merely settle for one interpretation. S/he thinks about other possible associations between tears and problems of living. So, what enables nurses to be able to look beyond the obvious are their skills in caring for the person/patient as an individual who has physical, psychological, social, environmental, and financial needs, not merely caring for their clinical/physical condition. The practical intervention to ease Pita's physical pain and provided an opening for the nurse to explore the reasons for Pita's emotional distress, without this interaction Pita's emotional needs may not have been addressed.

Because care often involves management of the person/patient's clinical condition, the relationship between nurses and people/patients is often established from that base. The fact that nurses care for people/patients in ways that are physically comforting symbolically establishes that they are caring human beings. Physical care is often the means through which emotional care is offered. People/patients come to know nurses as people who care about not only their clinical condition but also about how this condition is affecting them and their way of life in a very personal way.

Sometimes nurses believe that interpersonal skills are separate from other clinical skills, such as practical competence in administering medication. Just as people/patients cannot be separated into their component parts, neither can care be split into that which is physical and that which is not. Caring skills are as holistic as people/patients.

FAILING TO LISTEN

The above examples demonstrate how positive engagement with people/patients and relatives can be helpful. In some circumstances, health professionals fail to read the symbols of need or distress because they have a lack of skills or make value judgements about the person, as in the following example.

Molly has learning difficulties. She is 34 years old and stays at home with her mum Anne. This is Anne's worrying account:

Although Molly is 34 years old her ability to look after herself is limited. Molly's behaviour had changed over a few days. She's always had difficulty with verbal communication and I have become used to looking for other signs that let me know that she is unwell. Molly had become slightly more aggressive than normal for her and she was more lethargic than usual. Most days Molly is quite a handful even though she goes to a Day Centre to give me some respite, but this had changed – apart from some short outbursts she was quite docile. The morning I went to get her up she wouldn't – she just refused to get up. This was so out of character for her as she did like to go to meet her friends at the Day Centre. I was worried about her. I phoned the doctor's surgery and asked him to visit Molly at home.

When the doctor arrived it was a locum, our usual doctor was on holiday. I saw the doctor's facial expression change when he first saw Molly. He looked uncertain, almost as though he was frightened to go near her just in case he caught something (how often I have watched in despair, people look away or move in another direction when they see Molly). The doctor quickly examined Molly and asked her some questions. I tried to explain to the doctor that Molly at times got her 'yes' and 'no' responses mixed up, but the doctor didn't listen. He said, 'She appears to understand me fine.' When examining Molly's abdomen the doctor said this was swollen. Molly made no indication of discomfort or distress throughout the examination. The doctor asked her if she had been to the toilet recently to have her bowels open. Molly said no. The doctor said, 'I have fully examined Molly and I think it is only constipation. I cannot find anything else wrong with Molly, I think you are just worrying about nothing.' I told the doctor that I knew that Molly had been to the toilet the day before to have her bowels open as I had had to help her change her soiled underwear. At this the doctor said that I was just worrying too much and he was certain that after a couple of suppositories Molly would be 'right as rain'. I told him that I still felt unhappy with his diagnosis because I felt that there was something seriously wrong with my daughter. The doctor just smiled reassuringly and said, 'Let's wait until the suppositories work and we'll see.'

After the doctor had gone Molly just slept. The suppositories didn't work. I was beside myself with worry. I wanted to ring the doctor again but felt he might think I was just a nuisance. By the late afternoon I was so distraught that I rang the surgery again and asked to speak to the doctor. Another doctor from the practice came on the line. I was so relieved to hear the voice of someone who knew Molly. When I told the doctor how Molly was she said that she would come and see Molly after the surgery. When the doctor arrived she examined Molly again, asked me about the changes in Molly's behaviour and how long it was since Molly had been her 'normal self'. The doctor said that she wasn't happy with Molly's condition and although Molly was showing no signs of physical distress she felt that it would be best for Molly to be admitted to the hospital for tests.

When Molly was admitted to the hospital the tests identified that she had a perforated bowel and was very ill. Molly was lucky. She recovered. Had the doctor who knew Molly refused to listen to me too, then there is every possibility Molly might not have survived.

This account illustrates what happens when professionals fail to listen to either the person/patient or their carers. Had the first doctor who attended Molly listened and paid attention to Anne then he may have made a different decision. Instead he alienated her and gave the impression of only caring about what *he* believed was best.

FOCUSING TOO MUCH ON TASKS

Sometimes nurses neglect the interpersonal side of caring, although physical care is offered to people/patients (see Chapter 11). Consider the following, told by the relative of a person/patient:

I wasn't sure what to expect from the community nurse who came to visit us that day. Nerina, my wife, had already been through so much. The surgical repair to her back had gone all wrong. She contracted what seemed to me like every possible surgical complication. She responded poorly to the anaesthetic and took longer than usual to come out of it. She spent the night of surgery under constant surveillance by the recovery staff and they indicated that it was a bit 'touch and go'.

I was torn between staying with Nerina and returning home to be with my children. My mother was there at home with my children but, at age four and six, I felt that the absence of their mother in the home meant that they needed reassurance by my presence. At the same time I did not want to leave Nerina's side. So I stayed with Nerina, deciding that the children and my mum could cope without me.

Eventually Nerina came out of her anaesthetic sleep, but she went on to develop infections both in her surgical wound and her lungs. When I finally brought her home from hospital she was still very weak and ill. I felt extremely uncertain about my ability to care for Nerina at home. I helped with her care in hospital, but the staff were always there as a back-up. How was I going to care for her at home? The staff at the hospital reassured me that community care staff would visit us regularly to provide the necessary support to enable me to care for Nerina. With this in mind I eagerly anticipated the initial visit from the community carers. With this visit came the possibility of the assistance I felt I needed.

Terri, the first professional to visit us at home, seemed in a hurry even as she arrived. She did not take time to say much to me, or Nerina for that matter, and turned down my offer of a cup of tea. She seemed rushed and wanted to proceed straight away to changing Nerina's dressing. Terri seemed to know a lot about Nerina's condition and asked questions about the antibiotic medication Nerina was taking. The questions were quick and to the point. No time to expand, I thought, even though I knew Nerina had some questions about these medications. Terri didn't seem to have the time for any questions we might have, only her own. She skillfully and efficiently proceeded to change Nerina's dressing. As she did, she reviewed quickly what she was doing and why she was doing it. She explained that I would need to learn how to handle the dressing change. Terri went through numerous details about the dressing, all of which seemed important to me.

As I watched and listened, I thought, 'How am I ever going to be able to do this?' She proceeded with such skill and speed that I hardly had time to absorb all these details. I began to feel anxious about remembering everything. There was no time to review the details or have my questions answered.

'There,' she said, as she completed the dressing, 'that's all there is to it. You'll be right now', she said as she patted me on the back. She helped Nerina get comfortable in bed and began to pack up.

'But,' I said, 'I'm not sure I can actually do that dressing.'

'Of course you can', Terri replied. 'Just do what I did. There's nothing to it.' She repeated, 'You'll be all right, don't worry' and patted me on the back again. She told us that she would be returning to visit in two days time. She said goodbye to both of us and I showed her to the door.

'Thank you', I mumbled, more out of politeness than sincerity. Thank you for what? I thought to myself.

Nerina was resting when I returned from seeing Terri to the door. I went away from her room, sat down and tried to recall everything Terri had said about the dressing. I began to feel a bit panicked about remembering everything and still had so many questions in my mind. I felt a bit lost. Maybe next visit. . . .

Unfortunately, this account illustrates how easily nurses can focus on a task to the exclusion of all else. Terri's practical ability to change the dressing was without question. But her inability to relate to Charles and Nerina on an interpersonal level does raise questions. Taylor (1998) suggests that 'some nurses may choose to hide behind their professional masks. . . . Acting out the role of the nurse may serve to protect the hapless practitioner from the everyday battle-front of practical work, where emotional knocks and bruises may be the norm' (p. 74). Perhaps Terri had an extremely heavy caseload on the day she visited them. If this was the reason for her efficient yet diminished care, she could have acknowledged this by telling them she was in a hurry. Had Terri been sensitive to what Charles was expressing, she could have offered follow up in the form of a telephone call. Anything that indicated that she was interested in what he was experiencing may have helped.

Terri's lack of acknowledgement of how Charles was experiencing the situation, his doubts about changing the dressing after such a brief and rushed explanation, indicated a lack of awareness on her part. This lack of awareness for Charles' situation could indicate a lack of concern and regard for him. Instead of acknowledging Charles' concern, Terri brushed it aside with a false reassurance of 'You'll be all right'. In doing so, she not only failed to notice his concern but minimized it in a way that demonstrated that she did not care to understand. Terri's lack of insight, her inability to read the cues offered by Charles, demonstrates the impact on people/patients should nurses not develop an awareness of how their interactions and lack of interpersonal skills are affecting the people/patients and their carers. This emphasizes the need for nurses to develop their self-awareness skills. Chapter 4 deals explicitly with developing self-awareness, but the following section illustrates why it is important.

THE IMPORTANCE OF SELF-AWARENESS

Wayne is an experienced registered nurse who has worked for many years on an orthopaedic ward. Tom, a person/patient on that ward, came to symbolize one of Wayne's greatest frustrations as an orthopaedic nurse. Tom was addicted to pain medication and, although Wayne could understand intellectually that Tom became addicted as a result of medical intervention, he experienced an all too familiar sense of helpless frustration in trying to be of assistance to him.

Tom knew he needed to 'do something' about his addiction because his life had literally become his illness. When Tom's doctor suggested that he go 'cold turkey' in stopping the medication, Wayne could see the panic on Tom's face. He pleaded with the doctor to 'not let that happen again', as he had previously experienced the agony of abrupt cessation of his pain medication. As Wayne stood by Tom's bedside he too began to experience familiar feelings: helplessness at his inability to assist Tom, frustration at a system that allows addiction, and anger at both Tom and his doctor. Wayne knew he would be the one to experience Tom's suffering first-hand and he did not want to stand by helplessly. Part of him blamed Tom for getting himself into this predicament in the first place. After all, he was a responsible adult who should know better. All of these feelings created tension within Wayne and sparked a desire to detach from the situation.

Through reflecting on this experience Wayne began to realize that his anger was misdirected at Tom, through the interpersonal dynamic of 'blaming of the victim'. He began to recognize that his efforts to help Tom would be fruitless unless he aligned himself with him. Previously he lectured, coerced, cajoled, and detached himself from people/patients who were addicted. He began to realize that such responses kept him distanced and uninvolved. He decided that this time he would get involved and began to explore how he might be a resource to Tom. Wayne listened with a new openness to Tom's plight and plea for help and explored the possibility of assistance from the drug and alcohol team. When Wayne approached Tom's doctor with the idea of a referral to that team, his frustration mounted as he met with resistance. Through discussions with other nurses Wayne came to realize that he could initiate the referral. He mobilized help from the drug and alcohol team in assisting Tom with his withdrawal from pain medication. He formed an alliance with Tom that was based on understanding of his situation and tolerance for his predicament.

Wayne was astonished at his change in attitude toward people/patients who became addicted to pain medication. No longer did he feel annoyed and frustrated; no longer could he blame people/patients for the situation. He developed insight into his own frustration and a sense of empowerment in his nursing role. Most importantly, he grew to appreciate the importance of accepting people/patients as they are before trying to help them move to where they want to be. His self-awareness increased because he was willing to reflect on his own beliefs and values, and doing so benefited Tom.

CHAPTER SUMMARY

One of the most important messages of the chapter is that *there are no context-free rules about interacting with people/patients*. Nurses must consider a host of variables when they make contact with people/patients. Sometimes a discussion about feelings is suitable to the context, while at other times such discussions do not fit the context. The nurse and person/patient act and react to one another in order to define each other's role, presentation and the meaning of caring. However, this can only be achieved through the exercise of specific skills.

Guidelines about and specific skills for establishing interpersonal contact with people/patients are presented in the following chapters. However, each inter-action, like each person, will be unique and dynamic in its own right. The nurse must learn to attend to cues from the person/patient, relatives, colleagues and the general contexts of care in order to respond in a way that is sensitive and helpful.

REFERENCES

Hacking, M. (1981). Communication, dying and bereavement. *Nursing* (Oxford), 1, 1168–70.

Kagan, C., Evans, J. and Kay, B. (1986). *A Manual of Interpersonal Skills for Nurses: An Experiential Approach*. London: Harper Row.

Kagan, C. and Evans, J. (2001). *Professional Interprofessional Skills for Nurses*. Cheltenham: Nelson Thornes Ltd.

Maddux, R. B. (1988). *Team Building: An Exercise in Leadership*. London: Kogan Page.

Taylor, B. (1998). 'Ordinariness in Nursing as Therapy'. In R. McMahon and A. Pearson (eds), *Nursing as Therapy*. Cheltenham: Stanley Thornes.

CHAPTER 4

SELF-AWARENESS

INTRODUCTION

Nurses do not leave themselves behind when they enter a clinical setting. When caring for people/patients they not only use knowledge and procedural know-how but also what they think and feel, what they believe and value, and how they perceive themselves. Thus, personal repertoires and professional repertoires have direct bearing on interactions and relationships with people/patients.

In addition to knowledge and practical ability, nurses need to develop an awareness of how effectively they are using their skills, because such awareness enables them to evaluate their own performance. From a symbolic interactionist perspective, they are able to use the mirror held up to them in the form of person/patient reactions. They can engage in inner dialogue in order to reflect on what has occurred and is occurring within the care episode/relationship. Nurses who are able to evaluate their own performance are in a position to learn, grow and become more skilled and effective in their interactions with people/patients.

Traditionally, nurses are taught to ignore their subjectivity and to focus their attention on the person/patient. This may be interpreted to mean that nurses should disregard or forget themselves whenever they engage in person/patient care. By focusing on people/patients, at the exclusion of themselves, nurses run the risk of failing to recognize the significance of how *they* are affecting people/patients and how people/patients are affecting *them*.

The skills presented in the following chapters of this book can be learnt, developed and refined. Nevertheless, these skills are only as effective as the person using them. Each professional must employ the skills in a unique way. A professional who focuses solely on the skills without awareness of the ongoing actions and reactions within the relationship, without considering their contribution, runs the risk of a contrived performance that lacks spontaneity and relevance. For these reasons, skills of self-awareness, self-exploration and self-understanding are critical.

CHAPTER OVERVIEW

The chapter begins by outlining the nature of self and self-awareness. It describes how self-awareness is critical in understanding interactions between people/

patients and nurses. The next section connects self-awareness with personal growth. The chapter continues with an exploration of how the self is used positively within care episodes, and encourages the reader to assess her/his own repertoire, or personal/professional attributes. In order to become more self-aware, reflection and reflective practice are necessary. Both are defined and the processes in developing self-awareness are described. In particular, the sources of self-awareness are set out, followed by areas for self-exploration. While the attributes each person has that contribute to a sense of self are fluid, there are some characteristics that need to be developed and maintained. We outline these 'positive attributes' in the next section. Finally, the chapter ends by identifying the need to learn and practise skills that may be useful in specific interpersonal contexts, and by setting out how to self-assess before, during and after the application of these skills.

THE IMPORTANCE OF SELF-AWARENESS

In Chapter 1 we looked at how self was understood within a symbolic inter-actionist framework. We advocated thinking about the self, or sense of self, as something that is the product of our everyday interactions rather than as something given at birth. Our sense of self is derived from others' attitudes towards us and we use different behaviours (presentations of self) with different groups. For example your attire alters depending on the occasion, such as going for interview or out to a party; the greetings you give your mother differ to those you give a stranger. So, the self is constructed by: (a) being able to take the other person's role, by imagining what it is like to be in the other person's shoes; (b) by being able to interpret the response of the other person to the particular self that we are presenting, by noticing and thinking about the reaction of the other person to what we are saying or doing (or not saying or doing); (c) by the set of attributes that we notice or others distinguish in us. Thus, self is fluid. We do have a sense of self, self-awareness that perseveres. We are, after all, distinct in space and time, and at any time we have a set of attributes (a repertoire of beliefs, values, ideas, skills, experiences, feelings, behaviours) that we draw on and they influence our responses in certain situations. Self-awareness, or sense of self, is proportional to the degree that we are willing or able to reflect on:

- Our uniqueness: where we are in relation to others and how our unique position affects the other
- Our repertoires: through noticing our attributes, or noticing that others attribute qualities to us, and noticing how others are reacting to the enactment of our repertoires).

Thus, taking self as ever-changing encourages nurses to attend to the mutual relationship, not simply the person/patient in the relationship, where each person acts and reacts and interprets actions and reactions. When the focus is exclusively on the person/patient there can be mistaken assumptions and judgements about the person/patient that ignore the nurse's contribution. Consider the following account:

Sylvia is an experienced registered nurse who prides herself on her ability to care for seriously injured and impaired victims of brain damage. Peter had become one of those people/patients whom all the nurses on Sylvia's ward had come to dislike. He was labelled as unco-operative and difficult. Because some alleged his injuries had been self-inflicted, he engendered little sympathy from the nursing staff. They did not like caring for Peter and often complained bitterly to each other about their negative feelings toward him.

One day during change-of-shift report, Sylvia began to listen to her colleagues' complaints and negative judgements about Peter. She had been thinking about how some people/patients are labelled as difficult because of a journal article that she read. She came to realize that Peter had fallen into this unfortunate category. To her colleagues' relief and surprise she asked to be assigned to care for Peter. Little did they realize that Sylvia was challenging herself to try and understand Peter as a person rather than a label.

That day when she entered his room she noticed, for the first time, the frightened and uncomfortable look on this young man's face. His primary manner of communication was through blinking his eyes, as he had sustained an unstable neck injury. His hands were restrained because he was in the habit of pulling at tubes and equipment. Sylvia stood there for a moment, noticing and absorbing his situation.

Without even thinking she suddenly realized the cool temperature of the room and noticed that Peter had nothing more than a light sheet draped over his naked body. She looked at him and said, 'I bet you are cold'. His eyes blinked furiously in the affirmative. She immediately went to get him a warm blanket. The look of relief on his face was incredible. Throughout the entire time no one had noticed that Peter was cold. They did not notice because they had failed to perceive him as a person.

Sylvia no longer could say 'no' to the 'personhood' of Peter by thinking of him as a label. She began to question the dynamics that had led the nursing staff to label Peter and dismiss him as troublesome and difficult. Through reflection Sylvia had become more self-aware. She had become aware that the nursing self that she was presenting (in common with colleagues) was not helpful to Peter. Her awareness allowed her to put aside the labels used about Peter and to attend to his comfort needs.

This account highlights the importance of self-awareness: through active reflection and open acknowledgement Sylvia was able to take corrective action. Sometimes nurses try to deny the existence of negative person/patient labels, claiming that such evaluations are unprofessional and therefore unacceptable. They do so in the mistaken belief that nurses, by virtue of being professional people, can rise above their natural human tendency to judge, or that at least nurses can put such judgements aside so that they do not interfere with the provision of care. This shows a lack of self-awareness; a denial of the values, position, beliefs, preferred responses that one is operating with.

This is a vitally important point, as there is empirical evidence that professionals' judgements about people/patients can and do influence person/patient care. Self-awareness of the basis on which judgements are made becomes critical. For example, a recent study by Olsen (1997) found that the nurse's sense of caring and concern for people/patients was influenced by whether they thought the person/patient was responsible for the clinical situation. Nurses expressed less concern and sense of caring toward hypothetical people/patients who were seen to be responsible for their illness. Nevertheless, participants in the study did indicate they would make an effort to alleviate the person/patient's responsibility as a means of establishing a connection with them. In another study investigating actual behaviour of nurses and people/patients in their care, Carveth (1995) found nurses to be less supportive of people/patients who were labelled 'difficult', although the amount of time nurses actually spent with difficult people/patients was equal to the time spent with people/patients considered to be 'ideal'. Like the nurses in Olsen's 1997 study, nurses in Carveth's 1995 study tried to mitigate person/patient behaviour through the use of persuasion or coercion to change behaviour seen by the nurses as deviant.

The results of these two studies echo earlier studies that demonstrate how professionals' attitudes and interpersonal behaviour toward people/patients are affected by judgements made about people/patients. From a symbolic interactionist perspective, when a situation is defined as real it is real in its consequences. The judgements were based on person/patient characteristics such as the nature of the person/patient's disease, similarity of person/patient's and professional's values, social skills, ability to communicate and gratitude for care (Grief and Elliot 1994; Forrest 1989; Baer and Lowery 1987; Drew 1986; Armstrong-Esther and Browne 1986; Sayler and Stuart 1985; Kelly and May 1982).

Similarly, Johnson and Webb (1995a) found that nurses do judge the social worth of people/patients and that such judgements do have moral consequences. Nevertheless, their findings from a field study of nursing indicate that social evaluations of people/patients are not simply tied to personal characteristics of people/patients and their individual circumstances (for example, bearing responsibility for their illness). Referring to the process as 'social judgement' Johnson and Webb (1995a, b) describe a complex and dynamic system whereby evaluations of people/patients' social worth is negotiated and renegotiated throughout their interactions with nurses. That is, nurses' evaluations of people/patients can and do change over time.

The evidence suggests that it is more useful to encourage nurses to actively reflect on their evaluative perceptions of people/patients rather than ignore or deny that their judgements can and do affect care provision. Once negative evaluations are brought to conscious awareness, nurses can explore their meaning, and like Sylvia in the story, take corrective action if necessary. Reflection will not prevent negative evaluations, but it will assist nurses in challenging or altering them.

THE RELATIONSHIP BETWEEN SELF-AWARENESS AND PROFESSIONAL GROWTH

Nurses need to be able to evaluate how effectively they are relating to people/patients, and self-awareness as defined above is essential in this assessment. Evaluation of performance in the use of the skills presented in the following chapters is best achieved through the process of self-assessment. In assessing their performance, nurses begin with an awareness of how they are interacting with people/patients. Through consideration of their *intentions*, *actions*, *responses*, and *reactions*, nurses are able to evaluate their own performance in the interest of learning how to be more effective in each encounter with people/patients. However, each encounter is also an opportunity to extend the nurse's repertoire and depth of skills, encouraging self-growth. Understanding our behaviours and reactions to others' is not a simple task. The process of becoming more self-aware takes place over time and most of us will need some kind of support and help in developing it.

USE OF SELF AS PERSONAL AND PROFESSIONAL REPERTOIRES

In relating to people/patients, nurses are effective when they bring as much of themselves as possible into the relationship. In doing so, they are deliberately using themselves (their position in relation to the person/patient and their full personal and professional repertoires) for the benefit of people/patients. When nurses use themselves for the benefit of people/patients, they have a sense of agency. Self-awareness enables nurses to view themselves as human beings, with failures, faults, successes, and strengths, in different proportions in different contexts and at different times. They see themselves as people who have something to offer people/patients, and as people who can respond to the reactions of people/patients both to define themselves within the relationship and to define meaningful care. Engaging in Activity 4.1 allows the identification of repertoires.

Self-awareness versus self-consciousness

Completing Activity 4.1 often engenders feelings of self-consciousness and discomfort in people. This is because focusing on the self, especially the positive aspects, is usually a private affair, and 'seeing yourself on paper', even when it is not shared with anyone else, brings the private into the open, which often creates a sense of self-exposure and anxiety.

In bringing the self into awareness, even through an activity such as this, there is a danger of becoming preoccupied with self and uncomfortably self-conscious. Self-awareness is not the same as self-consciousness. There needs to be a balance between the self-consciousness that is experienced through focusing too much on self, and the lack of self-awareness that leads to alienation from the self. Achieving this balance is important for nurses because the risks of focusing too much on themselves are as great as the dangers of failing to take themselves into account at all.

Egan (1994) refers to the need to be 'productively self-conscious' when engaged in helping relationships. Productive self-consciousness has positive effects because it is the ability to be absorbed in an interaction, while simultaneously being aware of internal reactions and perceptions. It is the ability to raise self-awareness to a level that enhances reflection on the self, while not becoming so preoccupied with the self that there is a lack of ability to focus on the person being helped.

ACTIVITY 4.1

WHAT DO I HAVE TO OFFER TO PEOPLE/PATIENTS – MY REPERTOIRE?

 Process

1 Divide a blank piece of paper into two columns. In the first column record a description of those self attributes that you think are positive, ones you like about yourself. In the second column describe those self attributes that you would prefer to change, ones you do not always like about yourself. You do not need to share this list with anybody else – be as honest as possible with yourself.

2 From your list of positive attributes in the first column of your paper, reflect on how you could put these attributes to use in caring for and relating to people/patients.

3 From your list of negative attributes in the second column of your paper, reflect on how these may affect your relationships with people/patients, for better or for worse.

4 Write a brief summary of how your positive attributes might affect how you position yourself in relation to people/patients when delivering care. Do the same for your negative attributes.

Discussion

1 Which was easier: describing positive aspects of yourself or negative ones?

2 Which column contains more information?

3 Why do you think you negatively evaluate some attributes and positively evaluate others?

REFLECTION AND REFLECTIVE PRACTICE

We have outlined above how self-reflection is the route to self-awareness. More generally, reflection is an active exploration of personal experiences, consciously employed for the purpose of making sense of those experiences. Some people naturally engage in reflective processes, thinking deeply on life and their experiences of it. Other people may need guidance and assistance to be reflective. Professional carers are often encouraged to engage in reflection because their knowledge is embedded in practical experience.

A spirit of inquiry sparks reflective nurses to think about their actions as they are engaged in clinical practice. In this sense reflection is a way of functioning; it involves a here-and-now pursuit to make sense of the everyday world of practice as it is unfolds. This is reflection that 'looks on'. Reflection also involves thinking about experiences after they have occurred; this involves a there-and-then thinking process in order to use experience for the purpose of learning. This is reflection that 'looks back'. Reflection is also important prior to experience (Greenwood 1993) as nurses consider their intentions and plans for person/patient care. This is reflection that 'looks forward'.

Regardless of whether it occurs before, during or after clinical practice, reflection is a process for understanding and appreciating experiences (Clarke *et al.* 1996). This is especially true when experiences are novel and/or formidable. More importantly, reflection is a way of challenging and changing perspectives (Atkins and Murphy 1993), the purpose of which is to improve practice. Such improvements are aided and enhanced by linking reflections to theory. In this sense reflective processes accompany learning, encouraging nurses to develop theoretical understandings that will serve as guides for future action.

Nurses can reflect on various aspects of practice: the technical (for example, treatment regimes), the practical (for example, routines in care), the social and political (for example, how health care resources are expended) and the personal (for example, knowledge of the self) (Clarke *et al.* 1996). 'The focus of reflection is *the self* within the context of the specific practice situation' (Johns 1999: 242). In this respect the processes of reflection are closely related to increasing self-awareness. Nevertheless, a certain amount of self-awareness is required for reflection to occur in the first place (Atkins and Murphy 1993).

Processes for reflection

Effective reflection requires active strategies to support the process (Wilkinson 1999; Johns 1995). This means that most successful reflection is accompanied by structured activities such as keeping a professional diary or completing the activities in this book. Unless there is some means of tracking an individual's reflections over a period of time, sustainable professional growth through reflection may be difficult to ascertain.

In a study with first-year nursing students, Davies (1995) reports how students changed their views of their clinical nursing experience over the course of the year. Tracking these changes was possible through the use of reflective processes. What is most interesting from this study is that the person/patient emerged as the central focus of care for students, shifting from their initial focus on themselves.

With increasing frequency clinical supervision is considered by many as an ideal method to encourage and support reflective practice (Kim 1999; Fowler 1998). Clinical supervision, whether conducted individually or in groups of nurses, is aimed at using reflective processes for the purpose of improving the quality of nursing care. It has been shown to be useful in the development of interpersonal skills (Tichen and Binnie 1995) and in increasing self-awareness (Begat *et al.* 1997). The finding is unremarkable from a symbolic interactionist perspective. Clinical supervision is a means for the individual professional to read the reactions of peers to the presentation of the professional self that is naturally embedded in a case scenario. For example, the nurse outlines what s/he has been offering to a person/patient and the perceived successes and challenges. The supervisor(s) give feedback in relation to use of attributes, both clinical skills and other qualities, such as personal values, beliefs etc., thereby increasing self-awareness. (Clinical supervision is useful also for self-assessment as discussed below.)

Pitfalls in reflection

Despite its obvious benefits, reflection does have its potential pitfalls. It is important to remember that effective reflection will inevitably lead to anxiety (Haddock and Bassett 1997) because the process of reflecting involves change and challenge. It requires nurses to show a willingness to be challenged to view experiences in different lights and to reconsider what may be long-held and cherished beliefs. The anxiety and discomfort that accompanies effective reflection points to the need for support systems to be in place, for example, colleagues who serve as skilled facilitators and mentors (Foster and Greenwood 1998; Carr 1996).

Another pitfall relates to the difficulty of reflecting after an event has taken place. This difficulty is called 'hindsight bias' (Jones 1995), a term that describes the way people recall events that fit with the known outcome. For example, if a nurse were to interact with a patient who seemed distressed about a forthcoming procedure, only to discover that the distress involved another life event, then it would be difficult in retrospect for the nurse to recall that she initially associated the patient's distress with the procedure. Her recall of events would match what she now understands, not what she originally thought.

Taylor (1997) cautions nurses in the wholehearted embrace of reflection as a way of changing practice through empowerment and emancipation of nurses (see Chapter 11 also). The structural arrangements that are required for such emancipation may not be easy to attain, and reflection alone does not guarantee success in making such structural changes. In fact, reflective practices may result in nurses feeling less empowered by systems of health care delivery.

A final pitfall in the use of reflection is perhaps the most challenging of all in relation to beginning practitioners. It is that a nurse may need to be clinically experienced in order to benefit from reflection (Fowler 1998). This implies that the nurses who most need to learn in terms of clinical experience may be least able to benefit from the process of reflection. Nevertheless, structured reflection, especially under the guidance of a more experienced professional, is a useful way for beginning nurses to assess their own interpersonal skills and to improve self-awareness.

PROCESSES IN DEVELOPING SELF-AWARENESS

It is unlikely that any individual will ever fully know and appreciate all facets of her/himself. In any case, as argued above, the positions that people occupy and their collections of attributes alter over time and according to where they are and what they are doing. Nevertheless, nurses can develop their capabilities to engage in self-reflection, to perceive and accept input from others, and to openly disclose themselves to others to increase their self-awareness.

ACTIVITY 4.2

PERSONAL REACTIONS TO OTHER PEOPLE

Process

1   Recall a time when you reacted strongly to another person, either negatively or positively. On a separate piece of paper, record the circumstances and your reactions.

2   Reflect on why you think you reacted this way, and record this by completing the following sentence: 'I think I reacted this way because I . . .'.

Discussion

1   How did your reactions affect the way you related to this person?

2   What do you think and feel about the way you reacted?

3   What did you learn about your self-presentation?

Self-reflection

When considering how to increase self-awareness, the process of self-reflection often comes to mind. This often begins with noticing what elicits a personal response. 'Why did I react negatively when that patient told me he wanted to die? Why did I want to leave the room? Was it that I felt helpless, or unsure about how to respond? Do I believe that self-destructive thoughts are unacceptable? Have I ever felt this way before? Why did I find it so hard to listen to what he was saying? Why did I get so angry with the child when they hit me?' Engaging in such thoughts and feelings encourages nurses to discover more about themselves.

This activity may have uncovered emotional reactions to people/patients because feelings are bound to be a part of nurses' responses to people/patients. Personal emotions are aspects of self-awareness that may pose dilemmas for nurses because they are often taught, implicitly or explicitly, to keep their emotions under control. Nurses who allow emotions *to reach conscious awareness and focus on them* run the risk of losing control. Many nurses interpret the need to maintain control over their emotions to mean that they should be void of emotions. While a lack of emotional display in some situations assists nurses in managing such situations, a total lack of emotions prevents nurses from establishing interpersonal contact with people/patients (Lawler 1991).

Rather than deny their emotional responses, it is better for nurses to be aware of and reflect on such reactions. Without awareness, it is likely that these emotions will be expressed inadvertently to people/patients who will respond accordingly. Nurses who keep in tune with their emotional responses have a greater chance of maintaining true control than those who try to control emotions by ignoring them.

More importantly, the professional's feelings and reactions to people/patients serve a purpose – they provide useful information in measuring how the relationship with a patient is progressing. For example, anger and frustration toward a patient, when left unexamined, may lead to labelling that person/patient. It could be that the feelings of anger and frustration are a result of the professional's inability to understand what the person/patient is experiencing, a misreading of the situation. Perhaps the person/patient is not conforming to the professional's expectations of a 'good/patient'. A host of other possibilities exist. Self-reflection enables nurses to discover what their emotional reactions might be revealing about *their* relationships with people/patients. Personal thoughts and feelings triggered through interaction with people/patients are useful sources of information about oneself.

Input from others/interactive reflection

There are limits to how far self-awareness can progress and develop through the use of self-reflection alone. Natural 'blind spots', the ease with which self-reflective thoughts can be ignored, dismissed and defended, along with the tendency to protect the self through self-deception, pose barriers in the use of the reflective process.

Other people provide useful information through the way they react and respond. For this reason, another effective way to complement, not replace, self-reflection occurs when nurses attend to feedback from others, be it solicited or unsolicited. Feedback from good friends and peers is useful. Feedback from people/patients is another useful source of information, although nurses usually do not solicit it. A method that can aid the development of self-awareness through feedback from others and self-disclosure is known as the Johari Window (Luft 1969; Pfeiffer and Jones 1974).

It is through asking questions, receiving feedback and telling others about ourselves that our open pane (self-awareness) is expanded and potential within

Known to self	*Unknown to self*
OPEN Our conscious self – what we are aware of and what others know of us	BLIND Things that we don't know about ourselves but others can see more easily
HIDDEN Others cannot know this area unless we disclose it	UNKNOWN What we don't know about ourselves and what others don't know

The Johari Window

us used to the fullest. We will never achieve full self-awareness but we can constructively develop it to enhance our interpersonal relationships.

Input from people/patients

People/patients are not only expressing information about themselves when they interact with nurses, they also are expressing information about how they perceive the professional (Activity 4.3). People/patients reveal how they feel and what they think about the nurses who are interacting with them by the manner in which they behave. What they choose to discuss, how freely they disclose information and how comfortable they seem during an interaction are examples of input that people/patients provide about how they see the professional. The cues that indicate the effect nurses are having on them automatically surface throughout interactions. Nurses need to be receptive to such input from people/patients because this feedback informs them about themselves. In this regard, nurses need not actively solicit person/patient feedback.

ACTIVITY 4.3

PERCEIVING FEEDBACK FROM PEOPLE/PATIENTS

 Process

1   Reflect on a recent interaction with a person/patient. Record what happened between you and the person/patient.

2   Describe how this person/patient responded to you.

3   Through reflection on how this person/patient responded, try to determine what this person/patient was 'telling' you, about how they perceived you.

4   Discuss the situation and your experience with another participant.

Discussion

1   What are the various ways that participants interpreted how people/patients responded to them? What cues indicated these responses?

2   At the time of the interaction with the person/patient, how aware were participants that people/patients were actually revealing how they perceived the professional?

3   How many participants described negative/ineffective inter-actions? How many described positive/effective ones? What does this say?

Perceiving such input from people/patients begins with an awareness and understanding of its relevance. Next, nurses need to be open to receiving the information. Asking themselves questions such as 'What is it about me that enables people/patients to openly express their feelings?', 'Why is this patient telling *me* this?' and 'Have *I* inadvertently communicated that I do not wish to hear what this patient is saying?' enables nurses to become open to input from people/patients.

It is natural for nurses to ignore or reject input and feedback about themselves when this information lacks congruence with personal images (what nurses believe they are or want to be). Nurses who are feeling inept may not notice when people/patients reveal that they *are* quite effective. For this reason, feedback and input from others, especially people/patients, may challenge nurses to reconsider their current perspectives.

SELF-SHARING

Another process that is effective in increasing self-awareness arises out of a combination of self-reflection and interactive reflection (input and feedback from others). It is the process of self-sharing – the disclosure of personal thoughts, feelings, perceptions and interpretations by openly expressing them to others.

How self-sharing increases self-awareness

Self-sharing enhances self-awareness because it triggers (and therefore solicits) feedback from others, and also because it intensifies self-reflection. When internal thoughts, feelings and attitudes are made external through open discussion, they are often internally clarified, expanded and accepted. Sometimes self-sharing internally persuades nurses to challenge and alter their thoughts, feelings and attitudes. In this sense, self-sharing often transforms into a process of 'thinking aloud', and then having a dialogue with the self while using the other person as a sounding board.

At other times self-sharing enables nurses to test the validity of their current thoughts, feelings and attitudes. In 'testing' their internal responses nurses are asking others what they think or feel about these responses. This often leads nurses to reconsider their responses.

The relationship between self-sharing and self-awareness is a circular one (see Figure 4.1). While a certain degree of self-awareness is helpful to begin self-sharing, it is not vital. Through self-sharing, further input is received, both from others and from the self, which is then useful in increasing self-awareness.

Risks of self-sharing

Despite its potential value for increasing self-awareness, disclosing oneself to others is not always easy to do. There are many reasons for keeping oneself to oneself, choosing not to disclose. From a symbolic interactionist viewpoint, self-disclosure will inevitably elicit a response from the other – action brings reaction

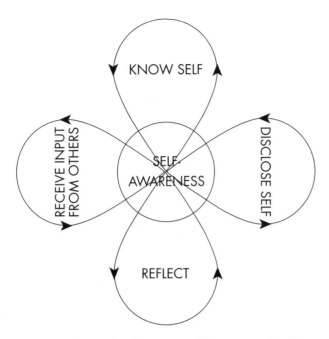

Figure 4.1 Relationship between self-sharing and self-awareness

– that cannot always be predicted. Activity 4.4 is designed to uncover some of the reasons why self-sharing may be difficult.

The major difficulty in disclosing self is the exposure that it brings. Once people are exposed, they often feel vulnerable, especially if the disclosure has been about problem areas or negative thoughts, feelings and perceptions. Offering and receiving such personal items is a transaction involving trust. There are risks of being rejected, being hurt and being challenged by others. This sense of vulnerability is not necessarily destructive to nurses, because of its potential to increase feelings of empathy with people/patients, who often feel exposed and vulnerable when they disclose themselves to carers. While there are obvious risks in exposing self, these are offset by its potential benefits.

The climate conducive to self-sharing

Because of the exposure and vulnerability that self-sharing can bring, it needs to take place in an atmosphere of trust and respect – trust in the sense that the disclosure will not be met with rejection, and respect in the sense that disclosed information will be regarded, not dismissed or ridiculed.

As a general rule, there is ease and comfort with disclosure when it is likely that personal thoughts, feelings and attitudes will be understood and appreciated by the other person. This is more likely to happen when the other person shares similar experiences. For this reason, nurses often benefit from disclosing themselves to other nurses (see Chapter 11). Through the process of self-sharing, nurses can be supported by their peers. They may also be challenged at times to reconsider their perceptions, thoughts and feelings.

ACTIVITY 4.4

DIFFICULTIES IN SELF-SHARING

Process

1 Working on your own, rank each of the following topics from 1–12, according to what is easiest for you to disclose about yourself (1) to what is hardest to disclose (12). Place these topics in the context of interacting with someone you do not know very well.

(a) Talking about my fears

(b) Sharing my hopes and dreams

(c) Discussing my family life

(d) Describing my previous health problems

(e) Stating what I dislike about other people

(f) Complaining about a mark on an assignment

(g) Expressing my political views

(h) Stating what I want or need

(i) Expressing confusion or uncertainty

(j) Describing how I like to be treated by others

(k) Complaining about being treated unfairly

(l) Telling others that I am not pleased about something they have done.

2 Review your answers to Step 1 and reflect on those items that you determined as easy to discuss (those ranked 1–5). Record your reasons for evaluating these items as easy to disclose.

3 Review your answers to Step 1 and reflect on those items you determined as difficult to disclose (those ranked 8–12). Record your reasons for evaluating these items as difficult to disclose.

4 Compare your responses with two other participants. Discuss your responses to Steps 2 and 3. Summarize what is easy to disclose and what is hard to disclose, focusing on your reasons why this is so.

5   This step lists some of the reasons for lack of self-disclosure. Working individually, rate each of these reasons in terms of how often it is true for you. Use the following descriptions:

■   Often
■   Sometimes
■   Rarely

If I tell others what I think and feel . . .

(a)   I may hurt them

(b)   They may take advantage of me

(c)   I may appear weak

(d)   I may become emotional

(e)   They may hurt me

(f)   They may talk to others about me

(g)   I may discover something about myself that I'd rather not know

(h)   They may use what I've said against me

(i)   I may discover problems I never knew I had.

6   Working in the same groups of three as for Step 4, discuss those items that you rated as 'Often' and 'Sometimes'. What similarities are there in your responses? What differences are there?

Discussion

1   What are the major reasons for reluctance to self-disclose?

2   What are the major disadvantages in self-disclosure? What are the major advantages?

3   How does self-disclosure promote self-awareness?

Self-disclosure with people/patients

Self-disclosure with people/patients (see Chapters 5, 6 and 7) is different from self-sharing. Self-disclosure with people/patients is employed as a therapeutic skill, and is therefore for the benefit of the person/patient, not the nurse. Although self-disclosure with people/patients may result in increased self-awareness in the professional, this is not its primary focus. The intent of self-disclosing with people/patients is to promote interaction and increase interpersonal involvement with people/patients through exchanging symbols of trust. The primary intent of self-sharing with people other than the person/patient is increased self-awareness in the professional.

AREAS OF SELF-EXPLORATION

It is important that nurses not only understand the processes for promoting greater self-awareness but also that they recognize those areas of themselves that are most relevant to the person/patient-care context. There are many facets of each professional's self that are woven together to create the sense of the person who is the health care provider. While many attributes of the self can be considered, those addressed in Activity 4.5 have the potential to affect the way that nurses approach helping people/patients.

Personal philosophy about health

Personal value systems, the 'shoulds' and 'ought tos' that direct individual behaviour, are part of all people's lives. These values and beliefs, which are a sub-set of the attributes of the self, assist a person in making choices and decisions about living. They provide direction about what is important, what matters, what is seen as significant and what is worthwhile. These values and beliefs are not static; they are altered, revised and adapted through life experiences. Nurses often find that their beliefs and values alter throughout their professional lives.

One aspect of personal value systems that is of particular relevance for nurses is their beliefs about health and helping. For example, nurses may feel less inclined to care for people/patients that they believe are responsible for their health problems (Olsen 1997).

Activity 4.5 is designed to make participants think about how they would approach helping other people on the basis of two central issues: *blame* and *control* (Brickman *et al.* 1982). Blame is the degree to which people are held responsible for causing their problems; control is the degree to which they are held responsible for solutions to their problems. Both involve questions of personal responsibility, and assumptions about personal responsibility have direct effects on the type of help offered.

Brickman *et al.* (1982) developed four models of helping based on the issues of blame and control (see Figure 4.2). The view from within the Medical model is that people are neither responsible for creating their problems, nor are they responsible for solutions to their problems. The Compensatory model operates from beliefs that people cannot be blamed for their problems, but are held responsible for doing something about them. Beliefs within the Enlightenment model are that people are responsible for creating their problems, but need to rely on others in solving these problems. The Moral model holds people responsible for both creating their problems and developing their own solutions.

Each stance results in an orientation to how to be of help to people/patients. When people believe the model to be real, it has real consequences. The Medical

ACTIVITY 4.5

BELIEFS ABOUT HELPING IN CLINICAL PRACTICE

● **Process**

1   For each of the following statements, record on a separate sheet of paper the response that most closely identifies your personal beliefs and attitudes. Use the following scale:

3   Basically, I agree with this statement
2   I am *undecided* in my opinion about this statement
1   For the most part, I disagree with this statement

(a)   People/patients should be encouraged to accept that they have contributed to their own health problems.

(b)   What happens in nurse–person/patient relationships is more the professional's responsibility than the person/patient's.

(c)   People are masters of their own destinies; solutions to whatever problems they have are in their own hands.

(d)   There are many social factors contributing to health problems that are beyond individual control.

(e)   Whether they realize it or not, people engage in behaviours that cause health problems.

(f)   Effective health education could prevent major health problems.

(g)   People/patients should be encouraged to find solutions and take action on their own behalf when dealing with health problems.

(h)   It irritates me when I hear somebody say that people/patients caused their own health problems; most of the time people can't help it.

(i)   Providing advice to people/patients is an essential aspect of effective health-care.

(j)   In my view of human nature, people are responsible for creating their problems.

(k)   People should be presented with options for health care so that they can choose what suits them best.

(l)   In recovering from an illness, it is essential that people/patients heed the advice of health-care professionals.

(m)   People/patients' health problems are most often of their own making.

(n)   Most people could change their problematic health habits if they really wanted to.

(o)   People/patients cannot be held responsible for causing their own health problems.

(p)   People/patients should determine their own goals when working with health-care professionals.

(q)   Most health problems are the result of the personal choices people make in conducting their lives.

(r)   I don't have much time for people/patients who won't follow the advice of knowledgeable health-care experts.

(s)   Diseases and illnesses are largely a result of biological and genetic factors, which are usually beyond individual control.

(t)   People/patients should place themselves in the hands of qualified health professionals who know best what to do about health problems.

Discussion

1   Reflect on your responses and consider whether you tend to hold people responsible for their health problems.

2   Consider your responses in light of whether you tend to think that people should take responsibility for their own health care.

3   In general, what do your responses reflect about your beliefs about health and health care?

model relies on expert advice and treats people/patients as passive recipients of assistance. People/patients are expected to seek and heed such advice and assistance. While people are not blamed for their problems, they may be blamed if they fail to cooperate with the solutions offered. Helping in the Compensatory model centres on the mobilization of needed resources, providing opportunities to compensate for what are seen as failures and weaknesses that are outside individual control. Acceptance of personal blame and a reliance on an external

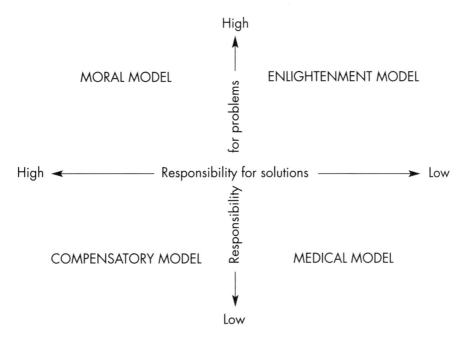

Figure 4.2 Models of helping (based on Brickman *et al.* 1982)

authority is the helping approach used in the Enlightenment model. The Moral model focuses helping on motivating people to change through persuasion, appeal, reprimand and reproach (Brickman *et al.* 1982; Cronenwett 1983; Corey *et al.* 1988).

In health-care provision there is likely to be a mixed application of these models, as illustrated in the following examples. Nurses might hold active smokers responsible for problems such as lung cancer, while lung cancer acquired from passive smoking usually does not bring such blame. In both of these situations people would not be held responsible for the possible solutions/ treatment for the lung cancer. Care would be provided to the active smokers (Enlightenment model), although some nurses may question the use of health-care resources on this population (Moral model). The victims of passive smoking might be approached using the Medical model, in which case they would not be held responsible for the cause or the solutions. A person with diabetes mellitus may not be held responsible for acquiring the disease, but will be expected to be actively involved in its control (Compensatory model). An actively suicidal person may be blamed for the problem and expected to find solutions, through effort and willpower (Moral model).

Help may not be effective if the person desiring help and the person offering help are operating from a different set of assumptions about personal responsibility (Brickman *et al.* 1982). For this reason, it is important that nurses not only realize their own orientation to helping and its underlying assumptions, but also that they are aware of and understand people/patients' orientations to helping.

Effects of personal values and beliefs

The professionals' personal values and beliefs directly affect their interactions with people/patients. They have the potential to restrict effective relationships with people/patients, however, they can also enhance these relationships.

One way that the professionals' values and personal beliefs may hinder effective relationships with people/patients stems from the fact that these values and beliefs often function as perceptual filters. Perceptual filters allow some aspects of people/patients' accounts to be accepted, while others are rejected. When values and personal beliefs function as filters, the skills of listening (see Chapter 5) are most affected. Cultural stereotypes (see Chapter 10), another possible hindrance in relating effectively with people/patients, often stem from values and personal beliefs.

Another way that personal values create interference occurs when nurses impose or project them onto people/patients, rather than keeping them in abeyance. When values and beliefs are imposed on people/patients, they are used as yardsticks for measuring people/patients. Whenever nurses make judgements about what people/patients 'should' or 'should not' be, there is a chance that they are evaluating people/patients in terms of their own value system. For this reason, nurses are encouraged to reflect on these types of judgements.

On the other hand, certain values and personal beliefs enhance and strengthen professionals' ability to relate to people/patients. For example, a personal belief that people are capable, worthwhile and dependable works in favour of establishing effective relationships with people/patients. Such beliefs help to create a climate of respect and regard for people/patients.

When relating to people/patients, nurses cannot be expected to abandon their values and personal beliefs, however they need to be able to distinguish their own philosophical stance from that of a person/patient. The more aware nurses are of their own values and personal beliefs, the less likely it is that interference will occur, and the more likely it is that the values that enhance effective relationships will be strengthened.

Expectations of nurses

Most nurses enter their role with some goal in mind (Activity 4.6). It might be to secure a job with the promise of sustained demand. It could be that part-time work is available. An advertisement in the local newspaper might have sparked interest in a health-care career in a 'Why not, I'm not doing anything else with my life?' fashion. Assuming there were options available, health-care roles are usually chosen because of an interest in people. In all likelihood this interest in people is directly related to a desire to be of help to them.

A common myth about health care is the belief that all benefits in health care are for the person/patient, never the professional. By focusing solely on their desire to help and to assist others, nurses fail to acknowledge the potential benefits of health care provision for themselves (Activity 4.7).

Activity 4.7 challenges the notion that nurses care solely because they are meeting the needs of people/patients. The 'ideal' nurse is often perceived as self-

ACTIVITY 4.6

EXPECTATIONS OF NURSES

 Process

1   Think of all the reasons why you chose your profession as a career. Record these on a sheet of paper. Do not place any identifying information about yourself on the paper.

2   Now complete the following sentences, recording your answers on the same sheet of paper.

    (a)   If I could do anything as a professional it would be to . . .

    (b)   In my role as a professional I see myself as . . .

    (c)   Nurses help others because they . . .

    (d)   My greatest disappointment as a professional would be if I . . .

3   Collect all the sheets of paper and distribute them among all participants.

4   Record, on a sheet of paper visible to all participants, all the reasons identified by the participants for choosing a nursing career. If a reason is given by more than one participant, record how many times it is stated.

Discussion

1   Discuss the responses to each of the items in Step 2 of the process. Remember, you are not discussing your own responses but rather the ones of the anonymous participant who authored the paper you received.

2   Do motivations to provide health care and expectations of the profession focus exclusively on helping others or are there references to personal gains and benefits?

sacrificing, and so 'other-oriented' that there is a denial of self. Such an ideal does not exist in reality.

Personal needs

Forming meaningful relationships with people/patients and assisting them with health issues and problems often has benefits for nurses as well as people/patients. For example, nurses derive satisfaction from seeing people/patients recover from

ACTIVITY 4.7

PERSONAL BENEFITS OF HEALTH CARE PROVISION

 Process

1 On a sheet of paper that only you will see, answer the following questions:

   (a) What does your profession do for you?

   (b) What do you personally gain through health-care provision?

   (c) What benefits are there for you in your profession?

   (d) How does health-care provision satisfy you?

2 From your answers and personal reflection, list personal needs that are met through health-care provision.

Discussion

1 How difficult was it for you to answer these questions?

2 What feelings did you experience while completing the activity?

3 Why is it important for nurses to realize that there are personal gains in health-care provision?

ACTIVITY 4.8

PERSONAL NEEDS THAT MAY INTERFERE

 Process

1 Use one of the following descriptions to rate questions (a)–(j):

   ■ Hardly ever
   ■ Sometimes
   ■ Most of the time

How often do I . . .

   (a) Let people take advantage of me because I am afraid to say no to their requests?

   (b) Focus on problems and negative aspects of a situation, so I fail to take into account the positive side of people and their strengths?

(c) Feel as if I must 'do something' to make other people feel better, to rescue them?

(d) Think I need to have all the answers when other people discuss problems with me?

(e) Worry about whether or not other people like me?

(f) Feel the need to be needed?

(g) Need to be in control of situations?

(h) Want other people to take care of me?

(i) Feel controlled by other people?

(j) Act as openly with other people as I want them to be with me?

2 Review your answers. If the majority of your answers are 'Sometimes', go back and change them to either 'Hardly ever' or 'Most of the time'. All of the items will be true for most people some of the time!

3 Identify the items that are 'Hardly ever' and 'Most of the time'. Reflect on these in terms of how these aspects of yourself may affect your relationships with people/patients.

Discussion

1 The items included in this self-assessment relate to three general areas of basic human needs: the need to feel attached to other people (included); the need to be in control; and the need for affection and affirmation from other people. Which one of these general areas of personal needs is predominant for you?

2 Discuss each of the three basic human needs and how, if they are predominant in a nurse, interactions and relationships with people/patients may be affected, for better or worse.

illnesses, especially when they know that they made a difference to the recovery. Does this mean that nurses meet their own needs through their person/patient relationships? A recognition and acknowledgement of the personal benefits of health care provision results in an affirmative answer to such a question. Nevertheless, there are obvious risks involved because the professionals' personal needs may interfere whenever relationships with people/patients are used as the *primary* source of meeting these needs (Activity 4.8). For example, relying on people/patients to satisfy the professional's need for personal recognition, appreciation and validation is fraught with danger. For this reason, nurses need to develop awareness of potential trouble spots, those personal needs that may interfere in their relationships with people/patients.

THE PROFESSIONAL REPERTOIRE: POSITIVE ATTRIBUTES

The focus of the preceding sections of this chapter has been on increasing self-awareness because self-awareness leads to self-understanding, self-challenge and self-change. Other than considering how different attributes of the self potentially affect relationships with people/patients, no effort has been made to evaluate them (or the person they characterize) in terms of right/wrong, good/bad or desirable/undesirable. No evaluation has been attempted because nurses must first develop awareness of 'what is' before considering 'what should be'. More importantly, the symbolic interactionist perspective suggests that the collection of attributes that may underpin a sense of self at time/place A may be different from the collection of attributes that are present at time/place B. However, despite this there are certain characteristics, personal beliefs, values, orientations toward helping, and skills that enhance nurses' abilities to relate effectively to people/patients. Indeed, as argued in Chapter 1, there are certain expectations of the nurse (of their professional repertoire) which, if absent, tend to disappoint patients. When they are present in the professional these characteristics help to facilitate interpersonal connections with people/patients because they help to create the necessary interpersonal climate for the development of person/patient–nurse relationships. The presence of this climate enables nurses to use effectively the skills and processes described in this book. If the facilitative climate is absent, the use of the skills may become hollow, mechanical and artificial.

From Activity 4.9 you may have discovered that people perceived to be helpful embody certain characteristics (what they are), demonstrate certain skills (what they do) and possess a degree of understanding about people (what they know). It is the personal characteristics associated with helpful people that are discussed here.

Characteristics that enhance the ability to be helpful include:

- Authenticity and congruence
- Respect and warmth
- Confidence and assertiveness.

Authenticity and congruence

To be authentic means that nurses behave in ways that reflect the collection of attributes they have available to them. Frequently, when nurses try to use the skills described in this book, feelings of awkwardness and lack of authenticity accompany their first attempts. This is especially true if the skill being tried is unfamiliar and foreign to the individual's current repertoire of skills. It is not part of the set of self attributes, although the value underpinning the skill may be

ACTIVITY 4.9

CHARACTERISTICS OF EFFECTIVE HELPERS

 Process

1 Think of someone in your life who you think is a helpful person to you, the person you go to for understanding, assistance and guidance.

2 Think about what this person is like. What personal characteristics do they possess? Focus on specific characteristics that are helpful to you. Describe these on a sheet of paper.

3 Now think about what this person does that you find helpful. What specific things does this person do? Describe these on your sheet of paper. Do not be concerned if there are similarities between the answers to Steps 2 and 3. In some instances they may be exactly the same.

4 Review what you have written. Briefly summarize what, in your opinion, enables this person to be effective in helping you.

5 Compare your descriptions with all other participants by compiling an overall description of a person who is helpful. Record this in a place visible to all participants.

6 Select key words from the description and record them.

Discussion

1 What are the similarities in participants' individual descriptions? What are the differences?

2 Focusing on the key words identified in Step 6 of the process, describe personal characteristics that are essential in being a helpful person.

3 Is there anything you would add to this list of personal characteristics?

present. For example, a person may be unskilled in challenging person/patient perceptions, yet believe that people have the potential for change through confronting a personal account. The nurse must tap into their authentic desire to help people/patients in order to overcome feelings of reluctance and awkwardness.

Congruence is related to authenticity because with congruence comes consistency between what nurses believe, how they feel and what they do. The skills described in this book are effective only if they are used in conjunction with an attitude that matches their intent. There is little point in pretending to listen through appropriate attending behaviour (see Chapter 5) if a nurse is not currently interested in what a person/patient is expressing. A listening posture without an attitude of genuine interest lacks congruence. Attempting to understand (see Chapter 6) without an open attitude to the uniqueness of each person/patient's experience also lacks congruence.

RESPECT AND WARMTH

With respect comes a deep concern for people/patients' individual experiences, an acceptance of their perspective and feelings. Respect emerges from the value that each human being has inherent worth and dignity. Under conditions of respect, people/patients are more likely to feel free in expressing who they are and what they are experiencing. When they are respected, people/patients are free to express themselves; they need not fear that they will be judged against a standard of what they 'should' be experiencing. They are empowered (see Chapter 10).

Holding personal judgements in abeyance (see Chapter 5) is one of the most striking ways nurses convey respect to people/patients. This highlights and reinforces the need for self-awareness. Unless nurses are cognisant of their personal values and beliefs, they may inadvertently judge people/patients against a personal value system.

Respect operates from an attitude of being 'for' people/patients. To be respectful is to assume the person/patient's goodwill (Egan 1994), to believe that people/patients are doing their best to cope, to adapt, to change. Respect upholds an inherent belief in people/patients' capabilities and resources. An attitude that is suspicious of people/patients' motives and behaviours lacks respect if suspicion is the nurse's first reaction.

This is not to say that nurses cannot or should not challenge people/patients to transform their view of a situation (see Chapter 8). Respect means not starting from the point of challenging, but rather developing an understanding of the situation (see Chapter 6), then intervening to promote change if this is required.

Warmth is a feeling and is conveyed primarily through nonverbal behaviour that demonstrates an active interest in and regard for people/patients. It is designed to put people/patients at ease with nurses because, through the expression of warmth, nurses convey friendliness, approachability and interest. In this way warmth is an active demonstration of respect because it conveys active concern. Warmth is not emotionally effusive or overly friendly behaviour. It cannot be feigned through insincere over-concern for people/patients.

Too much warmth creates a sense of false solicitude, lacking genuineness. People/patients might become frightened at the prospect of a nurse whose concern seems extreme, especially if this occurs early in the course of the relationship. Too little warmth distances people/patients because this gives an impression of lack of concern and regard. Judging the 'right' degree of warmth, especially in the beginning of a relationship with a patient, can only be achieved by paying careful attention to how the person/patient responds to the professional's demonstration of concern through warmth.

Confidence and assertiveness

Even when nurses are congruent and authentic, and able to convey respect and warmth, unless they also have an ability to express themselves confidently and assertively they may not be able to make interpersonal contact with people/patients. Knowing what to say and how to say it becomes inconsequential if nurses fail to use interpersonal skills because they are apprehensive and hesitant. Being confident and assertive is as important as being skilled and aware. High-level awareness and excellent technical ability are meaningless unless they are actually used when called for (Egan 1994). For example, nurses need to be assertive when they share perceptions and take the lead in exploring (see Chapter 6), and challenge people/patients to reframe their perceptions (see Chapter 7).

Assertiveness is most often presented as a means of resolving conflict, defending individual rights if they have been violated. However, conflict is not the specific focus here. In the general context of person/patient–nurse relationships, being assertive and confident means that nurses are able to take advantage of opportunities to make interpersonal contact with people/patients.

While nurses often recognize the need to be assertive when advocating *for* people/patients (for example, when another health professional or a family member is disregarding a person/patient's request), they often express concerns about being assertive *with* people/patients. Whenever nurses think 'I can't say *that* to a patient' they are experiencing concerns about what will happen. These concerns include a fear of upsetting people/patients, a discomfort with the expression of feelings, a perception that it is intrusive to ask personal questions and a reticence about delving into the subjective experiences of people/patients. Apprehensions such as these often inhibit nurses and may even restrict them from meeting their professional responsibilities to people/patients. For example, if a nurse is reluctant to explore a person/patient's apparent distress (out of fear of compounding that distress), vital information about the person/patient's experience may be missed or overlooked. The distress may in fact, represent an invitation to the nurse to ask questions.

The concerns that inhibit nurses are often based on faulty assumptions such as 'people/patients will become *more* upset if asked to discuss their distress', 'nurses should be passive and obedient' and 'it is impolite to discuss sensitive and personal matters with a relative stranger'. In becoming assertive with people/patients nurses need to overcome these concerns by challenging these assumptions.

First, nurses do not have the 'power' to 'make' people/patients more upset simply on the basis of bringing people/patients' distress into the open (although this is different from abuse of power, which is discussed in Chapter 7). When people/patients are distressed they are often relieved to share their emotional pain with an interested and understanding nurse. Rather than compounding their tension, open discussion can actually provide comfort. Second, while it would be impolite to discuss highly personal matters with a stranger in a social situation, person/patient–nurse interactions are different from usual social interactions. In caring for people/patients nurses need to discuss personal matters with people/patients because this is part of their professional responsibility.

There is more to assertiveness than just being able to bring up sensitive and sometimes troubling subjects. At times being assertive translates into making the decision 'not' to discuss something. For example, when a person/patient is coping by maintaining her/his emotions within manageable limits a nurse can make an active decision *not* to explore or focus on feelings. Additionally, the discussion of feelings requires trust between person/patient and nurse (see Chapter 6), and a nurse may choose to delay such discussion until trust is established. As long as the decision not to say something is based on an assessment of the situation, rather than the nurse's internal fear, assertiveness is present. Being assertive in relating to people/patients means that nurses have both the courage to say something and the wisdom to remain silent.

LEARNING THE SKILLS

The following chapters contain descriptions of a range of skills that enable nurses to interact effectively with people/patients. While theoretical understanding of the skills is a vital aspect of learning, understanding not accompanied by technical know-how in the use of the skills is insufficient. For this reason, learning the skills of interacting with people/patients is achieved most effectively through the performance of the skills.

Each nurse is encouraged to attempt each of the skills, see how they fit the particular health-care context and determine what alterations can be made to help them fit better. Some of the skills will be familiar and using them will come naturally because they already exist in the health-care provider's repertoire. Other skills will be foreign and nurses may feel awkward and unnatural when initially attempting to use these skills. Selecting some of the skills because they are comfortable to use and ignoring others because 'they don't feel right' limits practical learning opportunities and potential. The aim is to increase the repertoire of skills (as attributes). Having an extensive repertoire means that the nurse can select the skills that aid a presentation of self that is relevant to the specific care context.

The need to 'unlearn'

More than likely, the skills presented in the following chapters will be recognizable as everyday activities. For example listening (see Chapter 5) is a process that people engage in daily, whether it be effective or ineffective. Most people count listening as an attribute of self. This familiarity with some skills, however, presents a specific dilemma to nurses as they approach learning how to fit skills into a health-care context.

Because nurses have been interacting with other people all of their lives they may believe they already know how to talk to people/patients, and may be disconcerted to find out there is more to learn. But these familiar patterns of interacting may not be effective within the health-care context. As a result, some nurses may fail to recognize and appreciate the alterations that may be needed to make their interactions with people/patients more effective.

Learning how to use interpersonal skills within the health-care context is often a matter of 'letting go' of habitual and automatic ways of interacting, ways that have become comfortable. For example, offering advice and giving solutions is a common response to someone who presents a problem. In Chapter 6 this way of responding is shown to be less effective than a response that demonstrates understanding. If offering advice and giving solutions is their customary way of responding to those in need, nurses are challenged to refrain from their usual way of responding. The need to let go of familiar patterns and 'unlearn' ways that may have become entrenched presents a major hurdle in learning and developing effective interactive skills with people/patients.

Departing from the comfortable zone of usual and customary patterns of interacting and attempting new and unfamiliar ways initially results in feelings of falseness or being deskilled. Nurses may become confused by this apparent lack of authenticity, which has been discussed as a core condition for effective interactions. They may feel inept, clumsy and overly self-conscious as they struggle to let go of the familiar and to meet the demands of learning new ways of interacting.

Such feelings are often unavoidable during initial attempts in using any new skill and this highlights the need for continuous self-awareness. Through self-awareness, nurses come to appreciate what they are attempting in their interactions with people/patients, why they are attempting this and how it is affecting people/patients. Nurses are encouraged to promote their own growth as people and as health-care providers, and to challenge growth within themselves by trying various ways of interacting with people/patients, even when these ways initially feel awkward.

SELF-ASSESSMENT OF INTERPERSONAL SKILLS

Active and ongoing self-assessment is a strategy for reflection and is one of the most effective ways to increase interpersonal effectiveness as a nurse. Self-assessment draws on all of the processes for developing self-awareness that are described in this chapter. Nurses need to develop the ability to observe themselves as they participate in interactions with people/patients. This requires nurses to develop abilities to stand apart from themselves temporarily, and to tune their senses to recognize effective and ineffective interaction patterns. Observing feedback and input from people/patients, which indicates how they are responding to the nurse's attempts to interact, adds to this self-evaluation. Discussion with other nurses about relationships with people/patients offers opportunities to be both reassured and challenged. Finally, the sharing of motives, intentions, thoughts, and feelings, both with themselves and other nurses, offers further opportunities for growth in interpersonal effectiveness with people/patients.

Self-assessment has many advantages. First, through the process of self-assessment, 'mistakes', when made, are viewed as indicators for further growth and development, rather than outright failures. Nurses who can recognize when they either miss the point or could be handling an interaction more effectively have an opportunity to recover and move the interaction back on track. They can draw on their repertoire of skills and choose an intervention on a sounder basis than without self-assessment. When awareness is lacking, errors and omissions go unrecognized and future learning opportunities are missed.

Second, self-assessment has the advantage of using the nurse's first-hand experience in the interaction. Nurses who have participated in an interaction know best what happened. In this sense, 'being there' provides essential input. Nurses who 'were there' understand their own intentions or position during the interaction and can therefore evaluate an interaction in light of these intentions. In this regard, evaluation of performance is placed within the context of actual interactions, as opposed to employing rules that are context-free.

Finally and perhaps most importantly, developing the ability to assess self enables nurses to engage in continual learning. Through awareness and self-assessment, nurses come to understand their personal strengths and areas for improvement, and performance is evaluated in terms of these personal aspects. When every interaction is viewed as an opportunity for learning, nurses engage in continuous professional growth. In this respect, self-assessment, the evaluation of one's own performance, is considered an essential ability, even a skill in its own right.

Self-assessment is useful in evaluating interpersonal effectiveness after an interaction has occurred, and this is the most common way in which it is initially developed. When developed to its fullest, self-assessment also enables nurses to determine how best to approach a given situation *during* an interaction.

Approaches to self-assessment

Beginning and experienced nurses are encouraged to begin their self-evaluation with an assessment of how they are currently functioning with their interpersonal skills. Activity 4.10 is designed to increase awareness of current interaction patterns. It relies on the process of self-reflection, discussed earlier in this chapter, and is therefore an activity that should be completed in solitude.

In addition to reflecting on 'everyday' interactions, it is essential that nurses reflect on their interactions with people/patients. Interactions with people/patients are different from everyday interactions in the sense that nurses are often focused on being of help to people/patients. While helping others does occur during everyday interactions, this is not always the primary intent of such interactions.

In order to determine how best to approach situations with people/patients, nurses must be able to observe and reflect on the interaction while simultaneously participating in the interaction. The complexity of self-assessment is often overwhelming as a result of these demands. Because the ability to become a participant–observer during interactions can be quite cumbersome to manage all at once, it is often useful to sort the process of self-assessment into manageable units. Although the ultimate aim is to combine all units, first mastering smaller units helps develop the art of self-assessment. The following approaches and activities focus on these smaller units: observing, perceiving, reflecting, evaluating, and making alterations on the basis of the evaluation.

Reflection after interactions with people/patients

An effective approach to assessing performance, and one of the most commonly used approaches, is a reflective evaluation of an interaction after it has occurred.

ACTIVITY 4.10

ASSESSMENT OF CURRENT SKILLS

● Process

1   Observe your interactions for approximately ten days. Focus on situations in which you are aware of how you are interacting. These situations should contain interactions during which you felt you were effectively interacting with the other persons, and those that you felt were not as effective. These should be situations that illustrate how you typically communicate and interact with other people. Some examples of the type of situations you may observe include:

- Introducing yourself to a stranger
- Needing to clarify something that you have not understood
- Asking another person about themselves
- Speaking in a group
- Asking someone for a favour
- Wanting to say 'no' to a request
- Giving or seeking information
- Receiving negative feedback about yourself
- Explaining why you did or said something
- Disagreeing with someone
- Seeking assistance from someone
- Expressing concern for someone else
- Wanting to help someone else
- Demonstrating to someone that you care about them.

2   Record these situations as soon as possible after they occur. Include a description of what happened, what you thought about what happened and how you felt about what happened.

3   After you have recorded these situations for about ten days, review them in order to determine your major strengths when interacting with other people and those areas that you think you could improve.

Discussion

Write a brief summary of your interactions, using the following as a guide:

- What you observed about your interpersonal interactions (for example, 'I notice that I don't always listen when I am worried about what I am going to say')
- Your strengths and areas for improvement (for example, 'I am good at starting conversations with people I do not know')
- Your personal goals for improving your ability to interact and relate to others (for example, 'I would like to be able to seek clarification so that I'm sure I understand').

ACTIVITY 4.11

GUIDE TO SELF-REFLECTION

● **Process**

1 Describe (either through speaking or writing) an interaction in terms of what happened. Do not think about why it happened, just what happened between you and the person/patient.

2 Answer the following questions:

   (a) What did you say that was helpful to the person/patient?

   (b) What was your intent in saying this?

   (c) How did you know it was helpful?

   (d) What did you say/do that was not helpful to the person/patient?

   (e) What was your intent in saying this?

   (f) How did you know it was not helpful?

   (g) What could you have said that would have been more helpful?

   (h) What were you feeling during this interaction?

   (i) What do you think the person/patient was feeling during the interaction?

   (j) How would you have changed this interaction if you could do it again?

This approach to self-assessment is used after nurses have spontaneously participated in an interaction with a person/patient. Through reflection, nurses are able to identify skills that were used, assess the effects of these skills and, using person/patient responses and theoretical concepts as a guide, construct a probable explanation of why the skills were effective or ineffective.

Activity 4.11 is presented as a useful way for nurses to reflect personally on interactions with people/patients, be they positive or negative experiences.

Nurses may fall into the trap of being overly critical of themselves when they reflect on their interactions with people/patients, because they place pressure on themselves to 'do it right'. Rather than viewing interactions as opportunities for growth, nurses who want to 'do it right' perceive interactions as tests of effective performance. This view often stifles personal and professional development.

ACTIVITY 4.12

SELF-ASSESSMENT OF SPECIFIC SKILLS

Process

1 Identify which skill or set of skills is particularly difficult to understand or seems too uncomfortable to use.

2 Review the section of this book that covers this particular skill or set of skills.

3 During interactions with people/patients, look for opportunities when this skill or set of skills is appropriate to use, or notice each time you use the skill or set of skills during an interaction with people/patients.

Discussion

Each time you use the skill or set of skills:

1 Evaluate its effects on interaction with the person/patient.

2 Observe how the person/patient responds.

3 Reflect on how you felt and responded.

4 Make a note of the circumstances and immediate situation.

Whenever nurses are asked to reflect on their interactions, there is a danger that they will recall only those interactions during which they felt ineffective. For this reason it is important that nurses focus on positive, fulfilling and beneficial interactions, as well as those interactions that could have been more effective. Satisfying and successful interactions are as informative as those that are not.

Focus on specific skills during an interaction

At times nurses will want to develop a specific skill or related set of skills because they perceive these skills as difficult, uncomfortable to use or hard to understand. Under these circumstances an effective way to self-assess is to focus on these skills during an interaction (Activity 4.12).

Maintaining an ongoing record

The previously described self-assessment methods are most effective whenever nurses keep track of a number of people/patient interactions. Such a record is sometimes referred to as a 'journal' or 'diary'. In maintaining such a record, nurses are able to develop their understanding and use of interpersonal skills by referring to a variety of situations and circumstances. When a variety of situations are evaluated, comparisons and contrasts can be made and patterns begin to emerge. Keeping track of various people/patient situations, and various ways of interacting in these situations, enables nurses to formulate a more complete understanding than simply focusing on isolated events or isolated skills.

Soliciting help from other nurses

In addition to the self-reflection that the previous approaches encourage, it is useful for nurses to solicit feedback from other nurses about how they are interacting with people/patients. The questions in Activity 4.11 can be used to prompt information from your peers. The questions are exploratory. They refrain from passing judgement and encourage other nurses to reflect and determine how they are interacting.

This approach to helping other nurses is preferable to providing solutions and offering advice. When solutions and advice are given, nurses are not encouraged to generate their own solutions. Also, it is only the nurse who 'was there' during a given interaction who knows exactly what happened. Nurses who were not present yet receive a reported account of what happened are relying on the health care provider giving the account and are processing the information through their own filters. It is preferable for the nurse who 'was there' to process the interaction through her/his own perceptual filters because this approach has the greatest possibility for promoting self-awareness. Other nurses may offer alternative perspectives, thus encouraging a reappraisal of the situation, but it is best to begin with attempting to understand.

Pitfalls in self-assessment

The tendency to judge or evaluate their performance is often automatic, even natural for nurses. Nevertheless, a negative evaluation can be quite troublesome when the perceived stakes are great. In evaluating their interactions with people/patients, the stakes are often high for nurses because of a need to maintain a positive professional image. Most nurses will want to be effective in their interactions with people/patients, and performance judged as ineffective may threaten their professional image and professional esteem. For example, when nurses recognize that they have blocked or inhibited an interaction with a person/patient, they may find this behaviour unacceptable in a professional sense. In order to preserve and maintain a front as effective professionals, they may overlook, diminish, justify, or even reject flaws and mistakes in their performance.

Overcoming this potential pitfall is best achieved through recognition and continuous awareness that self-assessment is done for the purpose of professional growth and development. Continual reflection and evaluation of performance enables nurses to build on their experiences and learn from them. Through self-assessment nurses determine what was right or wrong, effective or ineffective about their interaction skills and patterns. Nevertheless, this evaluation is not the end point of self-assessment. Self-assessment is employed primarily for the purpose of seeking ways to improve. Thus, it is not simply an evaluative process but a learning process. A commitment to continual learning is an essential aspect of professionalism.

Another potential pitfall in using self-assessment is a tendency to gloss over performance, perceiving it globally as either all good or all bad. Focusing exclusively on positive aspects is as much a pitfall as focusing exclusively on negative aspects of performance. Nurses who can focus only on mistakes or flaws in their interactions with people/patients are being too harsh in their self-evaluation. Nurses who can focus only on positive aspects of their performance are failing to recognize areas for improvement and learning, which exist in the majority of situations.

The tendency to view performance globally as either all good or all bad is kept in check through the realization that most interactions will contain a mixture of positive and negative aspects. Whenever nurses can perceive only one type or the other, their self-assessment lacks accuracy and completeness. If this happens, nurses are encouraged to reflect further in order to develop a balanced view of evaluation.

A final potential pitfall in using one's self as the assessor of performance emerges whenever nurses lack understanding of the criteria on which to base their evaluations. A lack of understanding of how and why interpersonal skills are used is addressed through further reading and discussion about the theory of effective interactions in nursing. Additionally, nurses may need to solicit assistance from an external authority, for example, an experienced professional or an educator, in developing appropriate criteria on which to base their self-assessment.

CHAPTER SUMMARY

Nurses need to develop acute self-awareness whenever they engage in interactions and relationships with people/patients. Being self-aware means being able to identify reflectively the range of personal and professional attributes that the nurse has at a given time and in a given space. Without self-awareness, nurses run the risk of imposing their values and views onto people/patients. *Values that serve the nurse may be detrimental or useless to people/patients and lead to a misreading of the care episode.*

In order to increase self-awareness, processes of self-reflection are necessary. This chapter has reviewed three processes for developing self-awareness:

- Self-reflection
- Input from others
- Self-sharing

Nurses are encouraged to use these processes in their day-to-day encounters with people/patients. Reflection, both in solitude and through interaction with others, as well as self-sharing, enables nurses to meet the challenges of self-growth.

Self-awareness is the primary means through which nurses are able to evaluate their effectiveness in relating to people/patients. In every interaction, the nurse can respond to the feedback from the person/patient, using this as a means of deciding on the combination of attributes, the specific presentation of self that will be most appropriate.

REFERENCES

Armstrong-Esther, C. A. and Browne, K. D. (1986). The influence of elderly patients' mental impairment on nurse–patient interaction. *Journal of Advanced Nursing*, 11, 379–87.

Atkins, S. and Murphy, K. (1993). Reflection: a review of the literature. *Journal of Advanced Nursing*, 18, 1188–92.

Baer, E. and Lowery, B. J. (1987). Patient and situational factors that affect nursing students' like or dislike of caring for patients. *Nursing Research*, 36(5), 298–302.

Begat, I., Severinsson, E. and Berggren, I. (1997). Implementation of clinical supervision in a medical department: nurses' views of the effects. *Journal of Clinical Nursing*, 6(5), 389–94.

Brickman, P., Rabinowitz, V. C., Karuza, J., Coates, D., Cohn, E. and Kidder, L. (1982). Models of helping and coping. *American Psychologist*, 37(4), 368–84.

Carr, C. J. (1996). Reflecting on clinical practice: hectoring talk or reality? *Journal of Clinical Nursing*, 5, 289–95.

Carveth, J. A. (1995). Perceived patient deviance and avoidance by nurses. *Nursing Research*, 44(3), 173–8.

Clarke, B., James, C. and Kelly, J. (1996). Reflective practice: reviewing the issues and refocusing the debate. *International Journal of Nursing Studies*, 33(2), 171–80.

Corey, G., Coreu, M. S. and Callahan, P. (1988). *Issues and Ethics in the Helping Professions*, third edition. Belmont, CA: Brooks/Cole.

Cronenwett, L. R. (1983). When and how people help: theoretical issues and evidence. In P. L. Chinn (ed.), *Advances in Nursing Theory Development* (pp. 251–70). Rockville, MD: Aspen.

Davies, E. (1995). Reflective practice: a focus for caring. *Journal of Nursing Education*, 43(4), 167–74.

Drew, N. (1986). Exclusion and confirmation: phenomenology of people/patients' experiences with caregivers. *Image: Journal of Nursing Scholarship*, 18, 39–43.

Egan, G. (1994). *The Skilled Helper*, fifth edition. Monterey, CA: Brooks/Cole.

Forrest, D. (1989). The experience of caring. *Journal of Advanced Nursing*, 14, 815–23.

Foster, J. and Greenwood, J. (1998). Reflection: a challenging innovation for nurses. *Contemporary Nurse*, 7, 165–72.

Fowler, J. (1998). Evaluating the efficacy of reflective practice within the context of clinical supervision. *Journal of Advanced Nursing*, 27, 379–82.

Greenwood, J. (1993). Reflective practice: a critique of the work of Argyris and Schon. *Journal of Advanced Nursing*, 18, 1183–7.

Greenwood, J. (1998). The role of reflection in single and double loop learning, *Journal of Advanced Nursing*, 27, 1048–53.

Grief, C. L. and Elliot, R. (1994). Emergency nurses' moral evaluation of patients. *Journal of Emergency Nursing*, 20(4), 275–9.

Haddock, J. and Bassett, C. (1997). Nurses' perceptions of reflective practice. *Nursing Standard*, 11(32), 39–41.

Johns, C. (1995). The value of reflective practice for nursing. *Journal of Clinical Nursing*, 4(1), 23–30.

Johns, C. (1999). Reflection as empowerment? *Nursing Inquiry*, 6, 241–9.

Johnson, M. and Webb, C. (1995a). Rediscovering unpopular patients: The concept of social judgement. *Journal of Advanced Nursing*, 21, 455–66.

Johnson, M. and Webb, C. (1995b). The power of social judgement: Struggle and negotiation in the nursing process. *Nurse Education Today*, 15, 83–9.

Jones, P. R. (1995). Hindsight bias in reflective practice: an empirical investigation. *Journal of Advanced Nursing*, 21, 783–8.

Kelly, M. P. and May, D. (1982). Good and bad patients: a review of the literature and a theoretical critique. *Journal of Advanced Nursing*, 7, 147–56.

Kim, H. S. (1999). Critical reflective inquiry for knowledge development in nursing practice. *Journal of Advanced Nursing*, 29, 1205–12.

Lawler, J. (1991). *Behind the Screens: Nursing, Somology, and the Problem of the Body*. Melbourne: Churchill Livingstone.

Luft, J. (1969). *Of Human Interaction*. Palo Alto, CA: National Press Books.

Olsen, D. (1997). When the patient causes the problem: the effect of patient responsibility on the nurse–patient relationship. *Journal of Advanced Nursing*, 26, 515–22.

Pfeiffer, J. W. and Jones, J. E. (1974). *A Handbook of Structured Experiences for Human Relations Training*. La Jolla, CA: University Associates.

Sayler, J. and Stuart, B. J. (1985). Nurse–patient interaction in the intensive care unit. *Heart & Lung*, 14, 20–4.

Taylor, B. (1997). Big battles for small gains: a cautionary note for teaching reflective processes in nursing and midwifery practice. *Nursing Inquiry*, 4, 19–26.

Tichen, A. and Binnie, A. (1995). The art of clinical supervision. *Journal of Clinical Nursing*, 4(5), 327–34.

Wilkinson, J. (1999). Implementing reflective practice. *Nursing Standard*, 13(21), 36–40.

Part II

THE SKILLS

Part I of the book has offered a theoretical framework, symbolic inter-actionism, within which interpersonal relationships can be understood. Symbolic interactionism is a tool for nurses to use to understand the process of their encounters with people/patients and to analyse how these encounters sometimes seem to become stuck or unproductive.

In Part II we turn to helping nurses develop the skills that will assist them in being able to collaboratively define the meaning of care episodes with people/patients. Skills of listening, understanding, exploring, comforting, supporting and enabling all help nurses to 'read' situations with people/patients that they encounter. Of course, these skills are not used in isolation. They are interdependent. However, we have divided them in order to make them more easily learned. We have included numerous exercises in order to facilitate learning. Reading about a skill does not mean that the skill can be enacted. Sometimes the exercises require individual work and at other times learning is achieved through collaboration with colleagues.

Part II is a space where nurses can enlarge the set of attributes that make up their professional repertoire, try out their performances safely, with a view to enabling interpersonal interactions in the clinical sphere.

CHAPTER 5

ENCOURAGING INTERACTION:
LISTENING

INTRODUCTION

'It wasn't much, I mean, I really didn't do anything to help. All I did was listen.' Comments such as these, especially when expressed by nurses, fail to acknowledge or demonstrate an appreciation for the complexity and power of effective listening. 'Just listening' seems so simple, as if no effort is required, no expertise needed. The art of listening is knowing when not to interrupt a person/patient in the flow of their discussion. Sometimes when talking about difficult or sensitive topics, the person will pause to gather their thoughts and consider the situation; if the nurse intervenes at that moment the person may never reveal the underlying reason for the discussion, or indeed explore their worries and fears. It is for this reason that the nurse needs to enhance her/his listening ability.

Listening is powerful because it encourages people/patients to share their experiences; it validates people/patients as people with something to say; it promotes understanding between nurse and person/patient; and it provides the nurse with information on which to act. It is not nearly as 'simple' as it sounds on the surface. Quite a lot is happening when nurses 'just' listen. When nurses listen, *just* listen, they pay careful attention to what they hear and observe, they focus on what is explicitly expressed by the person/patient and they try to determine what the person/patient is meaning. Effective listening requires receptivity, sustained concentration and astute observation. All of this can hardly be summed up as 'not doing anything'. Nursing care is based on an understanding of people/patients' personal experiences of health and their responses to illness. In order to reach this level of understanding, nurses must first listen to what the person/patient says. To listen to the person/patient is one of the most valuable ways of ensuring that it is the person/patient's needs that are met and not the professional's. The skills of listening are fundamental and crucial to person/patient–nurse relationships. Listening permeates the entire relationship; if meaningful interpersonal connections are to occur, listening must be engaged in throughout every interaction.

Listening actively demonstrates nurses' presence with and interest in people/patients. Through listening, nurses orient themselves towards people/patients as people who 'are there'. Listening encourages people/patients to express themselves because it provides the necessary time and space for such expressions. Listening enables people/patients to experience being heard and accepted by nurses. Listening enables nurses to understand and appreciate people/patients' experiences. As such, it sets the stage for effective helping. Nurses base their responses to people/patients on what is perceived through listening. Once the stage is set, the players can enact their roles (the one helping and the one helped), but it is vital that the stage remains set throughout the relationship.

CHAPTER OVERVIEW

This chapter begins with a description of the process of effective listening, highlighting its complexity. Then the benefits of listening within the context of person/patient–nurse relationships are discussed. Because nurses need to listen with 'nursing ears', listening goals within the nursing-care context are explored next. The following section on mental preparation, the readiness to listen, focuses on how to become more receptive to people/patients by reducing potential interferences and distractions. A discussion of the skills of listening follows. These include attending, observing, perceiving, interpreting, and recalling. The chapter concludes with a description of how to evaluate whether listening has been effective.

THE LISTENING PROCESS

To truly focus on what the person is saying you must not only listen but also become attentive to the internal and external environment, consciously considering what is being communicated. Burnard (2001) identifies three hypothetical zones of attention that the professionals should consider to enhance their listening skills:

Burnard acknowledges that professionals will move freely between the three zones; however, he emphasizes the importance of becoming more aware of these to help improve the quality of interpersonal skills you use when carrying out care. Zone One is where the nurse focuses completely on the person/patient and what they are saying, while Zone Two is where nurses notice their own feelings and reactions before refocusing on what the person/patient is saying. Zone Three he identifies as the zone where the nurse makes assumptions about the person/patient's thoughts and feelings, for example, 'I know the person/patient isn't really feeling any pain. He won't admit he's getting better. He wants attention, that's all.' The problem with making such assumptions is that these get focused on the care setting, and then different care may be planned for the person/patient so that their needs are not met. Other assumptions may also stem from these interpretations that have not been checked. Linking this to the above example, the person/patient then may be refused analgesia, or may be labelled as a potential drug-abuser. It is for these reasons that Burnard recommends that nurses use their self-awareness skills and become aware of their focus of attention to enhance

The 'outside' experience (the external world)	The 'inside' experience (the internal world)
	ZONE TWO 'Attention in' focused on inner thoughts and ideas. The listener is distracted – does not listen fully.
ZONE ONE 'Attention out' – the whole of the nurse's attention is with the person/patient. The listener is really listening.	
	ZONE THREE Attention is focused on 'fantasy'. Perception is based on what is imagined to be the case. In this zone the nurse develops theories about the person/patient.

Burnard's zones of attention

listening and interpreting what is being said more effectively, rather than jumping to conclusions or making value judgements.

It is clear that listening is a complex process that encompasses the skills of reception, perception and interpretation of input. The process begins with input. Sights, sounds, smells, tastes, and tactile sensations are received through the sensory organs. The initial step is the reception of this input, predominantly through the eyes and ears. The ability to receive the input is dependent upon the listener's state of readiness, when receivers are 'turned on' and 'tuned in'. Next, the received input must be noticed as important; it must be actively perceived. During this stage of the process, external and internal distractions often interfere with accurate perception and create filters, which partially or completely block the input. Almost as soon as the input is perceived, the listener attaches meaning to it – an interpretation is made.

The meaning attached to a particular piece of sensory input is connected to the listener's memory, previous experience, expectations, desires, wants, needs, and current thoughts and feelings. For example, nurses working in a hospital unit know when they hear a particular buzz and see a light over a doorway to a person/patient's room (sensory input received and perceived) that the person/patient in that room has turned on the call light, requesting assistance (interpretation). To an outsider, the sound and sight of the call light activation may be received and noticed, but no particular meaning is derived unless there is a familiarity with how hospital units are equipped. If they are busy, nurses who notice the call light may interpret the person/patient's request for assistance as a nuisance (interpretation based on needs). Likewise, a nurse may decide that the person/patient requesting assistance is not in immediate need if this particular person/patient turns on the call light for minor reasons (interpretation based on experience and expectations).

Effective listening encompasses not only receiving sensory input but also perceiving it and interpreting its meaning. When nurses correctly interpret what people/patients are expressing, listening has been effective.

Hearing and listening

Listening and hearing are not the same. Any person with the apparatus for detecting audible tones can hear, but may or may not be capable of listening. People without hearing capabilities may be able to listen, while those with hearing capabilities may fail to listen. Listening involves paying active attention to what is being said; it is more than simply receiving sensory input.

Active and passive listening

Effective listening, the active process of taking in, absorbing and eventually understanding what is being expressed, requires energy and concentration on the part of the listener. Have you ever been in a conversation with somebody who claimed to be listening to you but was attending to another matter, for example, watching television or reading? No matter how much this person may try to convince you that they are is listening, it is not likely you will believe it, because they are not offering their full attention.

Hearing, without fully concentrating and attending, is passive listening. Active listening is listening for the purpose of understanding. Not only does it require the reception of sensory input; it also demands astute observation, undivided attention and the processing or interpretation of what is heard. It is important for nurses to show the person/patient that they are actively listening to what s/he is saying, by using minimal prompts such as head nods, 'yes', use of touch, and reflection of points being made, all of which let the person/patient know that you are taking in the information. While some people may be capable of listening to background music while reading or studying, this type of passive reception does not serve listeners well during engaged interpersonal interaction. Effective listening is only achieved in an active and involved manner. It cannot be done passively.

BENEFITS OF LISTENING

It is important that nurses understand the benefits of effective listening in order to appreciate more fully its power and helpfulness. The benefits can be described as those for the person/patient, those for the nurse and those for the relationship between them.

For the person/patient

Effective listening is consistent with the concept that nurses care about people/patients. When nurses take and make time to listen to what people/patients are expressing, they demonstrate genuine interest in and regard for people/patients. Listening is one of the clearest ways for nurses to convey respect for and acceptance of people/patients. By listening, nurses actively demonstrate to people/patients that what they have to say matters, that people/patients matter. Nurses give of themselves when they listen. People/patients feel worthwhile because they have been given the nurse's time, energy and attention. Listening reinforces the inherent worth of people/patients, and as a result, people/patients feel comforted because they are valued, acknowledged and validated. People/patients report that listening is an important aspect of what they want in a nurse (Webb and Hope 1995).

For the nurse

Any verbal response that nurses make is based on what is perceived through listening to the person/patient. Listening to people/patients enables nurses to receive information about people/patients, collect data on which to base nursing-care activities and reach deeper levels of understanding with people/patients. Being fully present with a person/patient, as would be evidenced through listening, has been linked to effective clinical decision-making in nursing (Doona *et al.* 1997).

Theoretical understanding of a particular clinical situation offers possibilities and probabilities, but listening to an individual person/patient's experience offers concrete, personally unique data on which to base responsive nursing care. For example, chronic illness often affects a person/patient's sense of self-worth (a theoretical possibility). But by listening to an individual person/patient's experience of and reactions to chronic illness, the nurse comes to understand concretely and specifically how this particular person/patient's sense of self-worth is, or is not, affected by the experience. Listening encourages people/patients to open up and tell their stories, and as a result, nurses are in a better position to understand patients more personally.

For the relationship

Listening encourages further interaction between person/patient and nurse. It is a catalyst in promoting trust in their relationship, because people/patients will come to know that they can rely on the nurse to 'be there'.

At times, listening with understanding is all that is needed in an interaction; it is an end in itself. For example, listening to a person/patient's expression of sadness in response to a loss may be just what the nurse needs to do in order to be of help. At other times, listening is a means to another end, a responsive nursing action based on understanding that is achieved through listening. For example, as a result of listening to a person/patient express a lack of understanding about a current medication regime, the nurse can explain why it is important, for example, to take medication prior to eating.

LISTENING FROM A NURSE'S PERSPECTIVE (PROFESSIONAL EARS)

The general benefits of listening in the professional-care context are important to appreciate; however, the benefits refer primarily to how meaningful interaction between person/patient and nurse is enhanced. What about the content of listening in the nursing-care context? When nurses listen, they need to listen for aspects of the person/patient's experience that are significant in the context of their nursing care. What should be the focus when listening to people/patients? What kinds of meanings and understandings are specific to the clinical practice setting? What particular aspects of people/patients' experiences are most relevant to the nurse? Listening with 'professional ears' is listening for specific professional-related meanings, and an understanding of these meanings forms the basis of listening goals within the professional context.

Activity 5.1 poses challenges because it suggests that certain limitations can be imposed on listening. Does listening with 'professional ears' mean that you should ignore, avoid or filter out aspects that are not directly related to professional concerns? Hardly, because this implies partial listening. While it is important for you to recognize what concerns you *as* a nurse, there is potential danger when listening goals are overemphasized. When this occurs, goals for listening become barriers.

Rather than perceiving these goals as limitations, it is better to think of them as focusing lenses through which to view people/patients. To take the analogy further, imagine looking through the lens of a camera and focusing on a particular subject within a scene. While the entire landscape is in view, the camera lens brings some aspects of the picture into sharper focus than others. Such is the case when using listening goals in the nursing context. While the entire 'picture', that is, the person/patient, is in view (received), some aspects are brought more sharply in focus (perceived), because these aspects have direct relevance to health care.

Another way to employ listening goals in your profession is to use them as orienting and guiding frameworks during the interpretation of received messages. Attention needs to be paid to the person/patient's entire message; however, the message is interpreted in light of the goals of listening. The message is perceived as is, but the meaning is interpreted using a professional framework. This framework, or orientation to listening, is then viewed as enhancing rather than limiting because it provides direction to the professional's listening – as in the following example.

> When he first met James Nott, Matthew, an experienced cardiac nurse, was completing the usual admission procedure to the cardiac surgical ward. He had to complete all the necessary observations of James' physical condition but, more importantly, he needed to get to know James as a person. As Matthew listened to his account of a lifelong problem with his mitral valve, he realized that James understood the implications of his scheduled valve replacement surgery. James told Matthew that he knew the surgery would need to be done some day. Naturally, James was concerned about the surgery itself, but he reassured himself in the knowledge that he was in the capable hands of an experienced cardiac surgery team. As he listened, Matthew began to realize the potential impact of the surgery on James' life. He was employed

ACTIVITY 5.1

LISTENING GOALS IN NURSING

 Process

1   Form small groups of about five participants.

2   Discuss the answers to the following questions:

(a) 'What do I need to know and understand about people/patients in order to care effectively for them?'

(b) 'When I am listening to people/patients, what is most significant for me to notice about what they are expressing?'

3   Record and compare your answers with other small groups.

Discussion

1   Do the answers to the questions provide any focus for listening in your profession? If so, what is the focus?

2   Are there aspects of people/patients' experiences that are more significant to your profession than other aspects? What are these?

3   What are the major goals of listening in your professional context? List them.

4   Listening with professional ears means focusing on goals. Compare your list in Step 3 with the following goals (presented in question form):

(a) What effects does the people/patients' current health status have on their daily living?

(b) How do people/patients interpret their health status?

(c) How are people/patients reacting to the health care they are receiving?

(d) How are they reacting to your professional approach in particular?

(e) How much do people/patients understand about their health status and health care? How much do they want to understand?

(f) Who or what is most important to people/patients? What do they value the most in life?

(g) What is worrying people/patients the most about their health status and health care?

as a night-shift supervisor of a large coal preparation plant, a position he worked hard to obtain and an achievement of which he was proud. Nevertheless, his job involved a great deal of walking around the plant and James noted his increasing inability 'to get around like I used to'. He was afraid that he might become disabled after the surgery, unable to continue in a job he obviously enjoyed. He understood the details of the surgery, recognized that it was necessary and accepted it. Yet he was worried about what it might mean to his future. In focusing on James' concern about the potential impact of the surgery, of what it might mean in terms of his daily life, Matthew was listening with 'professional ears'.

READINESS TO LISTEN

Effective listening requires a certain amount of mental preparation in order to achieve a state of readiness. A nurse's 'readiness to listen' is as important as the act of perceiving actively and fully what a person/patient is expressing. Even before messages are received, the conditions necessary for the reception of input must be realized. First, you must have the intent and desire to listen to people/patients. Positive intentions and desires alone, however, are not enough; they need to be conveyed to the person/patient. All too often nurses appear 'too busy', and therefore not ready to listen to people/patients. Scurrying around tending to the myriad of tasks that occupy a nurse's day communicates to people/patients that there is really no time to stop and listen. Focusing on tasks reflects a value that the tasks are more important than the person who is the person/patient. People/patients are left with the feeling that the nurse's time is too precious to interrupt.

Activity 5.2 highlights characteristics of effective listeners:

- Availability to interact
- Having the time to listen
- Not interrupting the speaker
- Not judging, evaluating, advising, or imposing their own ideas on the speaker
- Not merely listening for what they want to hear
- Showing an interest in what is being said
- Openness to whatever is being expressed

Effective listeners demonstrate readiness to listen.

Receptivity

In order for a television set to receive a signal or transmission, the set has to be tuned in to the correct frequency, so the signal can be processed. This analogy is useful in understanding the readiness to listen. Nurses must 'tune in' to people/patients' signals and adjust their receivers so that the messages are not only audible but also comprehensible. This involves the mental preparation of focusing concentration on a person/patient's messages and developing antennae to notice what a person/patient is expressing.

ACTIVITY 5.2

INDICATORS OF LISTENING

 Process

1   Think of someone in your life who really listens to you. Visualize this person. Reflect on your reasons for choosing this person. Why do you think of this person as one who listens? What does this person do that leads you to believe that they listen?

2   Record your thoughts and reflections about this person.

3   Now think of someone in your life who does not seem to listen to you. Visualize this person. Reflect on your reasons for choosing this person. Why do you think of this person as one who does not listen to you? What does this person do that leads you to believe that they do not listen?

4.   Record your thoughts and reflections about this person.

Discussion

1   Compare your recordings of each person, the listener and the non-listener. What differences do you note?

2   Summarize the major differences between people who listen and people who do not.

3   If working in a group, compare your summary with the summaries of other participants.

Tuning in to a person/patient's message is hard work. Some signals are easier to receive than others (Activity 5.2). At times, there is so much interference that the signal cannot be received at all.

Reducing interference

Interference stems from distractions that draw attention away from the person/patient and prevent clear reception of a message. Such distractions originate internally (from within the nurse) and externally (from outside of the nurse).

External interference

It is important to pay careful attention to the external environment when attempting to listen. For example, the sights and sounds of a busy, bustling

---

ACTIVITY 5.3

EASY OR HARD TO LISTEN TO

● **Process**

1 In small groups of about five to six participants, think about the subjects, topics, feelings and experiences that people/patients bring up with nurses. Consider as many as possible. List these.

2 Review the list and discuss whether the item is easy to listen to or hard to listen to, and mark each accordingly.

3 In small groups, compare lists and discuss similarities and differences.

Discussion

1 Were there any general areas that were assessed as hard? As easy? What are they?

2 On what basis were assessments of easy or hard made?

3 Are there any general trends and themes present? What are these themes? Divide these into easy and hard categories.

4 How might this assessment of easy and hard enhance or interfere with effective listening?

---

hospital setting often present many potential sources of external interference. The ringing of telephones, a variety of health care personnel coming and going, and people/patients being transported from one area to another are potential distractions. When nurses visit people/patients in their home setting, distractions such as the playful noise of small children and a radio or television may be sources of interference. It is not always possible to eliminate external sights, sounds and other stimuli, but attempts should be made to reduce them as much as possible when listening to people/patients.

In a hospital setting, drawing the curtains around a people/patient's bed not only provides a degree of privacy, but also decreases the number of external distractions and potential interferences. This simple act is effective in reducing the amount of visual distractions, but may not reduce the audible ones. Also, it sends a clear message to others that a meaningful activity is occurring.

Interruptions from other staff members can be particularly distracting – even the fear of being interrupted is a potential distraction. Nurses working together in a clinical setting need to be mindful of this; they should assess the need to avoid distracting another nurse who is engaged in an interaction with a person/patient.

Sometimes there are aspects of people/patients themselves that are sources of external interference. Examples of this kind of interference include: people/patients who speak in accents that are distracting to a nurse; who express themselves in a disjointed, rambling manner; or whose speech is barely audible and halting. In these instances, nurses can reduce the interference by attempting to put aside the distractions and concentrating carefully on what the person/patient is expressing.

In general, the reduction of external interference occurs whenever attempts are made to exclude the outside world. This is done by placing barriers between the outside world and the person/patient and nurse, or by consciously tuning out external noise.

Internal interference

When nurses are ready to listen, they are able to forget themselves for the moment. They allow themselves to be engrossed in the interaction with a person/patient and to notice and perceive what the person/patient is expressing. Internal interference, the nurse's own thoughts, feelings, preoccupations, or value judgements, are often more difficult to control than external interference. A noisy television set (an external interference) can simply be switched off in order to eliminate it as a source of distraction. Internal interferences cannot simply be switched off but can be recognized. Three kinds of interference are particularly important: (a) thoughts as internal interference; (b) value judgements as internal interference; (c) feelings as internal interference.

(a) Thoughts as internal interference

One common preoccupation that interferes with listening is the worry a nurse often feels about how to respond to the person/patient. 'What am I going to say to this person/patient?' 'What am I going to do for this person/patient?' Thoughts such as these are often related to a self-expectation that nurses must 'do something' in order to help people/patients. As a result, nurses become so preoccupied with their own anxieties that they fail to listen and perceive what the person/patient is expressing. An internal reminder that something is being done – 'I am listening to what this person/patient is expressing' – can help to draw nurses' focus away from their own thoughts and onto the person/patient. If something else can be done it will become evident *after* the nurse listens, with understanding, to what the person/patient is expressing.

Other thoughts that potentially interfere with listening include any preoccupations that the nurse may have at any given moment. These range from 'Have I remembered to defrost something to eat for dinner tonight?' to 'There is a waiting room full of mothers and babies and I am not going to have time to see each of them' to 'Ms Holmes will need pre-op medications soon. I wonder how long this conversation is going to last. How can I bring it to a close?' Sometimes these thoughts can be excluded from conscious awareness, while at other times they signal the need to attend to another matter, and then return to the interaction at hand. At yet other times, such thoughts are impossible to exclude from conscious awareness, but nurses pretend to be listening. It is far better to cease the interaction until such time that undivided attention can be given to a person/patient than to feign listening.

(b) Value judgement as internal interference

The natural tendency to judge what is heard as right or wrong, good or bad, interesting or boring is one of the greatest sources of internal interference when attempting to listen. This tendency is considered natural because it happens automatically, often without conscious awareness. 'That is a stupid way to react.' 'Mr Lyons should not be feeling this way.' 'What's she going on about – it's really nothing.' Such thoughts are judgemental, because they channel the person/patient's message through the nurse's personal interpretive filter. They interfere with listening because they close off possibilities that do not match the nurse's internal frame of reference.

What is heard may be evaluated negatively and rejected outright as unacceptable. Even if what is heard is evaluated in a positive light, it interferes with a nurse's ability to fully appreciate and understand the uniqueness of a person/patient's experience, because the nurse is still relying on a personal frame of reference.

While it is almost impossible to prevent valuative thoughts, an aware nurse recognizes them as stemming from a personal value system, and therefore is able to separate her/his own value system from the person/patient's value system. Personal judgements, once separated, can then be held in suspense, deferred and kept peripheral to the person/patient. Being non-judgemental is a near impossible goal to achieve; however, keeping one's value system separate and suspended is achievable. The most critical aspect of suspending judgement is the nurse's self-awareness (see Chapter 4).

(c) Feelings as internal interference

Sometimes internal interference stems from a nurse's lack of ability to cope with what the person/patient is expressing, for example, a feeling of despondency might overwhelm a nurse listening to the sorrow of a young mother dying of cancer. Nurses may fail to listen because of their own anxieties, and they may, unwittingly or unknowingly, either change the subject or avoid interacting with the person/patient altogether. There are times when nurses' own circumstances create a sense of vulnerability that prevents them from being fully present with a person/patient. But in the majority of times, nurses fail to listen to people/patients' stories that are distressing out of fear of not knowing what to say or how to respond. Not listening or even avoiding a person/patient for these reasons potentially compounds the person/patient's distress because it isolates and distances a person/patient from the nurse.

Nurses must remind themselves that listening to a person/patient's distress, no matter how disturbing, is comforting simply because it shows they are fully present and genuinely interested in the person/patient. Words spoken by nurses in an attempt to comfort may actually intrude.

When nurses become overwhelmed, and perhaps paralysed, by their own feelings as a result of what people/patients are expressing and experiencing, seeking support from other nurses is preferable to avoiding or emotionally abandoning the person/patient (see Chapter 11).

Once the state of readiness to listen is achieved, a nurse is available to be fully present during an interaction with a person/patient. Attention is focused and undivided, perceptual filters are open, antennae are up and interference is reduced. This state of readiness, when maintained throughout the interaction, not only enables nurses to listen, but also encourages further interaction.

THE SKILLS OF LISTENING

The groundwork involved in achieving the readiness to listen is an inward process initiated by nurses as they prepare both themselves and the environment. Readiness alone, however, is not sufficient for effective listening because two-way communication with a person/patient has not yet begun. This section explores the interactive nature of listening because the skills of listening are enacted through interchange with another person. The skills of listening are divided into five areas: attending, observing, perceiving, interpreting, and recalling.

Attending

Attending behaviour is the outward, physical manifestation of a nurse's readiness to listen. It communicates to the person/patient that the nurse is available to listen and accessible to interact. The outward behaviour of attending conveys the message 'Go ahead, you have my attention, I'm here with you now'.

The messages of attending are sent through nonverbal channels, predominantly body posture and eye contact. For example, nurses checking the flow of an intravenous drip line (no matter how casually), while attempting to listen, are not fully communicating their intent because they are not demonstrating attending behaviour to the person/patient.

Attending behaviour has two key elements: the spatial position of the nurse in relation to the person/patient, and the maintenance of eye contact. During Activity 5.4, the Bs probably altered their nonverbal behaviour by leaning forward and looking directly at the As when the conversation became more 'interesting'. They assumed the posture of attending.

While attending, nurses physically place themselves in a manner that promotes interaction between them and the person/patient. Attending behaviour demonstrates active interest in the person/patient. Egan (1994) presents general guidelines for attending, using the acronym SOLER, which stands for:

S   Squarely facing the person in a front-on presentation
O   Open posture, conveying an acceptance and openness to the other person
L   Leaning forward, demonstrating active interest
E   Eye contact maintained, including being at the same eye level as the other person
R   Relaxed posture, demonstrating ease with self, the other and the situation.

ACTIVITY 5.4

PHYSICAL ATTENDING

 Process

1   Divide the large group into three groups. Designate one of the three groups as As, one as Bs and one as Cs.

2   Distribute instructions to As, Bs and Cs. (These instructions can be found at the end of this chapter.) Do not share the instructions with participants who are not in the same group.

3   As and Bs should seat themselves according to the instructions. Allow enough room between each B so that they will not disturb other groups during the activity.

4   Cs should stand around the edge of the room and act as observers during the activity. Cs should follow the guidelines for observing as outlined in their instructions.

5   As and Bs now have a quiet conversation, following the instructions.

6   After five minutes, As and Bs stop the conversation and show each other their instructions.

7   Cs report their observations.

Discussion

1   How did the Bs' nonverbal behaviour change during the conversation?

2   What did the Cs notice about the change in the Bs' nonverbal behaviour, about two minutes into conversation?

3   What did the As notice about the Bs' nonverbal behaviour during the conversation?

4   What did the Bs notice about their own nonverbal behaviour during the conversation?

Attending promotes active engagement between nurses and person/patient, and encourages people/patients to continue expressing themselves.

Attending encourages further interaction between person/patient and nurse, while non-attending is discouraging. In Activity 5.5, person A probably did not wish to continue the conversation after person B began non-attending. No matter how intent a nurse may be on listening, without attending a person/patient will not be encouraged to continue.

ACTIVITY 5.5

ATTENDING AND NON-ATTENDING

 Process

1   Divide into pairs and designate one person as A and the other as B.

Instructions to A

2   Tell B about something exciting or interesting that has happened to you. Talk for about five minutes on the subject.

Instructions to B

3   Begin the interaction by assuming the attending posture, that is, face A, maintain eye contact, lean forward, and remain relaxed and open. After about a minute or two, start to lean back, fold your arms and look away from A. Focus on something other than what A is saying, for example, stare out the window, clean your nails, flip through a book. Do anything to violate the rules of attending. Remain silent, do not interrupt or change the subject, but do try to keep listening.

4   Stop the conversation after about five minutes.

Discussion

1   How did A feel during the interaction? What happened to A when B began non-attending?

2   How did B feel during the interaction? What happened to B when they began non-attending?

3   How did the conversation change when B no longer appeared interested?

However some words of caution about attending are needed. The intensity of attending is not always appropriate, because it is not always warranted by the topic at hand. Try assuming the posture during a conversation about the weather. You will note that intense attending feels awkward when the subject of the conversation is of little consequence. A discussion about the weather, unless there has recently been a significant event related to the weather, does not warrant such an intense listening response. This is important for nurses to bear in mind. There are times when people/patients discuss subjects that do not require the intensity of attending and for a nurse to assume the posture is not only awkward, but inappropriate.

The attending guideline about maintaining eye contact is another area that presents some difficulty, and caution needs to be exercised when applying this guideline. Unbroken eye contact is unnatural, awkward and even threatening because of the discomfort it creates. The head-on position of attending is criticized (Shea 1988) because it forces eye contact that is then difficult to break. When nurses are attending, it is important to bear in mind that occasional breaks in eye contact are not only natural, but also desirable in maintaining comfort and ease during the interaction.

Finally, an attending posture, which focuses on eye contact as one of its central aspects, may not be appropriate in some cultures. Maintaining eye contact can be a sign of disrespect when there are cultural norms about status. Looking directly into the eyes of a person who is of a higher status is unacceptable when these cultural norms are operating. Likewise, eye contact may vary with age and gender. Nurses need to be sensitive to how people/patients are responding to their attempts to encourage interaction through attending behaviour, and a large part of this sensitivity is awareness of age-related and cultural variances (see Chapter 10. 'Empowering interpersonal relationships').

Attending within the clinical context

In the clinical environment, it is sometimes difficult to assume the classic attending posture. Nurses must learn to adapt the attending posture to the realities of their particular clinical setting. It is not always possible to face the person/patient squarely. In a hospital situation, when people/patients are lying in bed and the nurse is standing nearby, the attending posture of squarely facing the other may be impossible to achieve. How can attending be demonstrated under these circumstances? Nurses need to physically situate themselves in such a manner to establish eye contact, maintain a relaxed stance and be close enough to interact in a meaningful manner, but far enough away to maintain comfort.

Standing at the side of the bed is preferable to standing at the foot of the bed. Although the foot position would allow a nurse to squarely face a person/patient, it may actually discourage interaction because it creates too much distance between person/patient and nurse, and places the nurse in an authoritarian stance. By placing themselves at the side of the bed, nurses are almost facing the same direction as the person/patient. Shea (1988) believes this position is actually preferable to the 'squarely facing' one, because it demonstrates that a nurse is attempting to view the world *with* the person/patient, sharing a common perspective.

While standing at the side of the bed, nurses are faced with the challenge of lowering themselves to the eye level of the person/patient, unless the height of the bed is at a level that places the person/patient at the same eye level as the nurse. Having a seat is the most logical way to meet this challenge. This also sends the message to the person/patient that the nurse intends to remain there, to interact. While seated, nurses are obviously accessible and available to the person/patient.

Awareness that being seated is preferable can pose a dilemma for nurses. There may be a shortage of chairs. If they seat themselves, they may be reprimanded or frowned upon by other nurses for not working hard enough. The hard work of listening to people/patients is often unrecognized and unacknowledged, especially in the hospital setting where so much 'other work' needs to be accomplished.

Silence

Obviously, when nurses are attending and listening to people/patients, they are silent. Silence plays a major part in effective listening and its value is important to recognize. To be silent and not interrupt a person/patient who is expressing themselves is a sign of respect and interest.

Silence can also go further in its helpfulness. Both person/patient and nurse may be silent for short periods of time. Silent moments are useful because they allow person/patient and nurse time to collect their thoughts and reflect on what has been expressed; they provide an opportunity for either person/patient or nurse to change the direction of the conversation; and they slow the pace of the interaction. Nevertheless, nurses frequently experience difficulty in remaining silent because of a felt need to say or do something.

There are times when silently being with a person/patient, fully attending and being fully present, is quite helpful. People/patients who are in severe physical pain may not wish to talk or be spoken to, but would like to have a nurse present. People/patients who are psychologically depressed may feel pressured to interact, and would benefit from a nurse's silent, undemanding presence. These two situations provide examples of contexts in which the silent presence of nurses is appropriate and helpful.

During a verbal interaction, it is important to ascertain when to allow the silence to proceed and when it is better to break the silence with speech or action. Nurses can employ some general guidelines when they are faced with the decision. First and foremost, silence should not be used as a substitute or excuse for not knowing how to respond or what to say. When used in this way silence could be interpreted by the person/patient as rejection or lack of interest on the part of the nurse. It is better for nurses to admit to feeling 'at a loss for words' under these circumstances. Silence is also ineffective if the person/patient expects or wants a verbal response from the nurse. Careful attention to the flow and direction of the interaction allows nurses to 'check its pulse', and perceive person/patient cues that indicate discomfort with the silence.

Silent periods also have limitations if they last longer than about 10–15 seconds (Cormier *et al.* 1986). When silence progresses beyond these time limits, the flow of the interaction may be stifled, rather than enhanced. Try this experiment the next time you are interacting with a person/patient: when a silent period ensues, check your watch and time it. You may be surprised how lengthy a 10–15-second period of silence actually feels. Next, evaluate whether or not the silence is of benefit to the interaction. Repeated experiments of this kind enable nurses to judge the length and usefulness of silent moments during interactions with people/patients.

Observing skills

Effective listening includes astute observation of the person/patient. A large part of listening is not only paying careful attention to what is expressed, but also how it is expressed. During listening, nurses have a good opportunity to observe the nonverbal aspects of the person/patient's expressions. Subtle and obvious cues about people/patients' experiences are better understood when nurses perceive people/patients' nonverbal behaviour. Nonverbal cues often shed light on the feeling aspects of a person/patient's experience. Feelings are most often expressed through facial expression, eye contact, body posture and movements, and other nonverbal behaviour. Such person/patient cues are signals for further exploration (see Chapter 6), but the nurse must first notice the cues. The noticing of cues and their initial interpretation occur in the context of listening.

No doubt, participants in this activity experienced a heightened awareness of the nonverbal indicators of feelings, because they were asked to determine what feelings other participants were expressing. Their perceptual antennae were ready for the reception of nonverbal input. It is beneficial for nurses to develop and maintain this degree of heightened perceptual awareness when interacting with people/patients. Heightened perceptual awareness enables nurses to be more astute in their observations. It makes them notice the way in which a person/ patient is relaying messages.

The inherent difficulty in accurately interpreting nonverbal messages is also demonstrated in Activity 5.6. This highlights and reinforces the need for nurses to check their perceptions through exploration (see Chapter 7). Noticing and observing nonverbal cues of people/patients is significant in the context of listening. The cues must then be validated by the person/patient as to their correct meaning, because listening enables nurses to observe them but not necessarily to interpret them accurately.

Perceiving messages

Attending demonstrates nurses' interest in listening to the person/patient and observing enables nurses to notice nonverbal cues presented by people/patients. People/patients are now encouraged and free to tell their account to an actively interested nurse, and the nurse is in a position to receive the person/patient's messages.

There are many facets to people/patients' accounts, including the actual content of the account, the related feelings and the general theme of the account. Each facet comes together to create a picture of the person/patient, the whole account. While it is vital that the nurse receives the whole account, knowledge of the various facets of messages guides a nurse's perception throughout the listening process.

The following account, related by a female resident of a nursing home, serves as an example of the various facets of an account:

> Michael, the diversional therapist, never pushes you to participate in his activities. He takes one look at you and knows whether you feel like participating that day. He'll say, 'Come along, and just watch today, okay?' He always has so many activities going, but you really don't have to do anything you don't feel like doing. That is what's so good about this place.

The content of this account revolves around the activities conducted by the diversional therapist. The feelings expressed are of contentment and satisfaction at

ACTIVITY 5.6

NONVERBAL EXPRESSIONS OF FEELINGS

 Process

1   Form groups of five to six participants and decide on a topic for discussion. The chosen topic can be of any nature, but it needs to be one about which participants can express emotions. Controversial topics are most effective, for example, euthanasia, abortion, IVF, rights of smokers, drug abuse, disabled persons' rights, genetic engineering.

2   Participants should reflect on their feelings or emotions in relation to the selected topic. Each participant records this feeling or emotion on a slip of paper. These slips of paper are not shared with other participants.

3   Participants should reflect on how they usually express their chosen emotion nonverbally.

4   In small groups now discuss the chosen topic. Throughout the discussion, each participant expresses their chosen feeling through nonverbal means only. Participants are not to express their chosen feeling in a verbal manner, that is, they cannot say how they feel.

5   Stop the discussion after about ten minutes.

6   Each member of a small group should record what feeling they believe was being expressed by each other member, as well as the nonverbal behaviour that led to this conclusion. Participants do not consult with any other members at this point.

7   Each group member takes a turn asking other members what feeling they thought they were expressing. After each states their conclusion, the member whose feeling was being discussed shows the other members the feeling recorded during Step 2. Continue around the small group until each member's feeling expression is discussed.

Discussion

1   On what basis did participants determine what feeling was being expressed? Would this differ between cultural groups, age groups or gender groups?

2   How accurate were the guesses about what feeling was being expressed? What discrepancies existed between what others interpreted and what the participant intended to convey? Why?

3   What does this say about the valid interpretation of nonverbal messages?

not being forced to participate in these activities. The resident uses her discussion of the diversional therapy programme as an illustration of the general manner in which residents of the nursing home are treated. The general theme is one of feeling respected by the way she is treated at the nursing home. The content (the diversional therapy activities) and its related feelings (happy and satisfied) come together to form the theme, the importance of having her wishes respected by others.

Notice how the resident speaks of herself in the second person, using the personal pronoun 'you' to indicate herself. When listening to people/patients it is important that nurses recognize use of the pronoun 'you' in people/patients' direct reference to themselves. In doing so, they are relating information about themselves, not another person. Perceptive nurses, who are in tune with people/ patients' expressions, notice this use of language and can more fully understand the themes of people/patients' stories as a result.

At times, people/patients directly express the content, feeling and thematic facets of their stories, as in the example about the diversional therapist. At other times, however, any or all of the facets are expressed indirectly, through implications, hints and cues. Either way, the various facets of the person/patient's account must be received and perceived by the nurse who is listening.

Perceiving content

The content of a message contains the objective, factual data about the topic being discussed and includes what is being discussed, who it involves, and when and where an event occurred. The content of a message is the account line. The following example, related by a female person/patient on an orthopaedic ward of a hospital, serves as an illustration.

> I had these pains in my Achilles tendon. I think it had something to do with playing tennis every day. At first I tried to ignore the pain, but it became so bad that I knew I had to do something. When I saw my local GP, he suggested cortisone injections, so I took the advice and had the injections. That was when the real trouble started. First my right leg started to give way, buckling on me. I fell a few times, and then the final time I fell, I really hurt myself. Now I'm told the right tendon has snapped, and here I am, needing to have it repaired. The whole thing has been going on for about six months now.

The content of this person/patient's account includes: pain, falling, the local GP, cortisone injections, injured Achilles tendon, the need to have the tendon repaired, and a time frame of the past six months.

Activity 5.7 highlights some of the difficulties inherent in listening. First, there is a tendency for the listener to add elements that are not directly stated. For example, the assumption is often made that the person speaking in account II is the mother of the child. It could be a primary care-giver of any relationship.

When nurses are listening, there is a tendency to make assumptions about what the person/patient is discussing. Sometimes these assumptions are accepted and even acted upon as if they were fact. When listening, it is important that nurses keep this tendency under check and recognize that further interaction is necessary to validate these initial assumptions (see Chapter 6).

ACTIVITY 5.7

LISTENING FOR CONTENT
(Adapted from Carkhuff 1983)

 Process

1   This activity lists seven person/patients' accounts, as told by them. Read each one *once* only. Then cover it up and try to recall the content of the account. If possible, have someone else read the stories to you aloud (once only).

2   Record as much of the content of the message that you can recall. In recalling content, think about the following: 'who' is being discussed, 'what' is being discussed, 'when' and 'where' did the 'what' occur, and 'why' it is being discussed. Record the content on a piece of paper using the headings who, what, when, where, and why.

Person/patient account I

I felt something really strange in my hip when I stood up yesterday. It began to really hurt and I was having trouble walking properly. Because it was Sunday afternoon I didn't want to bother anybody. So I took some aspirin, took it easy and went to bed early. The next morning when I woke up I rang my doctor. She said to go and have the hip X-rayed before I do anything else.

Person/patient account II

The day started off as usual. I fed him breakfast, and got him ready to go to nursery. I was getting ready to go to work, when he suddenly began rolling on the floor, clutching his stomach and writhing in pain. It took me a while to work out what was happening and I felt panicked inside, although I didn't let on. I knew it was something major, but had no idea what was happening. I rang my GP's surgery, and the receptionist said to come in straight away. I got into the car immediately and drove there.

Person/patient account III

I was outside doing the gardening when I suddenly realized I could not move my left arm. I looked at it, saw it was still there, but could not make it move an inch. My left arm was just hanging there. I walked toward the house, not knowing exactly what I was going to do. I sat down on the sofa to think, when I realized that I could move my arm again. Then I really didn't know what to do.

Cont.

Person/patient account IV

I have been really worried about him. He hasn't been himself for months. When he comes home from work, he has dinner and then just sits in front of the television. I can tell he is not really paying attention to it because he just stares. He doesn't even laugh at the funny bits of his favourite programme. When I ask what's wrong, he just shrugs his shoulders.

Person/patient account V

I know I should have regular cervical smears but I never seem to find the time. What with the kids, my job and everything I can't fit in a trip to my GP. Anyway, there is not cancer in my family. Maybe doing all those tests is just a way for the doctors to make money.

Person/patient account VI

All that chemo and radiotherapy really takes it out of me. I try so hard not to give in to feeling so tired. I go to my room and think, 'Oh, I'll just go close my eyes for a few minutes', and the next thing you know I have been asleep for a few hours. It's not fair on my kids because they need me to be there for them.

Person/patient account VII

I can't be bothered getting up in the morning. After my wife sees the children off to school she goes to work. I just feel so low. I took the pills the doctor gave me for a couple of weeks but they weren't working so I stopped them. I just feel everyone would be better off without me.

(*Note*: Suggested answers to this activity can be found at the end of this chapter.)

Discussion

1   In each account, which part of the content was easiest to recall? Which was most difficult? What difficulties did you experience in recalling the content of the stories?

2   How accurate was your recall of content, when you compare your results with those provided at the end of the chapter? (Do not become overly concerned if your answers do not match exactly the ones provided.)

3   Did you discover you 'read into' the stories, and added content that was not originally there? Were there aspects of the content that you deleted? Or distorted?

4   What methods did you find yourself using as you attempted to recall the content of the stories?

Perceiving feelings

When listening, the nurse must perceive the feeling aspects of the person/patient's account, the emotional reactions and subjective responses that accompany the content (Activity 5.8). People/patients often have strong emotional reactions to their health status and health care. The connection of feelings to content begins to complete the picture that is the person/patient's experience. At times, people/patients express their feelings directly. For example:

- 'I'm really worried about the operation'
- 'I am so pleased with the results of that test'
- 'I'm feeling a bit down and blue today.'

When expressed in a straightforward manner, people/patients' feelings are easy to perceive, as long as nurses are ready to listen and receive input. More often, feelings are not expressed so openly and directly. Feeling expression follows a more circuitous route, unlike content, which is often expressed in a straight-forward manner. Feelings are often hinted at, implied, inferred, and talked around rather than talked about. It could be that people/patients are reluctant to share their feelings because of uncertainty about how the nurse will react. This is especially true when trust has not yet been established between them. It could be that people/patients are unaware of, and out of touch with, their feelings. These are possible explanations for why feelings are expressed indirectly.

A more probable reason is that adults often try to conceal emotions, because they have learnt, through socialization, which emotions are appropriate to express in various situations (Nelson-Jones 1988). It may be that people/patients believe that feelings are not appropriate to share with nurses. But, no matter how much people/patients try to disguise or hide their feelings, their indirect expression is received by nurses whose perceptual antennae are ready to receive feeling messages.

There is, however, a word of caution about focusing on feelings. Research demonstrates that when nurses were perceptive to people/patients' feelings, the people/patients' distress increased (Reid-Ponte 1992). This could be because people/patients were encouraged to express emotions to nurses who were good listeners. There is evidence that nurses tend to over-estimate the degree of emotional distress people/patients are experiencing, when compared to what people/patients report (Hegedus 1999; Farrell 1991). That is, people/patients often do not perceive that their feelings are as significant as nurses think they are. The interpersonal dynamics at play are important to bear in mind when listening for feelings.

In listening for feelings, it is vital for nurses to suspend their personal judge-ments about what is acceptable and appropriate. Feelings, by their very nature, are often irrational, illogical and difficult to control. In order for nurses to be open to the perception of people/patients' feelings, they must hold the view that feelings are acceptable.

Open perception of feeling messages poses a challenge to nurses, not only because of the natural tendency to judge them, but also because of the way in which they are indirectly expressed. As described in the section on observing,

ACTIVITY 5.8

LISTENING FOR FEELINGS

 Process

1   Participants in a group take turns reading each person/patient statement aloud. Before each participant reads the statement they should think about a feeling to be conveyed along with the statement and then read it with the nonverbal cues that depict that feeling. Each participant records what they think the person reading the statement is feeling.

(a)   'I'm dying, aren't I?'

(b)   'Are you sure you know what you are doing?'

(c)   'That right leg won't ever be as strong as it used to be, no matter how hard I try.'

(d)   'I just wish I could be like I was before.'

(e)   'I've had enough. I just want to die.'

(f)   'Why can't anybody show me how to get out of this bed without pain?'

(g)   'I don't think my back will ever stop aching.'

(h)   'You have to be tough to be a nurse, don't you?'

(i)   'The labour didn't go the way I expected.'

(j)   'Have you ever done this procedure before?'

(k)   'I'm not sure I should be taking all those tablets.'

(l)   'I should have known better than to leave the cleaning liquid sitting out on the bench top. Now look what's happened.'

(m)   'My tummy is really hurting.'

(n)   'Why do people treat me different when I am in the wheel-chair?'

(*Note*: The answers to this activity can be found at the end of this chapter.)

> **Discussion**
>
> 1   Refer to the end of the chapter and compare your answers with those provided. Reflect on the differences between your answers and the ones provided.
>
> 2   If you are working in a group, compare your answers with other participants', following the reading of each person/patient statement. Discuss any differences in perception of feelings and try and determine why they are different.

feelings are often expressed nonverbally, and an observant nurse will pick up these nonverbal cues. Feelings are also expressed indirectly, through verbal means, and the perceptive nurse will notice them.

While there is a tendency to jump to conclusions and make assumptions when listening for content, there is an even greater danger of this when listening for feelings. Listeners tend to project their own opinions about what feelings are being expressed. This is partly because feelings are subjective by nature. The tendency is for the listener to perceive feelings on the basis of what they would feel, given a similar set of circumstances. To put oneself in the place of the other can be helpful in understanding (see Chapter 1), providing it does not limit interpretation. As with suspending judgement, nurses need to rely on their self-awareness in order to keep a balance.

Interpreting: listening for themes

The content of a person/patient's account and its accompanying feelings come together to form the general theme. Themes are the general point of the account, the consequences and implications of the content and feelings. It could be said that an understanding of the theme is the ultimate goal of listening, for once the point of each account is understood, the person/patient's entire experience comes into sharper focus (Activity 5.9). Nurses come to understand the theme of a person/patient's account by asking the following questions:

- What is the significance of the content and feelings?
- Why is the person/patient bringing this up at this time?
- How is this affecting the person/patient at the moment?
- What are the consequences of what the person/patient is expressing?
- What are the implications for the person/patient?

Understanding themes requires interpretation. This is always tentative at first and needs to be validated with the person/patient. After nurses have listened and attempted to understand, they are ready to respond. Perhaps the nurse's current understanding, achieved through listening, needs to be clarified, explored,

ACTIVITY 5.9

LISTENING FOR THEMES

 Process

1　Form pairs for this activity. Each member of a pair is to relate an account of something that has recently happened in their life. The account need not be earth-shattering, but it should be meaningful to the person telling the account.

2　The other person is to listen, attend and say little during the relating of the account. On completion, the listener states what they think is the theme. The person telling the account then validates (or invalidates) what the listener has interpreted as the theme.

3　Discuss any differences in interpretation.

Discussion

1　How accurate were the interpretations of the theme? What accounted for any inaccuracies?

2　What interfered with listening? What enhanced it?

and/or reflected back to the person/patient through paraphrasing. The skills needed to achieve any of these are covered in Chapters 6 and 7.

During this activity, it was probably easier for listeners to identify the theme if they had had a similar experience, that is, when the account had a sense of familiarity about it. Repeated listening and identification of themes enables nurses to attain a sense of familiarity with common person/patient themes. Listening with understanding becomes a valuable learning experience in accurately perceiving people/patients' stories.

Recalling messages

Sometimes the greatest challenge in listening is the recall of what people/patients have said. Accurate recall is important if understanding is to occur. Themes often become apparent only after numerous interactions with a person/patient. Nurses must rely on their ability to recall previous interactions and put them together with current ones.

People/patients' accounts are usually not as complicated as the one told in Activity 5.10. Nevertheless, this activity does highlight how easily stories become diminished, embellished and/or distorted. Recalling people/patients' accounts takes concentration and effort. If nurses find themselves asking people/patients to retell their accounts many times, people/patients may not believe that they have listened in the first place. When nurses listen and remember what they have heard,

ACTIVITY 5.10

RECALLING MESSAGES

 Process

1   Four volunteers are needed for this activity. They will participate in the relating of an incident that occurred during the night shift at a hospital. The details of the incident are provided below.

2   Two of the volunteers are to leave the room. The other two are to seat themselves in a place where all other participants can hear their conversation.

3   All other participants act as observers. They are to make notes of what is added, deleted and distorted each time the incident is reported.

4   The two volunteers who are in the room are to pretend they are in a handover report at the end of a night shift. One of them relates the following incident to the other by reading it aloud:

At about 2 a.m., Mr Smithers became confused and agitated. He got out of bed, went into the next room, over to Mrs Blue's bed, and began to tell her about how to grow azaleas. Mrs Blue became frightened, rang her husband on the phone, and asked him to come in immediately. She was so loud on the phone that all the other people/patients in the room were awakened. There was a recently admitted person/patient in bed 18. She reacted to Mrs Blue, tried to get out of bed and fell to the floor. In the meantime, Mr Smithers made his way off the ward and was heading toward the lift. Fortunately, another nurse was getting out of the lift and escorted him back to the ward. We contacted the Senior House Officer to come and see the new admission and Mr Smithers. He ordered X-rays for the new admission and a sedative for Mr Smithers. Now everybody is settled and back in bed. There were no major injuries, but it was a real circus here for a while. In the midst of all of the chaos, Mr Blue arrived, in response to his wife's request. We let him visit with her for about twenty minutes and now he's returned home. The incident report was completed and sent.

5   One of the volunteers, who is out of the room, is now called back in. The volunteer who received the report relates the incident to the volunteer who has come into the room, by retelling the account without reading it. No assistance is offered to the volunteer who is relating the account; they must rely on memory to recount the incident.

6   The remaining volunteer (who is still outside of the room) is brought back into the room, and the previous volunteer relates the incident by retelling the account. Again, no assistance is offered to this volunteer in retelling the account.

7   Each time the incident is retold, the observers are to record any additions, deletions and distortions made to the original account.

8   The incident report is now read aloud, as it was told originally.

Discussion

1   The participants who observed the activity should now relate what was added to the original account. What was deleted? What was distorted when the account was retold?

2   What accounted for the alterations that were made to the original account?

3   Volunteers should report their reactions to having to retell such a complex account.

people/patients are comforted to know that somebody has taken the time to understand them.

EVALUATION OF LISTENING

In the final analysis, nurses listen in order to respond in a manner that matches the person/patient's experience. Listening is considered effective when the nurse's response reflects understanding of what the person/patient is expressing (Activity 5.11). This is not to say that initial understanding (achieved through listening) will be entirely accurate. The nurse's interpretation is always tentative, awaiting correction, validation or further explication from the person/patient. Responses that shift the focus, change the subject or miss the point entirely do not indicate active listening.

CHAPTER SUMMARY

Meanings are derived, and initial understanding is achieved through active listening. Listening enables nurses to perceive the person/patient's reality, the world as the person/patient is experiencing it. After listening effectively, nurses are in a position to respond according to what is perceived. Listening engages both the nurse and person/patient. It is an essential and fundamental process in establishing effective relationships in nursing practice.

ACTIVITY 5.11

RESPONSES THAT INDICATE LISTENING

● **Process**

1   Each of the following person/patient statements has a variety of possible responses. Evaluate each response in terms of whether it indicates that the nurse making the response has listened. Record on a piece of paper a Yes or No on the basis of your evaluation. Do not evaluate how good or bad the response seems to you, or base your decision on whether or not you would actually make the response. Judge the response only in terms of listening, by asking yourself, 'Does the listener response indicate that the listener has heard the person/patient?' 'Does the response indicate an under-standing of what the person/patient has expressed?'

(a)   *Person/patient*

I don't think I'm going to make it. Am I going to die?

Responses

(i)   The power of positive thinking can really help a lot. Many people in your situation have survived because they refused to give up. Keep fighting. Where there is life, there is hope.

(ii)   What has happened to make you worried about it?

(iii)   I can't really say. You'll have to ask your doctor this question.

(iv)   We are all going to die sometime, but it's a frightening prospect when it stares us in the face.

(b)   *Person/patient*

Why is my blood pressure being taken so often?

Responses

(i)   We have to check your blood pressure frequently.

(ii)   It's doctor's orders.

(iii)   It is a general observation to keep a check on your vital signs.

(iv)   Is it worrying you?

(c) *Person/patient*

How long will I be in here?

Responses

(i)   As long as we think you need to be.

(ii) Let's discuss it with the doctor. If you think you're ready to go home, and the doctor is happy for you to go, then you can be discharged.

(iii) People who have the operation you are having usually stay in hospital about three days. That's the usual routine, if there are no complications.

(iv) What has your doctor said about this?

(d) *Person/patient*

Why me? Why do I have to be the one that suffers like this?

Responses

(i)   It is part of the usual course of this disease. If you tell me when you feel worse and better, I can help with the pain.

(ii) We all suffer some kind of pain during our lifetime.

(iii) It is just a bit of misfortune. You'll have better luck next time, I'm sure.

(iv) I wish I could answer that question. I'm not sure there always is a reason.

(e) *Person/patient*

I have contemplated suicide because I've hit rock bottom.

Responses

(i)   Are you thinking about suicide right now?

(ii) Things can't be that bad.

(iii) What's happened to you that you have hit rock bottom?

(iv) What exactly have you contemplated?

(f) *Person/patient*

What's going to happen when I come out of the operation?

Responses

(i)   We will look after you.

(ii) There's nothing to worry about. You will feel better than you did before.

(iii) Have you had a general anaesthetic before?

(iv) You'll be drowsy for a few hours, and depending on your level of pain, you will receive regular pain relief.

(g) *Person/patient*

I'm not sick, and yet I have to take all of these tablets every day.

Responses

(i)   It does seem a bit silly, doesn't it?

(ii) It could be that you don't feel sick because you are taking the tablets.

(iii) Which tablets are you taking?

(iv) How long have you been taking the tablets?

2. Now review each response for which you recorded a Yes. Evaluate each in terms of the major goal of listening, that is, the encouragement of people/patients to continue expressing their experiences. How encouraging is each?

3. Compare your answers with the ones provided at the end of the chapter.

ANSWERS TO ACTIVITIES

ACTIVITY 5.4: PHYSICAL ATTENDING

Instructions to A

You are going to speak to person B for about five minutes on a topic of your choosing. About two minutes into the conversation inform B that you are going to share a secret with them. Make sure you say that it is a secret, then proceed to share it with B. You will need to fabricate this 'secret', so prepare yourself by thinking of something really interesting to share.

Instructions to B

Seat yourself comfortably and place a seat facing you, for person A. Person A is going to talk to you for about five minutes. Act naturally during the conversation, while you listen to what A has to say.

Instructions to C

Person A and person B are going to have a conversation lasting about five minutes. You are to observe and note person B's nonverbal behaviour during the conversation. You do not need to actually hear what A and B are discussing. Pay particular attention to body posture, eye contact and other behaviours, which indicate B's level of interest in the conversation. Note especially any change in B's nonverbal behaviour about two minutes into the conversation.

See *Guidelines for role play*, p. 125.

ACTIVITY 5.7: LISTENING FOR CONTENT

Person/patient account I

Who: self (speaker), doctor
What: something happened to hip, difficulty walking
When: Sunday afternoon
Where: not stated
Why: reason for having the X-ray

Person/patient account II

Who: speaker, child, GP's receptionist
What: serious stomach pain, rang GP, drove to GP's surgery
When: beginning of a day
Where: GP's surgery
Why: explain the account, but not entirely clear

Person/patient account III

Who: speaker
What: unable to move left arm
When: not stated
Where: garden, then house
Why: don't know what to do

Person/patient account IV

Who: speaker, 'him'
What: he is not himself
When: 'for months'
Where: home, in front of television
Why: worried about 'him'

Person/patient account V

Who: speaker, GP
What: no time to have regular pap smears
When: not stated
Where: not stated
Why: questioning whether regular cervical smears are necessary

Person/patient account VI

Who: speaker
What: chemo and radiotherapy, feeling tired
When: now
Where: speaker's room
Why: can't attend to children

Person/patient account VII

Who: speaker
What: can't be bothered feeling low
When: now
Where: not stated
Why: Questioning worthiness in family role

ACTIVITY 5.8: LISTENING FOR FEELINGS

1   (a)   fear, anxiety, worry
    (b)   fear, anxiety, worry
    (c)   frustration, anger, resignation

(d)   sadness, anger, frustration

(e)   sadness, anger, resignation

(f)   anger, frustration

(g)   sadness, anger

(h)   fear, anxiety, apprehension

(i)   disappointment, frustration

(j)   apprehension, anxiety, fear

(k)   uncertainty

(l)   regret, guilt

(m)   worry, fear

(n)   disappointment, frustration

ACTIVITY 5.11: RESPONSES THAT INDICATE LISTENING

Note: The answer No indicates that the nurse responding has not understood/ acknowledged what the person/patient is saying, while the answer Yes indicates active reception of what the person/patient has said.

1   (a)   *Person/patient*: I don't think I'm going to make it. Am I going to die?
         (i)   No. The power of positive thinking can really help a lot. Many people in your situation have survived because they refused to give up. Keep fighting. Where there is life, there is hope.
         (ii)   Yes. What has happened to make you worried about it?
         (iii) No. I can't really say. You'll have to ask your doctor this question.
         (iv)   Yes. We are all going to die some time, but it's a frightening prospect when it stares us in the face.
     (b)   *Person/patient*: Why is my blood pressure being taken so often?
         (i)   No. We have to check your blood pressure frequently.
         (ii)   No. It's doctor's orders.
         (iii) Yes. It is a general observation to keep a check on your vital signs.
         (iv)   Yes. Is it worrying you?
     (c)   *Person/patient*: How long will I be in here?
         (i)   No. As long as we think you need to be.
         (ii)   Yes. Let's discuss it with the doctor. You need to decide if you think you're ready to go home. If the doctor is happy for you to go then, you can be discharged.
         (iii) Yes. People who have the operation you are having usually stay in hospital about ten days. That's the usual routine, if there are no complications.
         (iv)   Yes. What has your doctor said about this?
     (d)   *Person/patient*: Why me? Why do I have to be the one that suffers like this?
         (i)   No. It is the part of the usual course of this disease. If you tell me when you feel worse and better, I can help with the pain.
         (ii)   No. Everyone suffers some kind of pain during his or her lifetime.

> (iii)   No. It is just a bit of misfortune. You'll have better luck next time, I'm sure.
>
> (iv)   Yes. I wish I could answer that question. I'm not sure there always is a reason.
>
> (e)   *Person/patient*: I have contemplated suicide because I've hit rock bottom.
>
> (i)   Yes. Are you thinking about suicide right now?
>
> (ii)   No. Things can't be that bad.
>
> (iii)   Yes. What's happened to you that you have hit rock bottom?
>
> (iv)   Yes. What exactly have you contemplated?
>
> (f)   *Person/patient*: What's going to happen when I come out of the operation?
>
> (i)   No. We will look after you.
>
> (ii)   No. There's nothing to worry about. You will feel better than you did before.
>
> (iii)   No. Have you had a general anaesthetic before?
>
> (iv)   Yes. You'll be drowsy for a few hours, and depending on your level of pain, you will receive regular pain relief.
>
> (g)   *Person/patient*: I'm not sick, and yet I have to take all of these tablets every day.
>
> (i)   No. It does seem a bit silly, doesn't it?
>
> (ii)   No. It could be that you don't feel sick because you are taking the tablets.
>
> (iii)   Yes. Which tablets are you taking?
>
> (iv)   Yes. How long have you been taking the tablets?

GUIDELINES FOR ROLE PLAY

Role playing is one of the most commonly used experiential learning methods. Role playing is a process of acting 'as if' the situation is real. While it does not require formal drama skills, the participants' willingness to behave in ways that may be unfamiliar is essential if the action is to proceed.

Throughout this book various activities rely on this method. Whenever it is used, it is crucial that the following guidelines be presented to participants (on a whiteboard or circulate copies) who are enacting the role play. *Remember*: the onus is on the facilitator to present this information to the learners each time a role play exercise is introduced.

Before the action

1   Assume the role. Try not to let personal thoughts and feelings about the role interfere with your ability to adopt the role; accept it for what it is – an act designed to enhance learning. Take a few minutes prior to the action of the role play to 'put yourself' into the role.

2   Do not be concerned if you think you cannot enact the role because you are not good at dramatizing and performing. The purpose of role playing is to act naturally although you may be required to adopt a stance that feels different from your usual way of interacting with others.

3   Once you have assumed the role, let the action flow naturally. Do not overact or exaggerate your actions in an effort to be a good role player.

4   During the role play invent needed information, about yourself or specific details of the situation. Do not let the role play stop or flounder because you think you should know something; simply make it up in an effort to keep the action going.

5   It is acceptable, sometimes desirable, to change your ideas and attitudes throughout the role play. Even if your role prescribes certain attitudes and feelings, these may change as a result of the progress of the action. When this happens, let it flow naturally; do not cling to your original script.

After the action

1   Remain in the role and take a few minutes to discuss how you responded to the role and how it felt playing the role.

2   Make sure you clarify any information or detail that was fabricated in an effort to keep the action going.

3   Discuss any concerns you have about what others who participated in the role play may think or feel about you as a result of the role you have just assumed.

4   When the time comes, state aloud that you are no longer in the role and are returning to who you really are.

REFERENCES

Burnard, P. (2001). *Effective Communication Skills for Health Professionals*, second edition. Cheltenham: Nelson Thornes Ltd.

Carkhuff, R. R. (1983). *The Student Workbook for the Art of Helping*, second edition. Amherst, MA: Human Resource Press.

Cormier, L. S., Cormier, W. H. and Weisser, R. J. (1986). *Interviewing and Helping Skills for Health Professionals*. Boston, MA: Jones and Bartlett.

Doona, M. E., Haggerty, L. A. and Chase, S. K. (1997). Nursing presence: an existential exploration of the concept. *Scholarly Inquiry for Nursing Practice: An International Journal*, 11(1), 3–16.

Egan, G. (1994). *The Skilled Helper*, fifth edition. Pacific Grove, CA: Brooks/Cole.

Farrell, G. A. (1991). How accurately do nurses perceive people/patients' needs? A comparison of general and psychiatric settings. *Journal of Advanced Nursing*, 16, 1062–70.

Hegedus, K. S. (1999). Providers' and consumers' perspectives of nurses' caring behaviours. *Journal of Advanced Nursing*, 30, 1090–6.

Nelson-Jones, R. (1988). *Practical Counselling and Helping Skills*, second edition. Sydney: Holt, Rinehart and Winston.

Reid-Ponte, P. (1992). Distress in cancer people/patients and primary nurses' empathy skills. *Cancer Nursing*, 1(4), 283–92.

Shea, S. C. (1988). *Psychiatric Interviewing: The Art of Understanding.* Philadelphia, PA: Saunders.

Webb, C. and Hope, K. (1995). What kind of nurses do people/patients want? *Journal of Clinical Nursing*, 4(2), 101–8.

CHAPTER 6

BUILDING MEANING: UNDERSTANDING

INTRODUCTION

Understanding a person/patient's experience, that is, viewing the world from the person/patient's perspective, is one of the most central aspects of interacting and building relationships in nursing. Mutual understanding is the basis of meaningful interaction, and in the person/patient–nurse relationship, it is the nurse's responsibility to facilitate this understanding. Mutual understanding requires time, effort, commitment, and skill. It is challenging for one person to understand and appreciate another person's reality.

Effective attending and listening opens doors and aids the nurse's entry into the person/patient's world. The stage is set for a meaningful relationship, because interpersonal contact has been established. Listening enables the nurse to develop an initial understanding of the person/patient's experience. It is important to recognize that this understanding remains tentative, until it is either validated or corrected and altered through further interaction with the person/patient. The impressions formed in the process of listening are often partial, inaccurate and superficial. The nurse who acts immediately, without further interaction to check the accuracy of these impressions, risks attempting to build a relationship that lacks mutual understanding and providing help that is not necessarily congruent with the person/patient's needs. Taking time to understand a person/patient's experiences enables nurses to ground nursing care within a shared reality.

Listening is largely an absorptive activity, as nurses take in and process people/patients' stories. But at some point during an interaction, verbal responses must be uttered; the nurse usually has to say something. A variety of verbal responses are possible, however a response that promotes greater understanding between person/patient and nurse is most beneficial, especially in the early stages of the relationship. Responses that promote understanding not only demonstrate that the nurse has listened; they also convey a desire to comprehend the person/patient's experience more fully. Effective listening demonstrates open acceptance of the person/patient, and encourages the person/patient to interact.

Effective understanding encourages further interaction because it openly acknowledges the person/patient's experience, confirming its reality. Understanding responses check how effectively the nurse's perceptions and interpretations correspond to the person/patient's meaning. Because they build meaning, understanding responses deepen the relationship between person/patient and nurse.

CHAPTER OVERVIEW

This chapter begins with an overview of the ways in which nurses can verbally respond to people/patients. The various ways of responding are explained in depth, in order to demonstrate how they differ in intent and impact on the person/patient–nurse relationship. Understanding is shown to be the most appropriate way to respond when building this relationship. Understanding is viewed as the basis of the relationship, and the importance of understanding between person/patient and nurse is highlighted. The skills of understanding are covered next in the discussion. Paraphrasing is the major skill of understanding, and therefore is treated more extensively than the other skills. The other skills include: seeking clarification, reflecting feelings, connecting, and summarizing. Empathy is presented as a central concept in understanding. The concept of empathy is explained, and how the concept is integrated into caring practice is delineated. An analysis of how empathy is conceptualized in caring assists in the comparison of empathy with other related concepts, such as sympathy.

VERBAL RESPONDING

After actively listening to a person/patient and forming an initial impression, it is natural for a nurse to respond verbally. While it is important that responses be spontaneous and sincere, it is equally important that they be thoughtful, developed with intention and skilfully employed. The nurse's initial verbal responses set the direction for further interaction. Because there are a variety of possible ways to respond, nurses must ensure that their verbal responses move the relationship in a desired and intended direction. Choice of a response is based on insight into how it may affect the person/patient, the interaction and the relationship. A nurse who has this insight and awareness is in the best position to respond in a manner that both matches the current situation and realizes the response's desired intent. In regard to intent, nurses should consider what they need to know about people/patients and why they need to know it.

The initial phase of the relationship between person/patient and nurse is a particularly sensitive and critical time for responding, because, more than likely, the trust required for full person/patient disclosure is not yet firmly established. Responses that work best at this time are those that validate people/patients by acknowledging their experiences. Validating and acknowledging responses convey the nurse's willingness to understand the person/patient. People/patients will come to trust those nurses who can be relied on to understand.

Inadvertently, nurses may respond in a manner that suggests a lack of desire to understand. The following response, which denies the person/patient's experience, is an example:

Person/patient: I'm worried about how my family is going to manage without me.

Nurse: No need to worry, they'll survive without you. It'll do them good to realize how much you do for them.

While the nurse may have wished to encourage the person/patient with this response, it is likely that the response indicates a rejection of the person/patient's perception of the situation. By failing to acknowledge the person/patient's reality, responses such as these engender the feeling that the nurse does not want to understand. Compare the preceding example with the following:

Person/patient: I'm worried about how my family is going to manage without me.

Nurse: What is worrying you most about how they will manage?

Here the nurse provides acknowledgement and confirmation of the person/patient's reality. Responses such as this deepen interpersonal engagement and promote understanding between person/patient and nurse; as such, they build trust.

Most nurses develop habitual, routine and even stylized ways of responding to people/patients (Activity 6.1). The intent is usually to be of help or assistance to people/patients, but this intent may not be fully realized if nurses over-use one type of response and/or lack awareness of the impact of their responses. Goodwill and desire alone are not sufficient in the absence of awareness and direction.

WAYS OF RESPONDING

This section explores the various types of responses nurses might have to people/patients, based on categories developed by Johnson (2000). In this scheme, responses are categorized according to their intent, what they are designed to do or their purpose. On this basis, the majority of responses fit into one of the following categories:

- Advising and evaluating
- Analysing and interpreting
- Reassuring and supporting
- Questioning and probing
- Paraphrasing and understanding.

The categories include those responses that are significant – ones with the potential to have a critical impact on the interaction and the relationship. There are other possible responses that would not fit into any of these categories, for example, small talk about the weather. They are not included because they are

ACTIVITY 6.1

YOUR USUAL STYLE OF RESPONDING I

 Process

1   For each of the following statement(s) or question(s) (a)–(p), write a response. Do not spend too much time pondering your response, but do try to be helpful to the person speaking. Record a response that is typical of how you would usually respond.

(a)   A resident of a nursing home: 'I miss my wife. I don't know where she is. Where is she? Can you tell me?'

(b)   A relative of an unconscious person/patient hospitalized in intensive care: 'Mum is really going to be upset when she wakes up. She is going to kill us for letting her be in here.'

(c)   An adolescent person/patient during a routine health checkup: 'My folks keep pressuring me about the future. I don't have a clue about what I want to do.'

(d)   A first-time mother about to be discharged from a postnatal unit: 'How am I ever going to be able to manage this baby on my own?'

(e)   A person/patient to a community nurse during a home visit: 'I am so glad to see you. I have not been at all well lately.'

(f)   A person/patient, a young man, who is having regular haemodialysis: 'My girlfriend left me because she's afraid she might catch something and my best mate doesn't visit me any more because he hates the sight of blood.'

(g)   A resident of a hostel for the elderly: 'It's really boring in here. The days are so long and there's no one to talk to except the nurses, and they are always so busy.'

(h)   A mother during a routine visit at an early childhood centre: 'My husband left and I am having so much trouble managing on my own.'

(i)   A resident of a nursing home: 'It's hard when you grow old and your friends and family start to die. My children are great, but they have their own lives.'

(j)   A person/patient, a woman, during an outperson/patient clinic visit for a routine cervical smear: 'I am not really sure about having any more children. I'm 39 now and reckon I've pushed my luck far enough. I have two healthy children. Perhaps I should just leave it at that.'

(k)   A person/patient during a post-operative clinic visit: 'You know, I just take one day at a time. It's been two months since my surgery and I'm still not sure if I'll ever feel like my old self again.'

(l)   A person/patient during an admission interview in hospital: 'I've lived with arthritis for years, but lately I'm having more trouble than usual. I can hardly get out of bed in the morning and the pain is becoming unbearable.'

(m)   A resident of a hostel for drug and alcohol abusers: 'You can't possibly understand my needs. You never had this problem. How would you understand?'

(n)   A person/patient, a pregnant woman, during an antenatal visit: 'People are kind and concerned, but no one really knows what it is like to lose a child. It's the most painful experience imaginable. You never get over it.'

(o)   A person/patient, a man hospitalized for a myocardial infarction: 'I'm really worried about how my family will cope without my help. I have three small children, my wife works and we share all the household chores. Now that I've had this heart attack, I'm not sure how much assistance I can offer.'

(p)   A person/patient, a woman with learning difficulties: 'People talk to me as if I am an idiot, they seem to think I don't have feelings – nobody knows how much they hurt me.'

2   Reflect on each of your responses:

- What is your intention?
- What do you hope to achieve by responding in this way?
- How do you hope the person/patient will react to your response?

3   If you are working in groups, form pairs. One person now reads the statement or question and the other person reads their recorded response. The 'person/patient' reflects after each response:

- What is your impression of the nurse? Of the response?
- How has the response affected you?

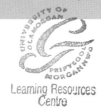

- How encouraged are you to continue the interaction?
- How much do you think the nurse understands your situation?

The 'person/patient' then shares these reflections with the 'nurse'.

4   The 'nurse' now shares her/his intention (Step 2 of the process) with the 'person/patient'. Make a note of the following:

- How similar is the nurse's intention with the effect on the 'person/patient'?

5   Continue to read each statement or question followed by its response and share the reflections.

6   Switch roles and complete Steps 3, 4 and 5.

Discussion

1   What differences are there between the 'nurses'' intentions and the 'people/patients'' impressions of the responses? How do you account for this?

2   Were there some responses that were more encouraging than others? Which ones were encouraging? and discouraging?

3   Which responses resulted in a negative impression on the 'person/patient', for example, 'the nurse does not understand', 'does not really care' or 'does not wish to discuss the topic'?

of less consequence to the overall relationship, although important in initially engaging with the person/patient.

Each way of responding may be helpful in its own right, and can be effectively employed within the context of the person/patient–nurse relationship. Nevertheless, each has a different intent, suggests a different type of relationship between person/patient and nurse and therefore has a different impact on their interactions, especially in the sensitive early stages. Some responses facilitate interaction better than others, so timing and an awareness of each type of response are crucial (Activity 6.2).

Advising and evaluating

This category includes responses that offer an opinion or advice, ranging from a mild suggestion to a directive about what the person/patient should do. Such responses are based on the nurse's opinions and ideas and therefore have an evaluative edge. Examples in this category include:

- 'It's best not to dwell too much on such things.'
- 'Try to relax and stop worrying so much, it doesn't really help.'
- 'Ask the doctor these questions.'
- 'Just tell your mother it's your life and you'll do with it what you want.'

Responses such as these are among the most common made by people who are trying to help. When nurses use this type of response they convey the message that they 'know best' and are in a position that is superior to the person/patient (Johnson 2000). Advice and evaluation carry the implication that people/patients are unable to know what to do, thus increasing their sense of vulnerability. For this reason, advising and evaluating responses run the risk of being met with a defensive reaction or a rejection of the advice. Have you ever told a friend what you think they should do to resolve a problem, only to be met with 'Yes, but . . .', or 'That's easy for you to say', or 'I already tried that and it didn't work'? When given as an initial response, advice rarely works because of its potential to produce a sense of inadequacy in the person/patient and the person/patient's need to defend against this feeling.

Responses that advise offer solutions about what ought to be done. As a general rule, it is better to reach a sound understanding of a person/patient's situation before launching into solutions. An advising response gives the impression that a person/patient's difficulties and problems are easily solved, that there is a 'quick fix'. Some situations are easily resolved but, more often than not, further elaboration is needed before answers are found (if any *can* be found). Advice-giving is better left until the nurse fully understands the person/patient's experience.

Just as it is difficult to listen without judging, it is equally difficult to curtail the tendency to evaluate and advise. The tendency of nurses to give advice reflects how many nurses perceive their role, as possessing knowledge and expertise. This perception often leads nurses to attempt to help people/patients by telling them what to do and providing answers.

While there are times when nurses offer expert advice to the person/patient, it is important that the person/patient's need and desire for such advice is established beforehand. Likewise, if advice is to be effective, it must be based on a clear understanding of the person/patient's experience. For example, explaining the usual course of events following anaesthesia and advising how to cope with 'waking up' is advice based on understanding of the situation. This is objective 'case knowledge' (see Chapter 1), which does not necessarily require interaction with the person/patient. In a more subjective situation, such as anxiety about impending surgery, telling a person/patient to relax is of little use unless the nurse takes the time to understand the nature of the person/patient's worry. Advice given without understanding runs the risk of being ill-timed or irrelevant.

Advising versus sharing information

Giving advice is sometimes confused with sharing information. While they are similar, sharing information is not the same as telling people/patients what to do. When they share information (see Chapter 8) nurses provide knowledge, alternatives and facts. When they offer advice, nurses provide specific actions to perform. Advice also involves reliance on the nurse's personal value judgements, while sharing information is free of such judgements.

Analysing and interpreting

A response that analyses and interprets reaches beyond what the person/patient has expressed into a deeper level of meaning. An interpretive response reads into people/patients' messages, giving the impression that the nurse knows how people/patients *really* feel or what they *really* think. Interpretations imply that a nurse knows more about people/patients than they know themselves (Johnson 2000). Examples of analysing and interpreting responses include:

- 'You really don't want to assume responsibility for your own health.'
- 'You are acting like most new mothers, worrying too much and being over-protective of your baby.'
- 'You are afraid that if you tell the surgeon how you feel about the operation, he will reject you entirely and drop you as a person/patient.'

Responses such as these delve beneath the surface and open up areas that the person/patient has not expressed directly. As with advising, interpreting may have a legitimate place, but as an initial response it is often too threatening to be effective in building the relationship. An interpretation, regardless of its accuracy, can be threatening because it confronts the person/patient with another reality, one that they may not be willing or able to face. Because such interpretations have a confronting edge, they are better left until the relationship has been established and the nurse has 'earned the right' to challenge in this way (see Chapter 8).

People/patients are more likely to accept interpretations from a nurse who has taken the time to understand their situation fully. It is unlikely that a nurse would know a person/patient well enough to make interpretations early in the course of their relationship. As an initial response, interpretations are intrusive and invasive and may impede the development of trust.

Reassuring and supporting

There is a definite place for realistic reassurance and support (see Chapter 8) in the course of person/patient–nurse relationships, and a nurse's approach needs to convey an overall attitude of support whenever interacting with people/patients. Nevertheless, a falsely reassuring response (the type discussed here) is one that glosses over and minimizes the importance of the person/patient's experience before that experience is entirely acknowledged and understood. In this respect, a falsely reassuring response is one that attempts to smooth the person/patient's discomfort, by making everything sound 'all right', regardless of the objective or subjective reality of the situation. It may convey a patronizing attitude or present the person/patient with a sense of unrealistic assurance. Examples of responses that falsely reassure and support include:

- 'A good night's sleep will do wonders for you.'
- 'There is nothing to worry about. It is only a minor procedure.'

■ 'Don't be silly, Mrs Jones, nothing will go wrong.'
■ 'You'll feel better after the operation and will get well soon.'

False reassurance may sound good on the surface but, more often than not, it is dismissive of the person/patient's reality; it lacks understanding. Reflect for a moment on how you feel whenever someone tells you not to worry about something that is causing you concern. Do you have an impression that this person is genuinely interested? Does this person demonstrate a desire to understand your concern?

The use of clichés is another example of responses that attempt to support and reassure. Some examples include:

■ 'It's always darkest just before dawn.'
■ 'Every cloud has a silver lining.'

Responses such as these, often said whenever people/patients express anxieties and concerns, fail to acknowledge the subjective reality of people/patients' experiences. They carry an implied judgement that people/patients' concerns are unfounded, even foolish. Because they discount the validity and significance of people/patients' feelings and perceptions, falsely reassuring responses sound as if the nurse is not really interested. Like premature advice, reassuring responses and clichés attempt to 'fix things' before they are fully clarified and understood.

Questioning and probing

A response that questions and probes is one which attempts to gather more information and explore the situation further. It indicates a need for elaboration and may ultimately lead to greater understanding. Examples of this type of response include:

■ 'What is worrying you most about the operation?'
■ 'Where is your pain?'
■ 'What have you tried to get to sleep?'
■ 'What do you think?'

Responses that question and probe indicate that nurses are trying to understand, but need more information to do so. Early in the course of the relationship, the nurse frequently employs questions in an effort to get to know the person/patient. Throughout the course of the relationship, questions are further employed to develop an even greater understanding of the person/patient's experience. Unless they are overused, responses that question and probe are quite useful if they are stated correctly and timed appropriately. There are other ways to explore aside from questioning and probing, and effective exploration involves the use of a variety of skills (see Chapter 7).

Paraphrasing and understanding

When nurses paraphrase, they share their understanding with the person/patient by rephrasing what the person/patient has expressed, using their own words

ACTIVITY 6.2

RECOGNITION OF THE TYPES OF RESPONSES

Process

1   There are five possible responses for the statements labelled (a(–(l). Read all five responses to the statement and decide on the response that most closely matches what you would say under the circumstances.

2   Determine which of the following categories best represents each response (record your answer on a separate sheet of paper):

E   Advising and evaluating
I   Analysing and interpreting
S   Reassuring and supporting
P   Questioning and probing
U   Paraphrasing and understanding

There is a response from each category in each set.

(a)   'I'm just so fed up with being sick and in pain. I'm tired of having to rely on the nurses all the time.'

Responses

(i)   'It's okay to rely on us. That's why we are here.'

(ii)   'You are an independent type of person who prefers to do things for yourself.'

(iii)   'All of this is really starting to get you down.'

(iv)   'Just relax and let us help you.'

(v)   'What is bothering you the most?'

(b)   'I never really looked after myself. Now look how I am suffering.'

Responses

(i)   'I don't know what you mean.'

(ii)   'Lots of people say the same thing.'

(iii)   'Well, you would have looked after yourself if it mattered to you.'

(iv)   'It's hard to look back with regrets, isn't it?'

(v)   'Sounds as if you're angry at yourself.'

(c)   'Don't bother with me. I am going to die anyway.'

Responses

(i)   'That sounds sad and depressing.'

(ii)   'Don't talk like that. You are not going to die.'

(iii)   'What makes you say that?'

(iv)   'It's not a bother to look after you. I am here because I want to help you.'

(v)   'You have given up hope because you are getting on in age.'

(d)   'I'm in so much pain all the time. I manage to get through the day all right, because I keep busy, but my backache prevents me from getting a good night's sleep. So I keep busy during the day, end up really tired, but then can't get the rest that I need. I'm getting more and more tired all the time.'

Responses

(i)   'Why don't you try some relaxation exercises to get to sleep?'

(ii)   'How often do you have a bad night?'

(iii)   'Keeping busy during the day helps with the pain, but getting enough sleep at night is more of a worry for you right now.'

(iv)   'Sounds as if you are letting the pain control your life.'

(v)   'I'm sure you'll be able to work something out once you become accustomed to living with the pain.'

(e)   'People think they want to live a long time, but I'm telling you, don't ever grow old. You'll end up in a place like this. It's boring and depressing. Look at everybody here, do they look happy to you?'

Responses

(i)   'Everybody feels a bit blue sometimes. Things will get better – you'll see.'

(ii) 'Come on, let's go for a walk. It's a beautiful day today.'

(iii) 'What's so boring and depressing about this place?'

(iv) 'You are approaching things with a negative attitude so, naturally, the whole world looks grim.'

(v)   'You're really not happy about being here, are you?'

(f)   'My wife died recently. I don't want to talk about it.'

Responses

(i)   'It does help to talk about these things.'

(ii) 'What do you want to talk about?'

(iii) 'You'll get over it in time, I am sure.'

(iv) 'Maybe you are the type of person who has difficulty letting people help you.'

(v)   'You don't feel like talking to me?'

(g)   'I know I should change my diet and alter my lifestyle. The doctor said I am a high risk for a heart attack. I've always been a bit of a go-getter, take after Dad in that respect. He had a heart attack at 50, so I guess I should do something – but I really don't know where to start.'

Responses

(i)   'Sounds as if you have been avoiding the inevitable. You know what to do, but don't want to face it. You could change if you really wanted to.'

(ii) 'Just try a bit harder to slow down and eat the right foods.'

(iii) 'You have an idea about what you should do, but are having trouble getting started.'

(iv) 'What do you think you should change first?'

(v)   'Worrying about it will only make things worse. I'm sure you can change.'

(h)   'I get so tired looking after David day after day. There is all the physical care, but I think the mental strain is the worst. I worry constantly about where he is and what he is doing. I think he gets a bit annoyed with my constant hovering over him. The worst thing is that I get no relief – it's so constant.'

Responses

(i)   'The constant worry is really getting to you and wearing you down. You just can't seem to get away from it.'

(ii)   'People in your situation often feel this way. It's a difficult problem to come to terms with.'

(iii) 'Try and put the worry out of your mind at least once each day. Make yourself a cup of tea, sit down and just relax.'

(iv)   'Is there ever an opportunity for you to get away?'

(v)   'There may be a bit of guilt in what you are saying. You probably keep thinking about the times in the past when you could have been more understanding and supportive toward David.'

(i)   'The least they could have done was warn me that Dad was going to be sedated. Those doctors didn't even tell me beforehand so I could have a quick visit with him. Now I need to leave the hospital without even speaking to Dad.'

Responses

(i)   'You sound like one of those people who likes to be in control.'

(ii)   'The doctors were really busy. Otherwise I am sure they would have told you.'

(iii) 'I can see you are frustrated and angry about not getting to talk to your Dad.'

(iv)   'If this happens again, I would say something if I were you.'

(v)   'What exactly did they tell you?'

(j)   'Mum was always there to look after us when we needed something. Now that she's sick, I guess it's our turn to look after her. It feels so strange and I'm not sure she will even let us do much for her.'

Responses

(i) 'Because you always had her to look after you, you wonder if she will let you look after her.'

(ii) 'Of course she will. Your mother is a sensible woman.'

(iii) 'You feel scared that you won't be able to switch roles with your Mum.'

(iv) 'Tell me more about it.'

(v) 'Just tell her she needs you now and she will have to let you take care of her.'

(k) 'What will happen to me if John dies. I don't know what I would do. I couldn't go on without him.'

Responses

(i) 'No need to worry about things before they happen.'

(ii) 'You're scared because you have allowed yourself to become too dependent on John and can't see how you'll make it on your own.'

(iii) 'What makes you think he won't make it?'

(iv) 'I suppose it's frightening to think you can't survive without John.'

(v) 'There is plenty of help around. You can join a social club in your area.'

(l) 'That surgeon explained everything about the operation, but I could not understand what was being said. I didn't even know what to ask.'

Responses

(i) 'You're scared to ask questions of the doctors because they are so powerful.'

(ii) 'So the surgeon's explanation was not quite enough for you to understand.'

(iii) 'What questions do you still have?'

(iv) 'The next time you see the surgeon, tell him you want some answers.'

(v) 'Don't worry too much, most people don't really understand the technical aspects of surgery.'

(*Note*: The answers to this activity can be found at the end of the chapter.)

Discussion

1 Compare your answers with those provided at the end of the chapter. Are there any types of responses that were difficult to recognize? Which are they? Review the section of the text that pertains to these.

2 In groups of five to six participants, discuss your answers. Are there any types of responses that other members had difficulty recognizing? Which are they? Discuss these until understanding of each type of response is achieved.

3 Review your responses to Step 1 of the process and determine whether there are some types of response you seem to provide naturally. Compare these results with the other participants in the group.

4 Discuss the reason(s) you tend to provide some types of response more than others.

instead of the person/patient's. Responses that paraphrase what the person/patient has expressed demonstrate that the nurse's intention is to understand the person/patient more fully. Examples in this category include:

- 'You are unable to sleep because of your uncertainty about the future.'
- 'You are feeling more relaxed now that you are in your own home.'
- 'It seems strange to you that you should have to keep asking the same questions over and over again.'

Responses that demonstrate understanding confirm and validate what people/patients have expressed, thus communicating nurses' genuine interest in and acceptance of people/patients. Through the use of the paraphrase, nurses share their understanding of people/patients' messages, in order to ensure this understanding is correct. Paraphrasing and understanding responses demonstrate that the nurse wants to follow the person/patient's meaning and will check to ensure this happens. They convey the message 'I won't assume I know what you mean or what you need until I am certain I know – and only you can tell me'. Early in the course of the relationship, this type of response is especially effective, because it places person/patient and nurse on equal footing and helps to build trust.

ACTIVITY 6.3

YOUR USUAL STYLE OF RESPONDING II

 Process

1   Refer to the responses that you recorded for Activity 6.1: Your usual style of responding.

2   For each of your responses, determine which type of response you used (that is, advising and evaluating; analysing and interpreting; reassuring and supporting; questioning and probing; or paraphrasing and understanding) and mark each accordingly. You may have used more than one category in a given response. If this is the case, include all categories used.

3   Tally the total number of times you used each type of response. Is there one type you used more than others? Reflect on the reasons for your apparent preference.

4   Have someone else determine which types of responses you used. Discuss any discrepancies and make a final determination of which type of response was used.

Discussion

1   Compare your tally with other participants. Is there a type of response that was preferred by a majority of participants? Discuss the results.

2   Which ways of responding seem to fit the perceived role of the nurse? Which do not?

3   How frequently was the paraphrasing and understanding response used? Discuss why this is the case.

All other categories of responses, except questioning and probing, are based on an assumption that nurses know what people/patients are experiencing and what is best for them. An understanding response attempts to validate or invalidate these assumptions. The meaning a nurse constructs from what a person/patient has expressed may not be what the person/patient actually meant. An understanding response is of value in preventing such lack of congruency; it addresses one of the most common problems in communication, which occurs when people do not realize there is sometimes a difference between what is meant and what is said and consequently misunderstanding what is meant.

The advising and evaluating type of response is one of the most frequently used when people are trying to be helpful (Johnson 2000). This is probably due to people's natural tendency to make judgements and offer opinions, especially when they are trying to be of help. There are times when being directive and prescriptive will be of help to people/patients, but there are risks if this approach is used exclusively or too extensively. When using advising and evaluating responses, nurses place themselves in the position of expert and may fail to acknowledge people/patients' expertise and capabilities in managing their own lives. People/patients are not encouraged to seek solutions that fit their unique experience but rather are offered solutions and answers.

Nurses often show a strong preference for the reassuring and supporting type of response (Activity 6.3). This is understandable because care is best given in a reassuring and supportive atmosphere. Nevertheless, a truly reassuring and supportive manner differs from glossing over the person/patient's experience with a reassuring cliché. Falsely reassuring statements may negate the reality of people/patients' experiences. Because of their failure to acknowledge and affirm the person/patient, such responses interfere with effective interaction between person/patient and nurse.

Two recent studies demonstrate how nurses respond to person/patient anxiety. The most common responses tried to cheer the person/patient up (reassuring and supporting) or offered an explanation about the symptoms (advising and evaluating). The least frequent responses demonstrated understanding (Motyka *et al.* 1997; Whyte *et al.* 1997). For more detail on these studies, see Chapter 8.

Ways of responding revisited

It is important to recognize that none of the categories is inherently good or bad. Each is appropriate at different times in the relationship and under different circumstances. The ultimate aim is for each nurse to develop as wide a repertoire as possible, and to use each type of response with awareness of its appropriateness and consequence. (Subsequent chapters cover the various types of responses, except the understanding type, which is the subject of this chapter.)

Understanding responses are most appropriate for building a relationship based on mutual meaning. They are effective in the early stages of the relationship and are also used throughout, as a natural reaction to active listening (see Chapter 5). Regardless of how effectively a nurse has suspended judgement during listening, the person/patient's messages are still processed through personal, interpretative filters. In processing people/patients' messages, nurses form impressions and reach conclusions about what people/patients are expressing and experiencing. These interpretations may not be entirely correct. If a nurse's interpretation of what a person/patient is saying is not shared actively and openly with the person/patient, potential misunderstandings are likely to go unchecked. In giving an understanding response nurses share their interpretations so that they can be validated or corrected. Such responses enable nurses to build meaning that is congruent with a person/patient's experience.

THE IMPORTANCE OF UNDERSTANDING

In order to be of help to people/patients, it is best if nurses operate from a vantage point within people/patients' experiences. When responding with understanding, nurses attempt to view the world from the person/patient's point of view. Nurses reach for meaning by asking. 'What is this person/patient experiencing?' 'What is the meaning of the experience for the person/patient?' 'Am I following . . . do I get the drift?' Understanding responses check the answers to such questions. The following scenario serves as an illustration:

Person/patient: It doesn't seem right that I am still in so much pain. My hip surgery was six weeks ago, and I still can't seem to get comfortable. Is it just me? I asked my doctor and she said, 'No, this is not unusual, so don't worry.' But I really don't know.

Nurse: It doesn't seem right to you that you are still in so much pain six weeks after the surgery.

Person/patient: Yes and no, because I really didn't know exactly what to expect.

Nurse: So, it's more that you don't know the usual course of events following hip surgery.

Person/patient: Yes, I mean all the doctor said was this is not *unusual*, so I'm still in the dark. I think I'm getting a bit neurotic about the whole thing.

Nurse: So, what you really want to know is how much pain is reasonable and to be expected six weeks after the surgery.

Person/patient: Yes, if I knew for sure that this is expected I wouldn't be so worried. What do you think?

Because understanding is achieved, the nurse can now proceed to act. The nurse can provide the person/patient with concrete information (see Chapter 8) about recovery after hip surgery. Exploration (see Chapter 7) of the exact nature of the person/patient's pain also may be warranted. Perhaps support (see Chapter 8) in pain management can be provided. The key is that the nurse is guided by the understanding that, for *this* person/patient, fear of the unknown is the central meaning in the expression.

Notice how the nurse's initial understanding response was not entirely accurate. The person/patient took the opportunity to clarify the meaning because the nurse's response indicated a desire to understand. The person/patient's final question, 'What do you think?' is indicative of their beginning trust in the nurse. The person/patient feels able to rely on this nurse because the nurse has taken the time to understand the situation.

Because each person/patient's experience is unique, another person/patient may have expressed similar thoughts for an entirely different reason. Here is a similar scenario, with a different person/patient:

Person/patient: It doesn't seem right that I am still in so much pain. My hip surgery was six weeks ago, and I still can't seem to get comfortable. Is it just me? I asked my doctor and she said, 'No, this is not unusual, so don't worry.' But I really don't know.

Nurse: It doesn't seem right to you that you are still in so much pain six weeks after the surgery.

Person/patient: It's not the pain so much, but the amount of medication I'm taking.

Nurse:	You think it might be too much.
Person/patient:	Well, yes, I take those tablets every four hours. Could I be taking too many?

As with the first scenario, the nurse may need to explore this situation further, or offer concrete information about the likelihood of taking too much pain medication. The illustrations show how different people/patients experience the same event. These scenarios exemplify the importance of achieving under-standing, which is based on the person/patient's view of the situation. While the situation is similar, each person/patient's experience of it is different. In each scenario, the nurse listens to the person/patient's view, comes to understand it and is then able to operate from a vantage point within the person/patient's experience. The nurse can now offer help, in the form of advice, information or reassurance that is specific to the person/patient.

Internal and external understanding

The understanding that is emphasized here is termed internal because it is grounded in the person/patient's subjective world and personal view of a situation. External understanding, on the other hand, is an objective view of a situation. In nursing, these external understandings are based on clinical information that is devoid of any specific person/patient (for example, a textbook case, referred to as case knowledge, see Chapter 1).

Nurses often become so focused on having the answers that they rely exclusively on an external understanding of the situation. An over-concern with 'What can I do?' often prevents nurses from asking 'What is this like for this person/patient?' This keeps nurses externally focused. There is a danger that care based solely on external understanding will be misguided, and will not take into account the uniqueness of the person/patient. In the scenarios given earlier, the nurse could have relied on an informed understanding of recovery following hip surgery, and not taken the time to understand *this* person/patient's experience of recovery.

Focusing externally can lead to premature and automatic solutions, which look to results and outcomes. Focusing internally meets people/patients where they are and offers a way of operating from within their experiences, before moving to solutions and outcomes. Advising, evaluating, interpreting, and falsely reassuring, in the absence of internal understanding, usually arise from externally focused approach. Both external and internal understandings are necessary. They can be combined to provide guidance in appreciating what is appropriate in caring for a particular person/patient.

Barriers to understanding

Many potential barriers exist when nurses are trying to understand a person/patient's perspective and frame of reference. The interferences that affect listening (see Chapter 5) are still active. The natural tendency to judge and evaluate must still be kept in abeyance. An even greater barrier is the tendency to jump to conclusions about what the person/patient is experiencing. Unless the person/

patient validates these conclusions, they remain assumptions. Unshared assumptions lead to unshared meaning.

THE SKILLS OF UNDERSTANDING

An interpersonal ability to build meaning through skilled interaction is as significant as an awareness of the importance of understanding. The skills of understanding are presented here in a particular order. Paraphrasing, seeking clarification, and reflecting feelings are used prior to connecting and summarizing. The final skill, expressing empathy, is viewed as the sum total of all other understanding skills (see Figure 6.1). The point at which the nurse can accurately express empathy is the point at which mutual understanding is achieved.

Paraphrasing

Paraphrasing is the backbone of understanding skills. When nurses paraphrase they restate what the person/patient has expressed, but instead of using the person/patient's words, nurses rephrase the person/patient's message in their own words and mode of expression. A paraphrase is a translation from the person/patient's language and manner of expression into the nurse's. Through the use of the paraphrase, nurses share their understanding of what people/patients have expressed.

Paraphrases acknowledge what the person/patient has said and demonstrate that the nurse has listened. They encourage further person/patient expression because they are confirming and accepting. Paraphrases, although statements,

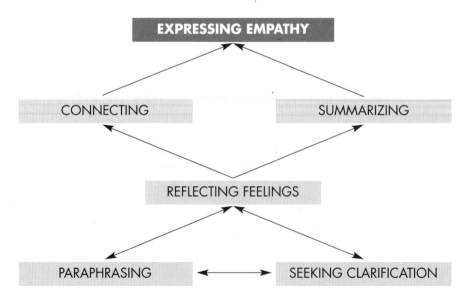

Figure 6.1 Hierarchy of understanding skills

contain an implied question, 'Is my understanding of what you are saying the same as what you mean to say?' They often begin with phrases such as:

- 'So, what you are saying is . . .'
- 'Would I be correct in saying that you . . .'
- 'In other words . . .'
- 'Let me see if I understand correctly . . .'

Beginning a paraphrase with phrases such as these brings the implied question into the open. However, it is not essential that paraphrases begin in this manner. A nurse may simply rephrase what the person/patient has expressed.

The value of the paraphrase is its ability to check the accuracy of the nurse's understanding of what the person/patient means against the person/patient's intended meaning. Use of the paraphrase is an effective way to prevent misunderstandings. Because people/patients hear the nurse's interpretation, they are afforded an opportunity to confirm or deny its accuracy.

Interchangeable responses

When paraphrasing, the nurse attempts to produce a response that is interchangeable with what the person/patient has expressed. An effective paraphrase neither adds to (additive response), nor detracts from (detractive response) what the person/patient has said.

Additive responses include comments on, explanations of, and opinions about what the person/patient is expressing. Analysing and interpreting responses are examples of additive responses. Although quite helpful when the goal is to increase the person/patient's awareness, additive responses do not necessarily facilitate the nurse's understanding.

Responses that detract are ones which shift the focus away from the person/patient or focus only on what the *nurse* thinks is important. Offering premature solutions and advice are examples of detractive responses. Paraphrases neither add nor detract; they are interchangeable with what the person/patient has expressed, and do not attempt to alter the meaning of that expression.

Accuracy in paraphrasing

Even though nurses attempt to make paraphrases interchangeable, there is still no guarantee that they will be entirely accurate (Activity 6.4). The meaning a nurse derives from the person/patient's expression may not be what the person/patient intended. This does not signal failure, because an inaccurate paraphrase allows the person/patient to correct the nurse's misinterpretation before progressing further in the interaction. In responding to a paraphrase, the person/patient has an opportunity to restate the meaning of an expression, amplify it or reiterate what was originally expressed. As long as nurses do not detract completely from the meaning, understanding can still be achieved through further interaction.

For this reason, it is important to state a paraphrase in a tentative manner, and closely observe the person/patient's response to it. Even when it is inaccurate, a paraphrase still conveys the nurse's desire to understand and willingness to engage in interactions that build meaning. The ultimate aim is to achieve similarity

ACTIVITY 6.4

PARAPHRASING – HAVE I GOT IT RIGHT?

 Process

1.   Form pairs for this activity, and designate one person as A and the other as B.

2   A makes a statement about a recent interaction with a person/ patient that was significant.

3   B responds with a paraphrase and begins with, 'So, in other words, what you are saying is . . .'. B is not to advise, judge, evaluate or probe. At the end of the paraphrase, B asks, 'Have I got it right?'

4   A confirms or denies B's paraphrase and then continues to discuss the situation. B continues to paraphrase each of A's statements, asking each time, 'Have I got it right?' This process continues until A is able to say to B, 'Yes, you have got it right, that's exactly what I mean.'

5   Reverse roles, with B relating a story and A paraphrasing.

Discussion

1   How accurate were the initial paraphrases? What was the response to an inaccurate paraphrase? How long did it take to achieve accuracy?

2   What were the effects of the use of the paraphrase on the inter- action? How did each participant feel during the interaction?

3   How was listening affected when you knew you had to para- phrase?

between what the person/patient means and what the nurse understands the person/patient to mean. This requires effort, time and the use of responses that work toward this aim. Mutual understanding must be negotiated between person/patient and nurse. The paraphrase works toward the goal of mutual understanding, because it enables meaning to be negotiated.

The paraphrase is effective in building meaning and, when used to this end, it results in greater understanding between person/patient and nurse. As with any skill, nurses must pay careful attention to how people/patients respond to paraphrasing. When the paraphrase encourages people/patients to elaborate on their experiences, thus enabling nurses to understand these experiences more fully, it is working toward its desired end.

Overuse of the paraphrase

Overuse of the paraphrase, in the absence of other skills, can be frustrating for a person/patient because the interaction may seem to be going in circles, with little forward progress. Continuous rephrasing of what the person/patient has said gives the impression that the interaction is 'going nowhere'. To prevent this, paraphrases need to be used with a mixture of other skills.

The aim and intention of the paraphrase must be borne in mind. An accurate paraphrase is a direct acknowledgement of what a person/patient has expressed. It serves as confirmation of the person/patient's reality. It conveys that the nurse is willing and able to view the person/patient's experience from the person/patient's frame of reference. All of this is done in order to deepen the relationship and encourage further interaction. When paraphrases stifle interaction, they do not meet their intended aim.

Reluctance to use paraphrasing

Despite the value of the paraphrase in building and negotiating meaning, there is sometimes a lack of appreciation of its use. Nurses are sometimes reluctant to employ the paraphrase out of a fear of appearing inept or poorly informed. They often think they 'should' automatically understand what people/patients are experiencing, and may feel foolish in not knowing. It is virtually impossible for nurses to fully appreciate what people/patients are experiencing until an effort is made to understand. Each person/patient's experience is unique, and subjective. To believe there is an objective reality that is applicable to all people/patients is unrealistic.

At other times, reluctance to employ the paraphrase stems from a fear of reinforcing a person/patient's negative state. For example, when people/patients express unpleasant emotions or self-destructive thoughts, nurses may fear that restating such negative experiences elevates them, giving them more status than they deserve. Nurses may believe that it is better to deny or dismiss them, avoid further discussion of them or try to talk the person/patient out of them. But avoidance alienates people/patients, giving the impression that nurses do not really care.

The paraphrase acknowledges the person/patient's reality, demonstrates acceptance of it and conveys the nurse's desire to understand that reality. This is not the same as agreement and reinforcement; eventually a nurse may challenge a person/patient and encourage the adoption of an alternative perspective (see Chapter 8). Another perspective cannot be introduced until the nurse shares the person/patient's current perspective and paraphrases work toward this shared understanding.

Seeking clarification

The skills of clarification are used whenever nurses are uncertain or unsure about what people/patients are saying. Under these circumstances, paraphrasing is not possible because the nurse is unable to get an adequate sense of what the person/patient means. Through clarification, nurses convey that they are trying to understand, and will not proceed until they are able to do so. Statements that clarify could begin with:

- 'I'm not sure I follow you . . .'
- 'That's not clear to me . . .'
- 'Run that by me again . . .'
- 'I'm not certain what you mean . . .'
- 'I don't follow what you are saying . . .'
- 'I'm having difficulty understanding that . . .'
- 'I'm a bit confused about . . .'.

Notice how the nurse takes responsibility for the lack of clarity and understanding. The intent and effect would be very different if statements such as 'You're not expressing yourself clearly' or 'That's not clear' were made. A properly phrased clarification is focused on a desire to receive a clearer message from the person/patient, a rephrasing, an illustration and/or amplification. It should not put people/patients on the defensive or lead to discomfort by creating the feeling that they have to justify themselves or provide rational explanations to nurses.

Clarification through questioning

Clarification is often achieved through the use of probing skills (see Chapter 7). However, the intention is not focused so much on exploration as it is on clearing up an area of confusion or ambiguity. An open question, such as 'What do you mean?', is a direct clarification. Nurses must use such a question with care and caution because of its potential to sound critical and accusatory (it could imply 'You are not making sense'). Intonation and other nonverbal aspects make the difference.

Restatement

At times a restatement of what a person/patient has said is an effective means of clarifying. The nurse simply parrots the person/patient's exact words, usually switching from the first person to the second person. The accompanying non-verbal intonation should indicate that the restatement is really a prompt, which is aimed at further amplification. Restatement is similar to one-word or phrase accents (see Chapter 7), except that in restatement the entire message is reiterated. An example of a restatement is:

Person/patient: I can't move my right arm.
Nurse: You can't move your right arm?

Sometimes nurses over-use restatement because they do not know what else to say. Over-use of parroting can lead to frustration on the part of the person/patient, so its use should be kept to a minimum. It should be used with the intention of reaching greater clarity and understanding, not as a substitute for lack of words.

Clarification through self-disclosure

At times, nurses clarify what a person/patient has said by sharin[...]
might feel, think and perceive the situation if they were the person/
example is: 'I'm not sure I entirely follow what it's like for you, but if
I'd be . . .' Care must be exercised when using self-disclosure, beca[...]
potential to shift the focus from the person/patient to the nurse. In [...]
disclosure in this manner the nurse is attempting to clear an area of confi[...]
detract from what the person/patient is expressing.

Reflecting feelings

Reflection is the mirroring of feelings expressed by people/patients. Because
feelings are often expressed indirectly, nurses translate the feeling aspects of a
person/patient's message into other words. In this sense, reflecting feelings is
similar to the paraphrase. Instead of rephrasing the actual words of the person/
patient, the nurse rephrases an indirectly expressed emotion. An example of
reflecting feelings is:

Person/patient: This darn leg won't get any stronger, despite all the physio.
Nurse: That leg is frustrating you, isn't it?

Reflecting feelings is useful because it conveys the nurse's recognition of
feelings and confirms the existence of emotions. More than any other area of the
person/patient's experience, feelings must be accepted as valid and real. Like the
paraphrase, the reflection of feelings must be stated tentatively, awaiting feedback
from the person/patient that either confirms or denies the accuracy of the nurse's
perception.

Reflecting feelings is verbalizing what a person/patient has implied, but this is
not the same as interpreting the person/patient's feelings. An interpretation
involves adding to the person/patient's expression, rather than bringing into
the open what was expressed indirectly. The nurse is still working with what
the person/patient has communicated, not providing an explanation of, or
judgement on, the person/patient's feelings.

In reflecting feelings, as in paraphrasing, nurses attempt to respond inter-
changeably with what people/patients have expressed. An interchangeable feeling
reflection matches both the type of feeling and its intensity. Frustration is
different from anger; feeling a bit blue is not the same as feeling despondent;
happiness is not equivalent to elation. Making the distinction between different
emotions and feelings requires an extensive vocabulary. A major difficulty in
reflecting feelings is a limitation of the language the nurse possesses for describing
feelings. Activity 6.5 below is designed to increase your feeling word
vocabulary.

When nurses are reflecting feelings, they must first identify the appropriate
feeling category. Most feelings will fit into one of the categories used in
Activity 6.5. Second, the intensity of the feeling expressed must be determined.
Once the correct feeling and its intensity have been decided, a word or phrase
that accurately describes the feeling is selected (Activity 6.6). The choice of

ACTIVITY 6.5

BUILDING A FEELING-WORD VOCABULARY
(Adapted from Carkhuff 1983)

 Process

1   Divide a blank piece of paper into seven vertical columns. Place the following 'feeling' categories at the top of each column:

Happy Sad Angry Confused Scared Weak Strong

2   In each column record as many words as you can that express the emotion. Phrases such as 'over the moon' can also be used.

3   Form groups of five to six participants and compare lists. Add words from other participants' lists that you have not already recorded.

4   Evaluate each feeling word on the list according to its intensity. Label each as high, medium or low intensity. For example: elated = high; happy = medium; pleased = low.

Discussion

1   In which feeling category(ies) was it easy to develop words and phrases? Which were difficult? Why are some categories easier to describe than others?

2   Which feeling category has the most words and phrases? Which the least? What do you make of this?

3   Compare the feeling categories that were hard and easy with the ones that have the most and least words and phrases. Is there any relationship? Explain.

4   Look at the language used in each of the categories. Are some feeling words and phrases more appropriate with people/patients in different age groups and from different cultural backgrounds?

5   What role does culture play in the evaluation of feeling word intensity?

6   Are there some words and phrases that you personally would not use under certain circumstances? What are they and why would you not use them?

ACTIVITY 6.6

REFLECTING FEELINGS

 Process

1   Refer to person/patient statements from Activity 5.8: Listening for feelings. For each statement, develop a response that reflects the expressed feeling. Refer to the list of words and phrases developed in Activity 6.5: Building a feeling-word vocabulary.

Discussion

1   Which feelings were easy to reflect? Which were difficult? What do you make of this?

2   Are there any feeling reflections you would find personally difficult to express? Why?

words must suit the age and cultural background of the person/patient (see Chapter 10).

A nurse's feeling-word vocabulary can be further built through interactions with people/patients by paying careful attention to the language used when people/patients express various emotions and feelings.

Because feelings are often expressed indirectly, through nonverbal means, inference and innuendo, nurses may first need to check their perceptions of how a person/patient is feeling before attempting to reflect the feeling accurately. Frequently it is better to check perceptions of feelings before proceeding to reflect them.

A word of caution about reflecting feelings

Some people/patients are more comfortable than others in discussing their feelings. Additionally, a discussion of feelings may enhance a person/patient's sense of vulnerability, because feelings are difficult to control and contain. When a person/patient is working hard at containing emotions, and prefers to keep doing so, it is insensitive for a nurse to proceed into a discussion that uncovers these feelings and focuses on them. Nurses must pay careful attention to a person/patient's reaction to the discussion of feelings.

Likewise, discussion of feelings should be left until trust has formed between person/patient and nurse. The extent to which a person/patient is relaxed and at ease with a discussion of feelings demonstrates the degree of trust that has been established. The nurse can use a feeling discussion as a means of determining how much trust has been established. This requires acute awareness and sensitivity to the person/patient's response.

ACTIVITY 6.7

CONNECTING THOUGHTS AND FEELINGS

Process

1 Refer to each person/patient statement in Activity 6.2: Recognition of the types of responses. Ignore the responses that are provided and develop one of your own that connects people/patients' expressed thoughts to their feelings. Use the format: 'You feel . . . when . . .' as a guide. Refer to your feeling-word vocabulary, developed in Activity 6.5, for ways to describe feelings.

2 Compare your responses with other participants.

Discussion

1. What differences are there in responses developed by various participants? Were there some responses that were the same?

2 In comparing connecting responses, how similar are the feeling portions? How different are they?

3 In comparing the connections between feelings and content, did some participants focus on content that was different from that of other participants?

Connecting thoughts and feelings

Chapter 5, on listening, differentiated listening for content and listening for feelings. In this chapter, the skill of paraphrasing is used predominantly to respond to content, while reflecting feelings responds to emotional states. While it is possible to perceive them separately, and even respond to them separately, people/patients' experiences include both content and feelings. Initially, nurses may choose to focus on one or the other when responding. Eventually, thoughts (content) and feelings (emotion) must be put together. Connecting skills are used for this purpose. When connecting, nurses can use the following format:

■   'You feel . . . when . . .'

Connecting thoughts and feelings adds depth to the nurse's understanding and moves the interaction in a forward direction. Through this response a nurse is moving into the area of fully understanding a person/patient's experience. Listening attentively and clarifying enables nurses to make the connection between people/patients' thoughts and their feelings. Again, it is necessary for the nurse to await feedback from the person/patient that confirms, denies or expands on the nurse's understanding.

Summarizing

Summarizing is the skill of responding in a way that reviews what has been discussed between person/patient and nurse. It is a brief, concise collection of paraphrases and feeling reflections that are accurately connected. Like other skills of understanding, a summary allows the nurse to check understanding by verbalizing it, then awaiting feedback from the person/patient. Summaries often begin with:

- ■ 'So, to sum it up . . .'
- ■ 'We have discussed so much, let me see if I can pull it together . . .'
- ■ 'Overall, I get the picture that . . .'

Summarizing is used most often to bring closure to an interaction, and serves as a final check of the nurse's understanding. When nurses use summarizing to bring closure to an interaction, it is important that they allow adequate time for people/patients to respond. As with other understanding skills, the person/patient needs an opportunity to clarify, expand on an idea or correct the nurse's misinterpretation.

There is an even more important reason for allowing adequate time following a summary. Frequently, people/patients present the most significant aspect of their experience just as the time draws near to close an interaction. In this case, the person/patient perceives the nurse's summary as a signal that time is of the essence, and uses the remaining time as a final opportunity for expression. This is not at all uncommon during person/patient–nurse interactions. An aware nurse recognizes and accepts this interpersonal dynamic, and allows time for its occurrence.

While closure is the most common reason to summarize, a summary is also effectively used either in the middle or the beginning of an interaction. When used in the middle of an interaction, a summary serves to open new areas of discussion by clearing the way for new ideas (Brammer and MacDonald 1996). When it is used at this point, summarizing serves as an exploration skill, that encourages people/patients to bring forward new thoughts and feelings. When it is used at the beginning of an interaction, summarizing serves to orient both person/patient and nurse to the current interaction by reviewing previous interactions.

EXPRESSION OF UNDERSTANDING

When nurses employ the skills of understanding (paraphrasing, seeking clarification, reflecting feelings, connecting and summarizing), in conjunction with effective exploration (see Chapter 7), they are in a position to know what a person/patient is experiencing from the personal perspective of the person/patient. This inside understanding involves knowing what is happening to that person, and even knowing what it is like to be that person. Knowing through vicarious experiences such as these is often referred to as empathy.

Empathy is the ability to perceive the world from another person's view, and to take on the perspective of another while not losing one's own perspective.

Empathy for nurses

Nurses have embraced the process of empathy as essential to caring practices (Pike 1990; Olsen 1991; Wiseman 1996; White 1997). As a result of being empathic, the nurse comes to know and understand the person/patient's experience. Developing empathic understanding is the process of exploring the person/patient's world, with the person/patient, in a non-judgemental manner, often without the offer of advice (Burnard 2002). This absorption of the person/patient's reality is one way that empathy is realized in the caring environment. Some of the first nursing theorists to discuss empathy (Triplett 1969; Zderad 1969; Travelbee 1971) emphasized the purpose of empathy as the promotion of rapport between person/patient and nurse. Rapport is built through mutual understanding and it is important that the person/patient feels understood by the nurse. Therefore nursing theorists who first discussed empathy also stressed the importance of the nurse communicating their understanding to the person/patient (Zderad 1969; Kalisch 1973; Gagan 1983).

Effects of empathy on the relationship

When communicating empathy, nurses respond with a direct, clear and accurate statement that reflects the core of the person/patient's experience. Expressing empathy is a skill that involves nurses sharing openly with people/patients that they understand their perspectives. Expressing empathy communicates this understanding, conveying both acceptance and confirmation of the reality of the person/patient's experience.

Empathic statements capture the essence of the person/patient's experience and move the relationship into a more intimate zone (Shea 1988). For this reason, empathy expression, especially in relation to people/patients' feelings, can be intrusive and prematurely intimate. Yet empathy expression in nursing is often equated with emotions. For example, White (1997) and Wiseman (1996) consider critical attributes of empathy to be recognition and understanding of the person/patient's feelings. Nevertheless, knowing the person/patient (see Chapter 2) in such an intimate way may not be appropriate or desirable.

An empathic statement exposes people/patients, laying their reality in the open. It can expose areas of weakness, uncertainty and vulnerability. A person/patient may not want this exposure, and sensitivity to the person/patient's reaction to an empathic statement is needed. If the person/patient wants to appear strong or maintain control, the nurse who is sensitive will accept this and move out of the intimacy that empathy can bring.

This move into intimacy is one reason that there are cautions in the nursing literature against a wholehearted, unquestioning embrace of empathy. Gould (1990) warns that it may be unrealistic and idealistic to expect nurses to be empathic with all people/patients. Diers (1990) says that empathy may not be always appropriate to the person/patient's situation. Gordon (1987) cautions against a danger in nurses projecting their own perceptions onto people/patients in an effort to be empathic.

It is for these reasons that timing is crucial when expressing empathy. If a nurse moves too quickly into empathic expression, a person/patient may feel invaded and inhibited. All the other skills of understanding should be used first, in order to establish understanding and build the relationship. When the person/patient demonstrates comfort with discussing feelings, has validated the nurse's paraphrases, confirms the connections made between thoughts and feelings and agrees with the summary, then the relationship is ready to move into the intimate zone of empathy. The point at which a nurse truly understands is the time to express empathy.

Another purpose of empathy

In addition to the promotion of rapport and understanding, empathy in nursing is considered a means of promoting personal change and growth within the person/patient (Pike 1990). This purpose of empathy relies on the nurse's objective analysis of the person/patient's experience and is based on a counselling model of helping that promotes more effective ways of living.

The counselling view of empathy in the nursing literature is based primarily on the work of Carl Rogers (Gould 1990; Morse *et al.* 1992a; Thompson 1996). Rogers, a psychologist who pioneered person-centred therapy, considered empathy to be an essential feature of the therapeutic counselling relationship (Rogers 1957, 1961). The humanistic philosophy that underpins Rogers' theory of counselling is consistent with person/patient-centred nursing care and the development of a therapeutic person/patient–nurse relationship. Therefore, it is understandable that nurses who first conceptualized the therapeutic nature of the person/patient–nurse relationship were influenced by the work of Carl Rogers.

Nevertheless, there is growing awareness and mounting criticism that a conceptualization of empathy in nursing that is based on theory borrowed from and developed for another discipline is inappropriate (Gould 1990; Morse *et al.* 1992a; Baille 1996). A counselling view of empathy, with its focus on encouraging a person/patient's personal growth, may not always be appropriate in a nursing situation unless the nurse is also a psychotherapist. Although nurses often interact with people who are experiencing change and transition, not all people/patients are in the process of personal growth. Nurses need to understand a person/patient's personal experience of illness (one purpose of empathy), but not necessarily focus on encouraging psychological growth and personality change (another purpose of empathy).

Description of empathy in nursing literature

In addition to empathy being recommended for different purposes, many authors claim empathy is poorly described in the nursing literature (Wiseman 1996; White 1997; Morse *et al.* 1992b; Gould 1990). The result is a weak theoretical understanding. Part of the difficulty lies in the fact that empathy is a complex concept. It 'may be seen as an ability, a communication style, a trait, a response, a skill, a process, or an experience' (Wheeler and Barrett 1994: 234).

In their review of the nursing literature on empathy, Morse *et al.* (1992a) identify four components of empathy. First is emotional empathy, which involves the subjective sharing of feelings. Next is cognitive empathy, which involves the ability to comprehend another's feelings from an objective stance. Third is moral empathy, or the inherent motivation to comprehend the experience of another. Fourth is behavioural empathy, which involves conveying understanding of another's perspective through communicating.

The four aspects of empathy that were identified by Morse *et al.* (1992a) can be compared to those described in Aligood's (1992) analysis of empathy. Aligood identifies two types of empathy: basic and trained. Basic empathy is an innate capacity to apprehend another's perspective, and can be likened to the emotional and moral components of empathy. Unlike basic empathy, trained empathy is learned. Trained empathy involves the cognitive and behavioural aspects of empathy, that is, standing back and analysing the person/patient's situation and communicating that understanding to the person/patient.

Empathy that is considered to be therapeutic most often includes the cognitive and behavioural components (Morse *et al.* 1992b), that is, trained empathy (Aligood 1992). Although empathy is a skill that can be taught (Wheeler and Barrett 1994), there is evidence that 'trained empathy', that is, the learnt skills of reflecting understanding to a person/patient, is not really sustained over time (Evans *et al.* 1998). While the communicative aspects of empathy can be taught, basic empathy is inherent. Nurses need self-awareness of their innate capacity for empathy so that they can build on their basic empathy and learn to express it.

Empathy and sympathy

Often a distinction is made between empathy and sympathy. Sympathy is viewed as 'feeling for' another person and empathy as 'feeling with' the other. Sympathy is often considered less desirable because nurses need to put their own concerns to one side and focus on the person/patient (Kalisch 1973; Pike 1990); these authors consider sympathetic responses to be focused on the nurse. In contrast Morse *et al.* (1992b) assert that because a sympathetic response is focused on the other (that is, the person/patient), responses such as sympathy and pity may be as comforting for people/patients as empathy. Florence Nightingale encouraged nurses to be sympathetic; so did Travelbee (1971). Still, nurses are encouraged to be empathetic, not sympathetic. What is the difference between sympathy and empathy?

Wispé's (1986) analysis of the distinction between empathy and sympathy may assist in answering this question. She asserts that in empathy we consider what it would be like *if* we were the other person; in sympathy we automatically (reflexively) know what it would be like *to be* the other person. In empathy we 'reach out' to that person; in sympathy we are 'moved by' the other. Sympathy urges action to alleviate the suffering of the other; empathy urges efforts to comprehend the consciousness of the other. Sympathy is a way of relating, while empathy is a way of knowing. We can send a sympathy card as an action; we do not send empathy cards.

Despite the useful analysis, the attempt to differentiate sympathy and empathy remains troublesome. The results of Baille's (1996) research into empathy has been criticized as confusing empathy with sympathy (Yegdich 1999), because the nurses in Baille's 1996 study described empathy as familiarity with the person/patient's situation because they had similar experiences. Perhaps what is at issue is not delineating one from the other but recognizing that both sympathy and empathy have a place in the caring environment. Just because they can be distinguished from each other does not mean one is more beneficial to people/patients than the other. In the clinical environment empathy is often touted as more beneficial, even though it has not been fully researched as to its effects on person/patient outcome. There is evidence that empathy decreases person/patient distress (Reid-Ponte 1992; Olson 1995) but other responses such as commiseration, pity and consolation serve to comfort people/patients (Morse *et al.* 1992b). More importantly, such responses are more engaging of the person/patient than the learned response of behavioural and cognitive styles of empathy that rely on objective analysis.

In their analysis, Morse *et al.* (1992b) use the criteria of engagement with the person/patient and focus on the person/patient as a way of determining what type of nursing response is of comfort to the person/patient. In a way, this approach sidesteps the sympathy–empathy distinction, but offers a useful way of determining the purpose of responses intended to be helpful and understanding. Those responses that engage people/patients and focus on them (as compared to responses that focus on the nurse and disengage the person/patient) are considered to be helpful because they are comforting.

Therefore, both sympathy and empathy can be employed for the purposes of helping and comforting people/patients. Sympathy will compel the nurse to act, while empathy will compel the nurse to understand. A sympathetic response to a person/patient's physical pain, followed by action to relieve the pain, is more appropriate than an empathic response, which merely confirms understanding that the person/patient is indeed in pain.

Expressing empathy

The purpose of expressing empathy should be borne in mind. Empathy is used to encourage the person/patient to continue expression, to provide direction to the nurse, to decrease the person/patient's sense of isolation, and to bond the person/patient and nurse in understanding. Often support and reassurance, direct aid and assistance, or advice or challenge follows the expression of empathy. At other times, empathy expression is an end in itself; it offers comfort and solace to people/patients – they know they are not alone because they are understood. See Chapter 8 for further discussion of empathy.

The frequency of empathy expression is also crucial. Short, precise empathic statements should be employed whenever nurses think understanding has been achieved. Too much empathy expression, especially early in the relationship, can sound paternalistic and superficial (Shea, 1988). Lack of empathy expression leaves people/patients with a sense of isolation, as if nurses do not care to receive their world.

The most congruent and compelling goal of empathy in caring, namely, for nurses to come to understand a person/patient's experience, is that nurses' actions are based on their understanding of the person/patient's situation. In the caring environment there is an obligation to act, not simply to understand, and acting without understanding may result in actions that are not helpful to people/patients. This is one possible explanation of why more experienced nurses in Reid-Ponte's (1992) study were less empathic than their less experienced colleagues.

ACTIVITY 6.8

EXPRESSING EMPATHY

 Process

1. Refer to Activity 6.1: Your usual style of responding.

2   For each statement or question, develop a response that expresses empathy with the person/patient's experience. Assume you have validated your understanding and have accurately understood the person/patient.

3   Compare these responses with the ones you originally developed when completing Activity 6.1.

Discussion

1   What differences are there between the responses you originally developed and the ones you have now developed?

2. Which took more time to develop?

    What risks are there in expressing empathy to people/patients?

4   What benefits are there in expressing empathy?

Clinical experience provides the knowledge to act, therefore experienced nurses may need to spend less time being verbally empathic in order to understand person/patient needs.

As a moral position, empathy demonstrates a commitment to understanding people/patients. In this regard its benefits are without question. What is questionable is whether cognitive and behavioural aspects of empathy should be given more credence because they are considered 'therapeutic'. They also have the potential to create more intimacy than is warranted by the person/patient situation (for example, the clinical/instrumental relationship described in Chapter 1), or disengage the person/patient because they are mechanical and objective when empathy is expressed in a formulaic manner such as 'I hear what you are saying'. Beginning nurses should bear these considerations in mind when employing the skills of understanding.

Reluctance to express empathy

At first, it feels awkward for nurses to express to people/patients what they are experiencing. The awkwardness is based on a false notion that it is presumptuous and arrogant, if not downright impolite, to openly state what another person is experiencing. When empathy is expressed with an attitude of 'let me tell you what you are experiencing', its basic nature has been violated. When employed in this manner, attempts at empathy expression will be met with defensiveness on the person/patient's part and will work against an effective relationship. Empathy expression is a confirmation, not an accusation. The nurse must remain sensitive and open to correction. When stated with too much certainty, empathy expression alienates rather than engages the person/patient.

CHAPTER SUMMARY

Understanding responses are used after nurses have received meaningful input from people/patients, during the process of listening. Once initial impressions are formed, understanding responses are employed to build meaning between people/patients and nurses. The skills of understanding are used to bring nurses in touch with people/patients' private and personal worlds. They allow nurses to be 'in tune' with people/patients.

Attending and listening to people/patients' reactions to understanding responses is essential and highlights the need for constant listening. People/patients may react to an understanding response by validating it, denying it, altering it, or expanding on it. Each of these person/patient reactions provides an opportunity for nurses to deepen their level of understanding.

It requires time and effort to truly understand another's reality. Nurses need to allow themselves time to think and reflect on how effectively they are understanding people/patients' experiences. They need to allow themselves enough time to respond with understanding to people/patients. This may also involve 'letting go' of familiar ways of responding, in favour of responses that reflect understanding.

ANSWERS TO ACTIVITIES

ACTIVITY 6.2: RECOGNITION OF THE TYPES OF RESPONSES

2 (a) (i)   S (reassuring and supporting)
         (ii)   I (analysing and interpreting)
         (iii) U (paraphrasing and understanding)
         (iv) E (advising and evaluating)
         (v)   P (questioning and probing)
    (b) (i)   P (questioning and probing)
         (ii) S (reassuring and supporting)
         (iii) E (advising and evaluating)
         (iv) U (paraphrasing and understanding)
         (v)   I (analysing and interpreting)
    (c) (i)   U (paraphrasing and understanding)
         (ii) E (advising and evaluating)
         (iii) P (questioning and probing)
         (iv) S (reassuring and supporting)
         (v)   I (analysing and interpreting)

(d) (i) E (advising and evaluating)
(ii) P (questioning and probing)
(iii) U (paraphrasing and understanding)
(iv) I (analysing and interpreting)
(v) S (reassuring and supporting)
(e) (i) S (reassuring and supporting)
(ii) E (advising and evaluating)
(iii) P (questioning and probing)
(iv) I (analysing and interpreting)
(v) U (paraphrasing and understanding)
(f) (i) E (advising and evaluating)
(ii) P (questioning and probing)
(iii) S (reassuring and supporting)
(iv) I (analysing and interpreting)
(v) U (paraphrasing and understanding)
(g) (i) I (analysing and interpreting)
(ii) E (advising and evaluating)
(iii) U (paraphrasing and understanding)
(iv) P (questioning and probing)
(v) S (reassuring and supporting)
(h) (i) U (paraphrasing and understanding)
(ii) S (reassuring and supporting)
(iii) E (advising and evaluating)
(iv) P (questioning and probing)
(v) I (analysing and interpreting)
(i) (i) I (analysing and interpreting)
(ii) S (reassuring and supporting)
(iii) U (paraphrasing and understanding)
(iv) E (advising and evaluating)
(v) P (questioning and probing)
(j) (i) U (paraphrasing and understanding)
(ii) S (reassuring and supporting)
(iii) I (analysing and interpreting)
(iv) P (questioning and probing)
(v) E (advising and evaluating)
(k) (i) S (reassuring and supporting)
(ii) I (analysing and interpreting)
(iii) P (questioning and probing)
(iv) U (paraphrasing and understanding)
(v) E (advising and evaluating)
(l) (i) I (analysing and interpreting)
(ii) U (paraphrasing and understanding)
(iii) P (questioning and probing)
(iv) E (advising and evaluating)
(v) S (reassuring and supporting)

REFERENCES

Aligood, M. R. (1992). Empathy: the importance of recognising two types. *Journal of Psychosocial Nursing*, 30(3), 14–17.

Baille, L. (1996). A phenomenological study of the nature of empathy. *Journal of Advanced Nursing*, 24, 1300–08.

Brammer, L. M. and MacDonald, G. (1996). *The Helping Relations: Process and Skills*, sixth edition. Boston, MA: Allyn and Bacon.

Burnard, P. (2002). *Learning Human Skills: An Experiential and Reflective Guide for Nurses and Health Care Professionals*, fourth edition. Oxford: Butterworth Heinemann.

Carkhuff, R. R. (1983). *The Student Workbook for the Art of Helping*, second edition. Amherst, MA: Human Resource Press.

Diers, D. (1990). Response to 'On the nature and place of empathy in clinical nursing practice'. *Journal of Professional Nursing*, 6(4), 240–1.

Evans, G. W., Wilt, D. L., Aligood, M. R. and O'Neil, M. (1998). Empathy: a study of two types. *Issues in Mental Health Nursing*, 19, 453–61.

Gagan, J. M. (1983). Methodological notes on empathy. *Advances in Nursing Science*, 5(2), 65–72.

Gordon, M. (1987). *Nursing Diagnosis: Process and Application*, second edition. New York: McGraw-Hill.

Gould, D. (1990). Empathy: a review of the literature with suggestions for an alternative research strategy. *Journal of Advanced Nursing*, 15, 1167–74.

Johnson, D. W. (2000). *Reaching Out: Interpersonal Effectiveness and Self Actualization*, seventh edition. Boston, MA: Allyn and Bacon.

Kalisch, B. J. (1973). What is empathy? *American Journal of Nursing*, 73, 1548–52.

Morse, J. M., Anderson, G., Bottoroff, J. L., Younge, O., O'Brien, B., Solberg, M. and Mellveen, K. H. (1992a). Exploring empathy: a conceptual fit for nursing practice? *Image: Journal of Nursing Scholarship*, 24(4), 273–80.

Morse, J. M., Bottoroff, J., Anderson, G., O'Brien, B. and Solberg, S. (1992b). Beyond empathy: expanding expressions of caring. *Journal of Advanced Nursing*, 17, 809–21.

Motyka, M., Motyka, H. and Wsolek, R. (1997). Elements of psychological support in nursing care. *Journal of Advanced Nursing*, 26, 909–12.

Olsen, D. P. (1991). Empathy as an ethical and philosophical basis for nursing. *Advances in Nursing Science*, 14(1), 65–75.

Olson, J. K. (1995). Relationship between nurse-expressed empathy and person/patient-perceived empathy and person/patient distress. *Image: Journal of Nursing Scholarship*, 27(4), 317–22.

Pike, A. W. (1990). On the nature and place of empathy in clinical nursing practice. *Journal of Professional Nursing*, 6(4), 235–340.

Reid-Ponte, P. (1992). Distress in cancer people/patients and primary nurses' empathy skills. *Cancer Nursing*, 15(4), 283–92.

Rogers, C. (1957). The necessary and sufficient conditions of therapeutic personality change. *Journal of Consulting Psychology*, 21, 91–105.

Rogers, C. (1961). *On Becoming a Person*. Boston MA: Houghton Mifflin.

Shea, S. C. (1988). *Psychiatric Interviewing: the Art of Understanding*. Philadelphia, PA: W. B. Saunders.

Thompson, S. (1996). Empathy: towards a clearer meaning for nursing. *Nursing Praxis in New Zealand*, 11(1), 19–26.

Travelbee, J. (1971). *Interpersonal Aspects of Nursing*. Philadelphia, PA: F. A. Davis.

Triplett, J. L. (1969). Empathy is . . . *Nursing Clinics of North America*, 4, 673–81.

Wheeler, K. and Barrett, E. A. M. (1994). Review and synthesis of selected nursing studies on teaching empathy and implication for nursing research and education. *Nursing Outlook*, 42(5), 230–6.

White, S. J. (1997). Empathy: a literature review and concept analysis. *Journal of Clinical Nursing*, 6, 253–7.

Whyte, L., Motyka, M., Motyka, H., Wsolek, R. and Tune, M. (1997). Polish and British nurses responses to person/patient need. *Nursing Standard*, 11(38), 34–7.

Wiseman, T. (1996). A concept analysis of empathy. *Journal of Advanced Nursing*, 23, 1162–7.

Wispé, L. (1986). The distinction between sympathy and empathy: to call forth a concept, a word is needed. *Journal of Personality and Social Psychology*, 50, 314–421.

Yegdich, T. (1999). On the phenomenology of empathy in nursing: empathy or sympathy. *Journal of Advanced Nursing*, 30, 83–93.

Zderad, L. T. (1969). Empathic nursing: realisation of a human capacity. *Nursing Clinics of North America*, 4, 655–62.

CHAPTER 7

COLLECTING INFORMATION: EXPLORING

INTRODUCTION

The skills covered in Chapters 6 and 7 – attending, listening and understanding – lay the foundation for effective interaction between person/patient and nurse because their use enables nurses to hear, perceive and reflect back what people/patients are expressing. Exploration, the subject of this chapter, moves the interaction beyond absorption and reiteration of people/patients' messages. Exploration opens new areas, focuses on selected areas and delves more deeply into a person/patient's total experience.

The process of exploration is one of searching, carried out for the purpose of discovery, detection, recognition, and identification. Successful exploration results in greater understanding between person/patient and nurse; it can be directed toward something in particular, or it can be open-ended, leading to the discovery of something unexpected, which is the case with interpersonal exploration carried out in the context of person/patient–nurse relationships. Collecting specific information from people/patients, the directed type of exploration, is necessary. Is Mr Green allergic to any medications? How long did Ms Geraghty sleep last night? Does Mr Nelson understand his special low-fat diet? Answers to such questions help guide care approaches and actions, and nurses need to know how to collect pertinent information from people/patients. Nevertheless, effective exploration in the caring context involves more than merely the collection of specific facts from people/patients. Open-ended, spontaneous inquiry, the other type of exploration, is also needed because it is the means by which a nurse can come to understand how a person/patient interprets health and illness. What are Mr Green's expectations about his pending surgery? What is interfering with Ms Geraghty's sleep? How different is Mr Nelson's special diet from his usual one? Exploring areas such as these is aimed at discovering ideas, thoughts, perceptions, feelings, and reactions experienced by people/patients. It is important that nurses come to understand people/patients' responses to health and illness, and effective exploration assists in this understanding.

Consider the following account:

> Martin Johnson spent his entire life in a rural part of the country. He felt very much at home 'on the land'. He disliked city life and avoided 'the big smoke' at all possible costs. Martin also had another aversion: visiting the doctor. He always put that off as long as he could. However, the obvious problems he was experiencing with his throat made it impossible to ignore his need of medical attention.
>
> When he was finally admitted to a large metropolitan hospital for major surgery, Martin felt very much out of place. However, coping with being in the city seemed minor in comparison to his worry about being ill and in hospital. He did not ask many questions of the surgeons when they came to explain his surgery, which included possible removal of his larynx (voice box). Martin listened as the surgeons explained what they would do, but did not think too much about what it meant. Being a man of few words, he did not ask for clarification.
>
> The night before his surgery, Lucille was the nurse caring for Martin. She felt an instant rapport with him, despite his quiet nature and the scarcity of words between them. As she explained to Martin what he could expect following the surgery, she slowly came to the realization that he did not understand that the surgery would affect his ability to speak. In fact, if the surgeons performed the laryngectomy he would not speak again. Although he had consented to the surgical procedure, he did not seem to appreciate the potential consequences for his life. Through exploring his understanding and desires, Lucille discovered that Martin preferred a shorter life with the ability to speak in favour of a longer life and the inability to speak. As a result of her exploration and understanding, Martin's surgery was cancelled and other treatment options were explored.

This account raises questions as to whether Martin's consent to the surgery was adequately informed and highlights the importance of coming to understand the person/patient's point of view. In turn, understanding the person/patient's point of view is reliant on effective questioning to ascertain the person/patient's perceptions and interpretation.

CHAPTER OVERVIEW

This chapter reviews the skills of exploration within the context of person/patient–nurse interaction. It distinguishes directed exploration, such as a formal interview, from the less formal, spontaneous exploration, which occurs as a result of a trigger or cue from the person/patient. Both types of exploration rely on the use of the same skills, and these skills are divided into the broad areas of prompting and probing. Prompting techniques include minimal encouragement; one-word/phrase accents; gentle commands; open-ended statements; finishing the sentence; and self-disclosure. The section on probing techniques covers open-ended questions and closed questions, and includes a discussion of when to use each type. The final sections review two processes of exploration: focused exploration and person/patient cue exploration.

PLANNED VERSUS SPONTANEOUS EXPLORATION

Planned exploration is directive, that is, the nurse controls the interaction by directing the flow and content of the person/patient's response. A good example of planned exploration is a formal interview conducted for the purpose of health assessment. Spontaneous exploration is responsive, that is, the nurse responds to something the person/patient has said or done (Activity 7.1). In planned exploration, nurses assume the lead and introduce the topics; in spontaneous exploration, nurses follow people/patients' leads. The distinction between planned exploration and spontaneous exploration is somewhat artificial because similar skills and techniques are used for both types of exploration. The distinction is drawn to highlight the different contexts in which nurses use exploration skills and techniques.

A common context in which nurses use exploration skills is when they conduct a health assessment. Most often nurses conduct health assessments when they encounter a person/patient for the first time, for example, on admission to hospital. Brown (1995) urges nurses to clarify the purpose of health assessments. If the purpose is to collect data about the person/patient's health status, then planned interviewing is appropriate. If the purpose of the health assessment is also to explore personal meaning of a person/patient's health status, then a less formalized, spontaneous exploration is appropriate. In nursing, both purposes are relevant. Nurses need to collect factual data about a person/patient's health as well as understanding the meaning of the health experience for person/patient. As a result, exploration is most effective when it is both planned and spontaneous. Brown refers to this style of exploration as 'conversational interviewing', which closely mirrors the balanced give and take of everyday conversations, as compared to the one-way, controlled structure of a formal interview in which 'questions impose an obligation to answer' (1995: 340).

Planned exploration

During planned exploration, the nurse directs and leads the search for information regarding pertinent aspects of a person/patient's 'health account' and current needs for professional care. Specific data collection is the primary purpose of planned exploration, and topic areas are introduced and explored on the basis of what the nurse needs to know in order to care for the person/patient. Nurses direct and often control this type of exploration.

Structured, planned exploration occurs in the beginning phase of the person/patient–nurse relationship, usually upon initial contact between person/patient and nurse. The manner in which exploration occurs during these initial contacts sets the stage for subsequent interactions and further development of the relationship by establishing the conditions for trust and openness. A nurse whose approach is authoritarian and rigid may convey a message to the person/patient that the nurse is in control, and obedience in answering the questions is expected. This might happen when the nurse becomes so focused on filling out the assessment documentation that people/patients are left with the impression that completion of the documentation is more important than them as people.

ACTIVITY 7.1

DEVELOPING EXPLORATORY RESPONSES I

● **Process**

Record how you would respond to each of the following person/patient statements. Do not concern yourself with how 'right' or 'wrong' your responses are, but do try to make them helpful to the person/patient. Assume that all statements are made to you, the nurse caring for the person/patient making the statement.

1   A hospitalized 65-year-old woman, who has recently undergone a total hip replacement: 'How am I ever going to manage on my own when I return home?'

2   A hospitalized person/patient speaking to a first-year nursing student: 'Do you know what you are doing? How much experience have you had?'

3   A twenty-year-old woman who is undergoing diagnostic tests on an out-patient basis: 'The doctor keeps evading my questions. What is really going on?'

4   A mother of a five-week-old baby during a routine visit to an early childhood centre: 'I wish I could get a decent night's sleep like I used to.'

5   A long-term resident of a nursing home: 'I can't stand being here. There's nothing to do and no one ever comes to visit me.'

6   A twenty-year-old man who is hospitalized with a fractured femur, following a motor vehicle accident: 'Why do these things always have to happen to me? All the bad things like this happen to me.'

7   A hospitalized person/patient, during medication rounds in hospital: 'I think all of these tablets are really making me sleepy.'

8   A hospitalized person/patient during morning care: 'I have asked the doctors how long they think I have to live, but they keep avoiding the question. Will you tell me, please?'

9   A hospitalized person/patient during morning nursing rounds: 'I'm so glad to see you. Those nurses on the night shift just don't help me.'

10 A 70-year-old man in an out-patient clinic, following consultation with the doctor: 'If what the doctor says is true, I don't see the point in going on and suffering . . . better to just end it now.'

11 A 16-year-old girl who is hospitalized suffering from anorexia nervosa: 'I am not going to eat that – greasy food like that makes me want to vomit!'

Discussion

1   Each of the statements presented in the process section indicates a situation that requires further exploration by the nurse – more information, clarification and/or elaboration is required. Review your responses and decide which of your responses do in fact explore the person/patient's statement. Mark these with a tick.

2   Write a new response for those not marked. Try to make this revised response an exploratory one.

(*Note*: This activity will be further developed in Activity 7.10 Developing exploratory responses II.)

Likewise, over-concern with the techniques of exploration may interfere with a nurse's ability to fully attend and listen to people/patients' replies.

The nurse needs to bear in mind the potential of this type of exploration to disempower the person/patient, so they should always consider using spontaneous exploration alongside planned exploration in every situation, as the person/patient is continually sending out verbal and nonverbal cues (see Chapter 2).

Spontaneous exploration

This type of exploration occurs when nurses pick up and follow through in exploring a person/patient cue. People/patients often express their needs to nurses in indirect, disguised ways (Macleod Clark 1984), not because they want to keep the nurse guessing but because people/patients perceive that an indirect message poses less of a threat to nurses. How nurses respond to these messages or cues from people/patients helps to shape the direction of their continuing relationship. This type of exploration tends to be person/patient-controlled and person/patient-led. The nurse follows the person/patient's lead instead of the person/patient following the nurse's lead.

Spontaneous exploration is important to the continuing relationship between person/patient and nurse because it affirms that the nurse is attending and listening to the person/patient. It deepens the relationship and communicates the nurse's continued interest in the person/patient's welfare, because it is a concrete demonstration of the nurse's ongoing concern for the person/patient.

The difference between planned and spontaneous exploration

In both types of exploration, information is collected and greater depth of understanding is achieved, but the process is different because the roles of leader and follower are reversed. In the real world of person/patient care, this distinction

Table 7.1 Planned versus spontaneous exploration

Planned exploration	**Spontaneous exploration**
Directive	Responsive
Nurse-led	Person/patient-led
Prescribed format, usually	No prescribed format
Information solicited	**Meaning sought**
Topic areas determined by the nurse	Topic areas introduced by the person/patient
More questioning techniques (probes) used	More exploratory statements (prompts) used

in the types of exploration may not be obvious, because there is give and take between nurse and person/patient. The roles of leader and follower are continuously shifting.

Whether leading or following, nurses utilize similar skills and techniques, although the type and frequency of skills used may be different, for example, more questioning techniques are employed in planned exploration than in spontaneous exploration. Planned exploration, such as the formal interview, often follows a prescribed format, even if the sequence is altered; spontaneous exploration has no set format. Planned exploration aims to solicit fairly standard information, while spontaneous exploration is more a search for meaning and for a person/patient–nurse relationship in which more information and feelings can be shared. The differences are highlighted in Table 7.1.

The summary of this activity will most likely show that the second interview (with no questions used) created more anxiety. The interviewer in these circumstances often feels uncomfortable and sometimes even selfish. Nevertheless, the type of information obtained when no questions are asked is often more personal, focused and meaningful in getting to know the interviewee. Asking no questions usually results in more reciprocal sharing during the interview and this eventually leads the interviewer to a greater understanding of the interviewee on a personal level. The first interview usually collects a lot of facts about the interviewee, but does not really uncover subjective opinions and ideas. The first interview usually covers more breadth, while the second one covers more depth.

Questions tend to focus on the collection of information and are associated with formal interviews. Exploratory statements tend to focus more on reciprocal sharing of ideas, opinions, beliefs, and feelings, and reflect a conversational style of interacting. Each type of exploration yields different types of information; how information is collected affects what information is gleaned.

THE SKILLS OF EXPLORATION

As demonstrated in Activity 7.2, exploration can be accomplished with or without the use of questions. This section divides the skills of exploration into two major categories: prompting and probing. Prompting skills are exploration techniques that are statements; probing skills are exploration techniques that are questions.

Prompting skills

Verbal prompts are a means of instigating further interaction and serve to assist the person/patient in elaboration and expansion of partially expressed ideas. Prompting skills include:

- Minimal encouragement
- One-word/phrase accents
- Gentle commands
- Open-ended statements
- Finishing the sentence
- Self-disclosure.

Minimal encouragement

Minimal encouragement is expressed by verbal responses such as 'uh huh', 'mm hum' and 'yes'. Often they are utterances that are not really classified as words, yet convey messages, such as 'I'm with you', 'I'm following what you are saying' and 'I want to hear more'. They are signals that acknowledge the person/patient's verbalization and encourage further elaboration. Visualize a person on the telephone who keeps repeating 'Yes' and 'uh huh'. Although you cannot hear the person on the other end of the line, you can ascertain that the person on this end is encouraging the other person to carry on the conversation. A person talking on the telephone uses minimal encouragement extensively because nonverbal messages are limited. In face-to-face communication, minimal encouragement reinforces attentive listening, but is not really a substitute for it. Attentive and active listening (see Chapter 5) is, in itself, an effective prompt because it conveys messages similar to those of minimal encouragement.

Sometimes minimal encouragement is used without conscious awareness, even when active listening is absent. If this is the case, the verbal and nonverbal messages are incongruent. Because of this incongruence, minimal encouragement, without attentive listening, would probably not prompt further interaction. Try it in a conversation. Keep uttering 'uh huh' while not really attending and listening to the other person. Eventually the person speaking to you either gives up or tells you, 'Hey, you're not listening to me!'.

Minimal encouragement works best when people/patients are willing and able to continue the interaction. When people/patients are having difficulty verbalizing their experiences, more explicit prompting and probing techniques need to be employed.

One-word/phrase accents

One-word/phrase accents are the repetition of key words or phrases, and are an effective way to both extend and focus the interaction. The choice of which word or phrase to repeat is important because it determines the direction of the exploration; it becomes the focus. It is best to repeat words or phrases that are judged to be the most central or critical. The following example illustrates the uses of accents:

Person/patient: My son won't be visiting me while I'm here in hospital.
Nurse: *Won't be* visiting?
Person/patient: Yes, he says he can't stand the sight and smells of the hospital.

Notice how the accent encourages the person/patient to expand the initial comment. Nurses effectively use the accent to explore what they perceive to be the most significant part of the person/patient's statement. Had the nurse repeated the words 'your son?' the interaction may have taken a different direction. In this regard, one-word/phrase accents are controlled by the nurse, although they are always in response to what the person/patient has said. If a person/patient does not elaborate, a nurse should follow the person/patient's lead and end the discussion.

ACTIVITY 7.2

WAYS OF EXPLORING: QUESTIONS VERSUS STATEMENTS

 Process

1   Form pairs for this activity. The participants in a pair should not be well known to each other. Designate one person as the interviewer and the other as the interviewee. If the number of participants is uneven, form a group of three, with the third person acting as an observer.

Interview I

2   The interviewer is to find out as much as possible about the interviewee by asking questions only. The interviewer is not to make any statements during the interview. This interview is to last five minutes.

3   After the interview, each of the participants records a summary of the information discussed, as well as the reactions and feelings experienced during the interview. Observers (if used) record what type of information (for example, factual, opinions, feelings) the interviewer actively solicited, as well as general impressions about the comfort level of participants in the interview.

Interview II

4   Interviewer and interviewee now reverse roles. Conduct a second interview, but this time the ground rule is that no questions are to be asked during the interview. The interviewer is to learn as much as possible about the interviewee by making statements only. This interview is to last five minutes. The observer records the specific strategies used by the interviewer during the interaction.

5   After the interview, each of the participants records a summary of the information discussed, as well as reactions and feelings during the interview. Observers (if used) record the type of information that was solicited during the interview, as well as general impressions about the comfort level of participants in the interview.

6   Before proceeding to the discussion section, participant pairs should discuss their reactions to the activity with each other.

Discussion

On a board visible to all participants, record the answers to the following discussion questions, using the grid in Figure 7.1 as a format.

	Interview I: all questions	**Interview II:** no questions
Interviewer reactions		
Interviewee reactions		
Type of information		
Strategies used		

Figure 7.1 Grid for Activity 7.2

Discussion questions for Interview I

1   What were the reactions of the interviewer to the first interview?

2   What were the reactions of the interviewee to the first interview?

3   What kind of information was discussed during the interview? How much was learnt about the interviewee during this interview?

4   Observers (if used) report their general impressions of Interview I.

Discussion questions for Interview II

5   What were the reactions of the interviewee to the second interview?

6   What were the reactions of the interviewer to the second interview?

7   What kind of information was discussed during the interview? How much was learnt about the interviewee during the interview?

8   Observers (if used) report their general impressions of Interview II.

Gentle commands

Gentle commands (Shea 1988) are explicit requests for information or elaboration. Although specific topics are often introduced with gentle commands, they are open-ended because they allow the person/patient to determine the direction and flow of the response. Examples of gentle commands include:

- 'Tell me about your family.'
- 'Can you describe that in more detail?'
- 'Tell me more.'
- 'Let's talk about that further.'
- 'Tell me what it's like for you to be in hospital.'
- 'Go on, say what's on your mind.'

In response to the first example, 'Tell me about your family', people/patients can choose whatever they wish to share about their family. One person/patient could say how many children she has, while another may focus on relationships with his extended family. The gentle command is directive in one sense yet allows the person/patient to control the direction in another sense.

Gentle commands should always be said in a way that allows people/patients to maintain a sense of control; they should not be demands. Although the idea of commanding people/patients to tell the nurse something sounds a bit harsh, the qualifier 'gentle' must not be forgotten. 'Gentle' means that the command is stated as an interested request for more information, rather than an order to speak. The qualifying phrase 'Can you?' is often placed before the command for this reason. 'Can you tell me about your family?' sounds less harsh than, 'Tell me about your family'. Technically, the addition of 'Can you' turns the statement into a closed question, and a person/patient can simply respond 'Yes' or 'No' without any further elaboration. In general, this does not happen because the underlying message that the nurse wants to hear more than a simple 'Yes' or 'No' is usually understood.

The gentleness of the command is conveyed primarily through nonverbal messages. Practise a few of the examples cited, using a variety of vocal tones and facial expressions, and include the qualifier 'Can you?' at the beginning of the statement. Note that the words can sound harsh if said in a controlling, demanding manner. Nevertheless, if gentleness is put into the tone and facial expression, such commands are quite effective in exploring people/patients' experiences.

Open-ended statements

Open-ended statements provide a broad introduction to topics for discussion and are sometimes referred to as 'indirect questions' (Benjamin 1969). They indicate to a person/patient that the nurse would like to hear more about something and provide an open invitation for the person/patient to speak about a topic. Examples of open-ended statements include:

- 'So, this is the first time you are having surgery.'
- 'I wonder how it is being sick when you've been so healthy all of your life.'

- 'I hear from your family that you are quite the athlete.'
- 'You've been giving yourself insulin injections for a few years now.'

It is clear from these examples that the nurse making the statement is interested in hearing more about the topic that is introduced, and desires the discussion to proceed further. Open-ended statements are invitations to people/patients to say more, if they choose to accept the invitation. In this way open-ended statements are similar to gentle commands, because they allow the person/patient to determine the direction and depth of the interaction. Open-ended statements are often a good way to begin an interaction, because they introduce a topic, but still allow the interaction to take various directions. While they introduce a topic, they do not control the direction of the conversation.

Finishing the sentence

This exploration technique is similar to open-ended statements. Instead of completing a sentence the nurse begins it, then trails off with an expectation that the person/patient will finish the sentence (Carnevali 1983). Examples of finishing the sentence include:

- 'So you're most worried about . . .'
- 'And when you are in pain you usually . . .'
- 'Today has been . . .'
- 'What you really would like to know is . . .'

To be effective, finishing the sentence relies heavily on an inquisitive, anticipatory facial expression, which lets the person/patient know that the nurse has not had a lapse in memory or become preoccupied with other thoughts or activities. The nonverbal message, conveyed through facial expression and body posture, communicates that the nurse is awaiting completion of the sentence by the person/patient.

Self-disclosure

Sometimes the most effective way to encourage people/patients to explore their experiences with nurses is for nurses to share their own thoughts with a person/patient. Through self-disclosure, nurses open an area for exploration by stating their own reactions, feelings or thoughts. Self-disclosure must always be honest. There is little point in nurses fabricating information about themselves in an attempt to make people/patients open up. Self-disclosure is not the same as giving an opinion or a valuative judgement. Examples of self-disclosure as an exploration technique include:

- 'If I were in your place, I'd be angry.'
- 'I don't handle pain all that well.'
- 'I think I'd be wondering, what is wrong with me?'

Self-disclosure lets the person/patient know that the nurse is not afraid to be open. When used in the context of exploration it serves as a trigger for the person/patient to expand and elaborate, because it creates a climate of safety.

It works well as an exploration technique with people/patients who seem reluctant to reveal themselves. While self-disclosures is utilized here as a means of encouraging exploration, a complete discussion of it can be found in Chapter 8.

Probing skills

The techniques of asking questions are probing skills. Carefully worded and well-timed questions frequently provide the backbone of effective exploration and interviewing (Activity 7.3). Questions come in different varieties, yielding different responses and taking the interaction in different directions, depending on the type used. Both planned and spontaneous explorations combine the various types of questions. There are two major types of probing skills: open-ended questions and closed questions. Closed questions have two subtypes, which are particularly relevant to exploration within the nursing context: focused and multiple-choice questions.

Open-ended questions

Open-ended questions are those that require more than a one-word response, such as 'Yes' or 'No', thereby encouraging more elaboration in the answer (Activity 7.4). Examples of open-ended questions include:

- 'How did you sleep last night?'
- 'What concerns you most about the surgery?'
- 'What types of food do you enjoy eating?'
- 'How was your visit to the out-patient department?'

Open-ended questions begin with interrogative words such as who, what, when, where, why, and how. Not all questions beginning with these words are open-ended, for example, 'Where do you live?' is a closed question, while 'Where do you see yourself in five years time?' is an open-ended question. Questions that are open-ended often yield more information than closed questions because their replies include more detailed expansion and elaboration. Additionally, open-ended questions allow more flexibility in response than closed questions. In answering open-ended questions, people/patients can highlight what is most relevant to their experience and therefore retain a sense of control in the inter-action. Nevertheless, an open-ended question, no matter how well-stated, can pressure people/patients to disclose personal matters before they feel trusting enough to share their inner experiences. Because open-ended questions often probe more deeply than closed ones, nurses need to be mindful about the level of trust established before delving too deeply into the person/patient's experience.

Closed questions

Closed questions are those that are usually answered with a simple 'Yes', 'No' or some other one-word response. They control the direction of the conversation and limit the amount of information that is shared or obtained. If closed questions are over-used, an interaction begins to resemble an interrogation and can result in a person/patient feeling put on the spot because, short of refusing to answer or lying, the person/patient often feels obliged to answer direct questions posed by a nurse. Examples of closed questions include:

- 'Have you been in hospital before?'
- 'Do you wear glasses?'
- 'Is your wife coming to visit you tonight?'
- 'Do you have any children?'
- 'When did you last have something to eat?'

Closed questions can also differ and can be categorized as (a) focused, closed questions, and (b) multiple-choice questions.

(a) Focused, closed questions

At times, it is necessary for nurses to ask closed questions that are focused and directed at obtaining information about a specific clinical situation. These questions are based on the nurse's clinical knowledge and experience. Without them, important and even vital information may be missed (Shea 1988). Examples of focused, closed questions include:

- 'Are you feeling nauseous?' (to a person/patient recovering from anaesthesia)
- 'Do you ever feel dizzy when you get out of bed quickly?' (to a person/patient whose blood pressure is low)
- 'Is your mouth dry?' (to a person/patient taking medication that produces a dry mouth as a side effect)
- 'Are you allergic to any medication?' (to a person/patient who is being prescribed a new drug).

Each of these examples is a closed, focused question that is appropriate under the circumstances. The trigger for these closed questions is the nurse's awareness and understanding of what is pertinent to explore in a given clinical situation. People/patients may not recognize the significance of their clinical symptoms and therefore feel reassured by such questions. An open-ended question may not yield the information needed or reveal progress in a particular direction.

(b) Multiple-choice questions

Multiple-choice questions are another form of specific, closed questioning that is based on the nurse's understanding of a particular clinical phenomenon. In multiple-choice questions, the nurse provides options to the person/patient in an attempt to obtain an answer to the question 'Which of these is correct?' A good example is when a nurse tries to obtain a complete description of a person/patient's pain. An open-ended question such as 'How does the pain feel?' or even 'How would you describe the pain?' is often met with responses such as 'It feels like pain, it hurts' or 'I don't know, pain just feels like pain'. A multiple-choice

ACTIVITY 7.3

CONVERTING PROBES INTO PROMPTS

 Process

Questions (probes) are often over-used as a means of exploration. This activity challenges participants to turn closed questions into exploratory statements (prompts). Table 7.2 demonstrates how this is accomplished.

Table 7.2 Converting probes into prompts

Closed question	Open-ended question (prompt)	Exploratory statement
Are you feeling all right?	How are you feeling?	Tell me how you are feeling.
Will it help to make you more comfortable if I rearrange your pillows?	What would help you to be more comfortable in the bed?	Perhaps if I rearrange your pillow, you'll be more comfortable.
Did that medication help to relieve your pain?	How did that medication help in relieving your pain?	You had your pain medication 30 minutes ago, I see.
Do you want your sponge now?	When would you like your sponge?	You can have your sponge now or later.
Would it help if I stayed with you a while?	How would you feel if I stayed with you a while?	Perhaps if I stayed with you a while it would help

1 Make a list of closed questions pertinent to the nursing context. Divide a piece of paper into three columns and place the closed questions down the left column.

2 Convert each of these questions into an exploratory statement by first making the closed question into an open-ended one. Place these in the middle column of the page.

3 Now convert the open-ended question into an exploratory statement, a probe. Place these in the right column of the page.

Discussion

1 Which of your closed questions were easy to convert to exploratory statements? Which were difficult? Were there any that you found impossible to convert?

2 Review each of the exploratory statements and discuss how making a statement instead of asking a question would alter the interaction between nurse and person/patient.

3 Would you obtain different information from an exploratory statement? If so, is the information obtained more relevant?

4 Which of the exploratory statements seem appropriate to the topic being discussed? Do any seem inappropriate or foolish?

5 Can you imagine yourself using the exploratory statements? Why? Why not?

ACTIVITY 7.4

QUESTIONS AND STATEMENTS FOR CONDUCTING AN INITIAL ASSESSMENT

 Process

Each of the topic areas in Step 1 is an aspect of a person/patient's history, completed on admission to hospital. During the gathering of information regarding a person/patient history, the nurse explores specific areas in order to collect data about the person/patient's functioning and experiences. The manner in which the data are collected depends on the nurse's ability to explore effectively. The wording of the questions and exploratory statements affects not only the type of information collected but also the amount and quality of that information.

1   For each of the following topic areas, develop and write an open-ended question. The first one is completed to provide an example of how to undertake this activity.

Topic area	*Open-ended question*
Perception of hospitalization:	■ What do you anticipate will happen while you are in hospital?
	■ What are your expectations of this hospital stay?
Understanding of current health status	■ How is your illness affecting your lifestyle?
Social/living situation	
Activities of living	
Nutrition/eating habits	
Sleep and rest patterns	
Elimination patterns	

2   Now develop an exploratory statement for each of the topic areas.

Discussion

1   Which way of exploring – questioning (probing) or making statements (prompting) – seems more effective in collecting information in each of the identified topic areas?

2   Do some topic areas lend themselves more to exploratory statements than others?

question is helpful under such circumstances. In posing a multiple-choice question, the nurse asks, 'Is the pain burning, grabbing, crushing, pinpoint, dull, or sharp?' This type of questioning about pain yields specific information about the nature of the person/patient's pain. In the example provided, the nurse uses knowledge of the various types of pain to focus and direct the exploration.

Open-ended versus closed questions

As a general rule, open-ended questions are more effective as exploration techniques than closed questions, because responses to open questions are more elaborate and encourage expansion of ideas through the addition of subjective opinions and beliefs. They also allow the person/patient to direct the interaction and therefore the nurse who asks an open-ended question is likely to hear what is most significant to the person/patient at the time.

Does this mean that closed questions should be avoided? Not necessarily, because closed questions have a legitimate place in the context of person/patient–nurse interaction. The choice between open-ended and closed questions depends on what information is being sought, by whom, with whom, in which context, and to what end. In making the decision to use one type or the other, nurses must consider their relationship with the person/patient as well as the need for specific information. For example, when a nurse wants to know whether a person/patient can tolerate aspirin, they might begin by asking 'Have you ever used aspirin?' Then, if the answer is affirmative, questions such as 'How much?', 'How often?', 'For what reason?', and 'What effects were noted?' may follow. Asking open-ended questions such as 'How do you experience aspirin?' or 'What do you think about aspirin?' are nonsensical and inappropriate to the content being explored and the information required. On the other hand, a question such as 'How was your first pregnancy?' is appropriate in exploring an experience as personal and unique as pregnancy. Nevertheless, questions such as 'How do you feel about being pregnant?' probe too deeply if person/patient and nurse have not established a trusting relationship. Questions need to probe at a depth that is appropriate to the level of trust between person/patient and nurse.

The decision about which type of question to use should be based on an under-standing of each type of questioning. Table 7.3 compares the two types of question and provides useful guidelines for the selection.

If the open-ended type is selected as more suitable, the next choice is which open-ended question is best, given the circumstances. In most instances, questions beginning with 'Who', 'What', 'Where', and 'When' yield factual, objective data; while questions beginning with 'How' yield more personal, subjective information. For example, 'What surgery did you have in 1978?' will yield a factual answer such as 'I had my appendix removed'. If this is followed by a question such as 'And how was that surgery?', exploration of the person/patient's subjective experience of the surgery is achieved. This general guideline is not a hard and fast rule; for example, 'What were your feelings about the surgery?' is a question that probes on a personal level. The focus of the question is as important as its type.

The most effective exploration will include a combination of both open and closed questions, as illustrated in the following interaction:

Table 7.3 Comparison of open-ended and closed questions

Open-ended questions	Closed questions
Yield information and facilitate elaboration	Yield information and limit elaboration
Allow person/patient to determine the direction of the interactions	Focus the person/patient in one direction
May not be useful when specific information is required	Are useful in obtaining specific information
Probe subjective experiences and may threaten person/patient if trust is not established	Maintain interpersonal safety by keeping the interaction on a less personal level

Nurse:	Have you ever had surgery before? [Closed]
Person/patient:	Yes, once before.
Nurse:	What happened that you needed surgery? [Open]
Person/patient:	I had my appendix removed when I was ten years old.
Nurse:	Were you in hospital? [Closed]
Person/patient:	Yes.
Nurse:	How was that hospitalization? [Open]
Person/patient:	Fine, the nurses were great, my Mum was with me the whole time and I don't remember being in any pain.
Nurse:	So, you have good memories of that? [Closed]
Person/patient:	Yes.
Nurse:	What do you expect will happen this time in hospital? [Open]
Person/patient:	Well, I am a lot older, so my Mum won't be here the whole time. I am a bit worried about the pain.
Nurse:	What worries you most? [Open]
Person/patient:	That nobody will be able to help me with the pain . . . I am a bit of a baby.
Nurse:	The nurses are here to make sure you are not in pain. You do realize that? [Closed]
Person/patient:	Yes, I guess . . . but I don't know what you will do to help.

Notice how, in this interview, the nurse moves between closed and open-ended questioning and each question is appropriate to the content and the purpose of the interview. During the interaction, the nurse gathers objective data (previous experience with surgery) as well as subjective data (the person/patient's personal experience of the surgery). Open and closed questions are not inherently good or bad, because their 'goodness' or 'badness' depends on what information is being sought, and for what reason.

Pitfalls in the use of probing skills

Despite the fact that questions are neither good nor bad in themselves, there are some common pitfalls in the use of questioning, including some types of question that are best avoided altogether. Common pitfalls include (a) over-use of questions, (b) continuous multiple questions, (c) the 'why' question and (d) the leading question.

(a) Overuse of questioning

The most common pitfall in probing is the overuse of questioning. Asking too many questions during an interaction can interrupt and confuse the person/patient (Benjamin 1969). Overuse of questioning runs the risk of continually shifting the focus of the interaction. Additionally, it has the potential to convey the message that the nurse is in an overbearing position of authority. In order to be effective, questions need to be mixed with exploratory, prompting statements.

(b) Continuous multiple questions

Another pitfall in questioning is the use of multiple questions, asked in succession, without allowing time for a reply from the person/patient, for example, 'How did you sleep last night? Did the sleeping tablet help? Was there too much noise?' While this manner of questioning sounds a bit ridiculous, it does occur in person/patient–nurse interactions (Macleod Clark 1984). Asking multiple questions in succession is counterproductive to the exploration process. If a question is asked, the nurse needs to ensure that enough time is allowed for the person/patient to respond before proceeding.

(c) The 'why?' question

The 'why?' question is a tricky one because often in the nursing context the answer to 'why?' needs to be sought. 'Why does Mr Kendall experience so much pain, even after maximum pain relief is administered?' 'Why is Ms Holmes having so much difficulty breast-feeding her baby?' While it is important to uncover the reasons for such occurrences, asking the question 'Why?' directly of people/patients can have a negative impact, and may not be the most effective way to find the answer (Activity 7.5). This is partly due to the fact that the question 'Why?' often creates anxiety and a defensive reaction. It implies that people/patients have to justify and explain their actions and feelings, or that something is not right about their actions and feelings. Imagine you are about to administer a medication to a person/patient and another nurse approaches you and asks, 'Why are you giving that medication now?' Your internal reaction may range from, 'What's it to you?' to 'Oh no, maybe I've made a mistake!' Perhaps your colleague just wants to know if the person/patient receiving the medication is still experiencing pain. Somehow, your reaction to the 'why?' question does not acknowledge such a well-intentioned motive on your colleague's behalf. Instead, you become defensive or anxious.

The reaction to 'Why?' is often defensive because the question has a way of sounding like a negative evaluation. This may be due to experiences in childhood such as when Mum asked, 'Why did you spill the milk on the floor?' as she stands there, hands on hips, looking and sounding quite cross. It quickly becomes apparent to the child that Mum is not the least bit interested in why the milk was spilt. (Does she want an explanation about gravitational force?) The message

ACTIVITY 7.5

EFFECTS OF 'WHY?' QUESTIONS

Process

1   Form pairs for this activity. Designate one person as A and the other as B.

2   A discusses an experience that produced a strong feeling reaction.

3   B listens attentively but keeps asking 'Why?' whenever A brings up a feeling. B is to embark 'on a mission' to uncover the reasons behind A's feelings and reactions.

Discussion

1   A reports his/her response to the interaction by answering the question, 'How did it feel to be constantly asked why?'

2   B reports his/her response to the interaction by answering the question, 'How did it feel to keep asking why?' What did B notice about A's reactions?

conveyed by the 'Why?' question in this instance is, 'Don't do it again, I get cross when milk is spilt'. This possible socialization as to the interpretation of the 'Why?' question, and the potential defensiveness produced by it, are reasons for avoiding its use in person/patient–nurse interaction.

Frequently the 'Why?' question is asked in an attempt to explore feelings, for example, 'Why do you feel sad, Kate?' The use of the 'Why' question in this instance assumes that Kate knows why she feels sad, and that these feelings have a rational basis. People/patients often do not know why they feel a certain way, but may think they need to justify or rationally explain their feelings when asked 'Why?' Again, the reaction may be a defensive one, a justification of feelings. In general, it is best to avoid the 'Why?' question altogether. It is often counter-productive to exploration because of its potential to close off further interaction (Activity 7.6).

(d) The leading question

Another type of question to avoid is the 'leading' question (Activity 7.7). Leading questions are not exploratory but rhetorical, because they have an implied answer and are often designed to confirm what nurses think they already know. Examples of leading questions include:

■   'You're all right, aren't you?'
■   'Why don't you just co-operate with us?'

ACTIVITY 7.6

ALTERNATIVES TO 'WHY?'

 Process

The following person/patient statements have the potential to elicit a 'Why?' question from nurses. Read each and record an alternative to 'Why?'.

1   Person/patient (who has been on renal dialysis for a long time and is awaiting a renal transplant): 'I want to stop dialysis.'

2   Person/patient (who is awaiting results of diagnostic tests): 'I had a really bad night's sleep because I'm so worried.'

3   Person/patient (who is a recently arrived resident of a nursing home): 'How would you like being stuck in here? I hate this place and just want to die.'

4   Person/patient (who has recently undergone coronary artery bypass surgery): 'I really thought I was going to die this morning.'

5   Person/patient (who has been told she should have a hysterectomy): 'I can't possibly spare the time to have this operation.'

6   Person/patient (who has recently taken an overdose): 'I don't want any treatment. My family will be better off without me!'

Discussion

1   Did you find you were tempted to ask 'Why?' in response to each statement?

2   Review your alternatives to the 'Why?' question. Are any of them 'Why?' in disguise, for example, 'How come?' or 'What makes you feel that way?'

3   What type of exploratory response did you develop? Are any of the responses exploratory statements?

4   Compare your responses with those of other participants. How much variety exists between the responses?

5   Try to use some of your responses with other participants playing the role of person/patient. Ask the person who is playing the role of person/patient to describe the effects of each response.

ACTIVITY 7.7

RECOGNIZING TYPES OF QUESTIONS

Process

Classify each question according to its type, using the following key:

A Closed question
B Open-ended question
C Leading question
D Disguised 'Why?' question

1 What makes you feel scared?

2 How are you feeling today?

3 What is your doctor's name?

4 Do you really enjoy drinking heavily?

5 When does your pain get worse?

6 Are you interested in seeing a volunteer from Alcoholics Anonymous?

7 What are your reasons for refusing your medication?

8 What kind of nurse do you think I am?

9 You really don't want any more pain medication, do you?

10 What did the doctor say?

11 Did that medication help with the nausea?

12 How do you like your breakfast tray to be arranged?

13 How did you go with physiotherapy today?

14 What makes you say that?

15 How old are your children?

16 How was the visit with your family last night?

17 Did you sleep well after having the sleeping tablet?

18 When are you going to stop bothering the other people/patients?

19 Are you worried about having sexual relations after your heart surgery?

20 Don't you think you had better try to stick to your diet this time?

21 How do you usually manage your diabetic diet?

22 Are you still hurting your baby by smoking while you are pregnant?

23 What would help you to be more comfortable?

Note: The answers to this activity can be found at the end of this chapter.

- 'Are you really going to ring the doctor at this hour of the night?'
- 'Is your anger really justified?'
- 'What's making you so hard to get along with?'
- 'You really don't want any more medication, do you?'

Leading questions are not really questions at all. They are statements in disguise, 'dressed up' to look like questions. Like the 'Why' question, they have a tendency to put the other person on the defensive because they usually contain a value judgement. It is far better to make a statement than to pretend to want an answer to a question that does not really have one. Review the previous examples of leading questions, turn them into statements and note the difference.

FOCUSED EXPLORATION

The skills of exploration can be employed effectively in the process of focusing an interaction between person/patient and nurse. The process of focused exploration deepens the nurse's general understanding of the person/patient's experience by concentrating on a specific aspect. This process of focusing is sometimes referred to as 'funnelling' (Burnard, 1989), because of the way in which it continues to narrow the topic being explored. Any of the various exploration skills identified can be employed in the process of focusing. The following interaction, from a postpartum maternity ward, is an illustration of focusing:

Nurse: How are you today? [Open question]
Person/patient: OK, I guess.
Nurse: You guess? [One-word accent]
Person/patient: I didn't sleep very well last night.
Nurse: Couldn't sleep, huh? [Closed question]
Person/patient: No, I kept worrying about my baby.
Nurse: What, in particular, was worrying you? [Open question]
Person/patient: The paediatrician was here last night to examine him and he noticed his high-pitched cry.
Nurse: And? [Minimal encouragement]
Person/patient: Well, the doctor said it was probably nothing to worry about because it was most likely due to some swelling in my son's brain as a result of the labour. I was in second stage for a long time, you know.
Nurse: Yes, it might clear up in a few days. I have seen babies with that cry before, and it was due to temporary swelling that went away after a few days. But, it doesn't really stop the worry, just because you know it might be nothing. [Open-ended statement]
Person/patient: What is most worrying is that the doctor said it could be a sign of brain damage.
Nurse: And that's what has you most worried? [Closed question]
Person/patient: Yes. I kept asking the doctor what else besides temporary swelling could be causing the cry. Now I'm sorry I asked. I might have been better off not knowing. There's nothing I can do now but worry and wait.

Notice how the nurse in this interaction begins broadly then keeps focusing and narrowing the conversation. This is accomplished through the use of a variety of exploration skills. The nurse chose to focus on what s/he perceived to be the most significant aspect of the person/patient's messages. The focusing process serves to highlight and elaborate on a particular topic.

PERSON/PATIENT-CUE EXPLORATION

People/patients frequently communicate their needs, desires and feelings through indirect messages, indicating what they are experiencing by hints, suggestions and implied questions (Macleod Clark 1984). Indirectly, people/patients are requesting a response from the nurse by presenting these communication cues.

Cues are small units of information that are part of a larger, more complex phenomenon (Carnevali 1983). They indicate a need for further exploration of the phenomenon. They signal the need for exploration much like a green light at a traffic intersection signals drivers to proceed. Effective exploration of person/patient cues, like all exploration, leads to further data collection and greater understanding between person/patient and nurse (Activity 7.8). Sadly, nurses frequently either fail to acknowledge person/patient cues or even actively discourage further exploration of them (Macleod Clark 1984).

Cues and inferences

A cue is a unit of sensory input, a sight, sound, smell, taste, or touch, that is perceived as important to be noticed. For example, during an interaction, the nurse notices that the person/patient keeps fidgeting with the bed clothes. By noticing this piece of information, the nurse has perceived a cue.

Almost without awareness, meanings are assigned to perceived cues as a way of making sense of what is experienced. The meanings attached to cues are inferences, conclusions drawn from the cues. Inferences are based on knowledge, previous experience, expectations, and needs. For example, fidgeting with the bed clothes may be interpreted as a sign of general anxiety or discomfort with the interaction. Nevertheless, inferences are usually formed on the basis of more than one cue. The combination of fidgeting with the bed clothes, startling easily, pressured speech, nonstop talking, and foot tapping are person/patient cues that may lead to an inference that a person/patient is anxious.

It is impossible not to make such interpretations about what is perceived; inferences are automatic. What is possible is to differentiate a cue (concrete data), from an inference (the interpretation of the data) (Activity 7.9).

Once inferences are recognized by the nurse, they need to be validated with the person/patient in order to determine if they are correct. In the example of fidgeting with the bed clothes, if the person/patient admits to feeling anxious, the inference is validated. It is important not to jump too quickly to a conclusion about person/patient cues. Further exploration is usually the most appropriate initial response to a person/patient cue.

ACTIVITY 7.8

EXPLORING PERSON/PATIENT CUES

 Process

1   Think of an instance, real or imagined, in which a person/patient presents a cue, indicating the need for further exploration and/or elaboration (for example, a facial grimace, possibly indicating pain). Record this person/patient cue on a slip of paper, providing any information that would be of assistance in understanding the situation (the setting and circumstances).

2   Collect the slips of paper and redistribute them to other participants in the activity.

3   The contents of the slips of paper are then read aloud to all participants. Each participant develops and records an exploratory response, using any type of exploration technique.

4   Form groups of five to six participants and share exploratory responses in this group. Each small group discusses the various exploratory responses and selects the one that is most appropriate as an exploration technique. These are then read aloud to the rest of the participants.

Discussion

Discuss each person/patient cue and responses selected by the small groups. During the discussion, use the following questions to evaluate the responses, bearing in mind that the purpose of the response is to explore the cue presented by the person/patient:

1   Which exploration technique was used?

2   How effective is the response in exploring the cue?

3   In which context would this response be most appropriate?

4   What purpose does the exploration serve? Is it helpful? How?

5   Could you actually say this to a person/patient? If not, why not?

ACTIVITY 7.9

CUES AND INFERENCES

 Process

Determine whether each of the following statements is a cue or an inference.

1　Answered interview questions completely.

2　Uninterested in the interview.

3　Changed the topic when asked about her family.

4　An open person.

5　Sleeping quietly.

6　Shallow, rapid respirations.

7　Doesn't understand prescribed medications.

8　Keeps asking questions about diagnostic tests.

9　No eye contact during the interview.

10　Speech is pressured.

11　Puzzled expression on her face when I asked her about the surgery.

12　Doesn't know what to expect.

13　No visible signs of distress.

Discussion

1　Compare your answers with those of other class participants. Are there any differences in the answers?

2　If differences exist, discuss the item(s) and decide what makes them inferences or what makes them cues.

3　Compare your answers with those provided at the end of this chapter.

Note: The answers to this activity can be found at the end of this chapter.

Communication cues

When nurses prompt and probe during the process of exploration, many verbal and nonverbal cues are elicited because the exploration itself triggers the cues. A straightforward, closed question such as 'Have you ever been in hospital before?' may elicit numerous cues about the person/patient's experience in hospital. The person/patient's tone of voice may change, their rate of speech may accelerate, they may disclose feelings and reactions to previous hospitalizations. In this instance, the exploration triggered the cues and the cue is a trigger for further exploration. This spiralling effect is common in effective exploration.

Person/patient questions as cues

Often person/patient cues come in the form of questions asked of the nurse. Person/patient questions that are difficult to answer, yet require a response from the nurse, are examples of cues needing further exploration. For example:

- 'Am I going to die?'
- 'Is Dr Nelson a good surgeon?'
- 'What would you do if you were in my place?'

Questions such as these, which put nurses on the spot, are difficult to answer but equally difficult to ignore. Perceiving person/patient questions as cues for exploration is useful because this enables nurses to respond effectively. Further exploration helps to uncover what is really on the person/patient's mind. The first example, 'Am I going to die?', can be explored by stating, 'That's difficult for me to answer, but I am curious about the question'. This open-ended statement indicates the nurse's willingness to hear more about what the person/patient is experiencing. Think 'exploration' whenever people/patients pose questions that either have no answer or are difficult to answer (Activity 7.10). It is preferable to do this rather than ignoring the question or changing the subject, which could happen when nurses feel put on the spot and uncomfortable.

Cue perception

Person/patient cues must be noticed and perceived if they are to be of use in exploration. Complete attending and active listening keep nurses open and receptive to cue recognition. Attending to how a person/patient reacts and responds to the environment, and the situation at hand, is a skill in itself (see Chapter 5).

Often, nurses perceive subtle communication cues from people/patients on the basis of a 'gut' feeling, hunch or intuition that the person/patient is trying to tell them something. Cue perception involves not only noticing how the person/patient is responding, but also trusting such 'gut' reaction about what might be going on. In the following situation, a nursing student relates such a hunch in discussing her observations of a young man, close to her own age, who had recently become a paraplegic:

> He kept joking around all morning about the MRI that was scheduled that day. I was quite comfortable with the banter because I like to joke around a lot too. He kept asking me, in a silly, almost childlike way, if I would be coming with him to 'hold his hand' when he had the procedure. Although I joked back about him being a 'big boy' now and stuff like that, I had the feeling he might have been scared about the test. I wondered how much he really understood about what was going to happen. I guess I am especially sensitive to this because, as I said, I often joke around, especially about things that are really upsetting me.

A hunch such as this is often an indication of a need, however well disguised it is by a person/patient. The nursing student perceived the possibility that this person/patient was trying to express a need by interpreting the cues that he was presenting. She identified an opportunity for further exploration.

Cue exploration: sharing perceptions

Person/patient cues can be explored using any of the skills described in this chapter, but one of the most effective ways to explore cues is through an open-ended statement, in which nurses state their own perceptions. Open-ended statements allow nurses to validate their observations and interpretations of the cue, by sharing them with the person/patient. In the preceding scenario, an effective way for the nursing student to explore her hunch would be to say, 'Hey, all joking aside, I get the feeling you may be a bit uptight about the MRI'. This open-ended statement shares the student's perception with the person/patient, attempts to validate the perception, and therefore opens the interaction to exploration of the cues. Open-ended exploratory statements, which share the nurse's perceptions, usually begin with:

- 'I notice that . . .'
- 'I get the feeling that . . .'
- 'I'm wondering if . . .'

These sentences are then completed by a concrete description of what the nurse has observed, perceived and/or interpreted from the person/patient's messages. This is an effective way to validate a cue and explore it further because it acknowledges the person/patient's message, encourages further discussion of the person/patient's experience and demonstrates the nurse's willingness to listen.

However a word of caution about sharing perceptions is needed. The danger in exploring in this manner is that the nurse may fall into the trap of being a pseudo-psychoanalyst, always looking for hidden meanings and motives. People/patients present cues in an attempt to communicate to nurses, so the question nurses must ask themselves is 'Do I get the feeling this person/patient is trying to tell me something?', rather than 'What's really behind this person/patient's behaviour?' It is a subtle yet important distinction.

DEVELOPING EXPLORATORY RESPONSES II

 Process

1   Refer to your responses in Activity 7.1: Developing exploratory responses I. Label each of your responses according to the skills outlined in this chapter. You may have used more than one type of exploratory response.

2   Determine if you have a tendency to use one type of exploratory response in preference to the other types.

3   If you tend to ask closed questions, make these open-ended.

4   Do any of your questions begin with 'Why'? If so, find an alternative.

5   Turn your exploratory questions into exploratory statements. What possible effects would these changes have on the interaction with the person/patient in the situation?

NURSES' CONTROL IN EXPLORATION

Previously in this chapter planned exploration was differentiated from spontaneous exploration. In planned exploration the nurse leads and takes charge of the direction and focus of an interaction. In spontaneous exploration the nurse follows the person/patient's lead, usually through the clarifying and probing person/patient cues. The same skills are used in both type of exploration, although not to the same extent. For example, closed questions may be more prevalent when the nurse is leading and one-word/phrase accents may be more prevalent when the nurse is following (Activity 7.11).

At the heart of the difference between spontaneous and planned exploration is the notion of who is in control. Control in the context of person/patient–nurse interaction refers to who dominates in determining the flow of information exchange (Kristjanson and Chalmers 1990). When the person/patient is in control they dominate. The reverse is true when the nurse controls the interaction.

Ideally, a balance is achieved when both person/patient and nurse share control of interactions. Nevertheless, is there any evidence to support the ideal? Answers to this question can be found in research studies in which verbal communication between nurses and people/patients as they interact in clinical settings is analysed (for example, Macleod Clark 1984; Wilkinson 1991; Hewison 1995). Analyses of person/patient–nurse interactions in studies such as these reveal that nurses 'block' and 'control' interactions through a variety of strategies. Some of these strategies included focusing on tasks, exerting power over people/patients,

ACTIVITY 7.11

PERSON/PATIENT INTERVIEW

 Process

1 Each participant is to obtain a blank admission assessment form from a health-care agency. Review the form and determine the most appropriate way to explore each area with a person/patient.

2 Form groups of three and designate one person as A, another as B and the third as C.

3 A conducts a person/patient assessment interview with B acting in the role of person/patient. C acts as observer. A informs B about the setting and the circumstances of the person/patient interview. C records the types of exploratory skills used by A during the interview by keeping a record of the name of each skill used.

4 C now interviews A, who plays the role of person/patient. B is now the observer. Continue as per instructions in Step 3.

5 B now interviews person C, who plays the role of person/patient. C is now the observer. Continue as per instructions in Step 3.

Discussion

1 What types of exploratory skills were used during the interviews? Were some types used more frequently than others?

2 Were there areas of the assessment documentation that lent themselves to the use of a certain skill more than other areas? If so, what are these areas? Which skills seemed most appropriate for these areas?

3 How did it feel when you were in the role of person/patient? Did you think you had enough opportunity to tell your story? Did you think the nurse got to know you as a person during the interview?

4 When you were the nurse, what was easy to explore? What was difficult? Were there any areas you thought were not covered adequately? How well did you come to understand the person/patient during the interview? What would you change in the interview, if you had the opportunity?

5 What generalizations can be made from the activity, in terms of conducting interviews between people/patients and nurses?

spending little time actually talking to people/patients, and even avoiding interaction with people/patients. In community-based settings, Kristjanson and Chalmers (1990) found that interactions were either nurse-controlled or jointly controlled by person/patient and nurse, but no interactions were controlled by people/patients.

Although the results of the studies cited in the previous paragraph suggest that nurses do not pick up person/patient cues and that they control interactions, other studies suggest that when nurses are expert they are alert to person/patient cues (Johnson 1993) and offered opportunities for people/patients to introduce issues that were affecting their lives (Brown 1995).

While the evidence on whether nurses control interactions is inconclusive, there are helpful guidelines that can be ascertained. These guidelines include the need for nurses to be alert to the cues of people/patients and to be able to follow such person/patient leads. Likewise, nurses will at times control the interaction when they are obtaining specific information. Self-aware nurses who reflect on their interactions will notice whether they tend to be controlling in their interactions. In today's climate of person/patient-centred care, nurses need to consider ways in which to effectively use their interactions to ensure that this is achieved (see Chapter 10 for a further review of these issues).

CHAPTER SUMMARY

The process of exploration is one of the most important aspects of person/patient–nurse interaction because it not only provides the means by which information is obtained but also demonstrates the nurse's active regard for understanding the person/patient's experience. During planned exploration, nurses focus on what is most significant for them to know about people/patients. During spontaneous exploration, nurses focus on what is most significant to the person/patient at the time. Both types of exploration require the use of effective questioning (probes) and exploratory statements (prompts). When used in conjunction with other interpersonal skills, exploration helps to shape effective and facilitative person/patient–nurse interaction and leads to greater understanding.

ANSWERS TO ACTIVITIES

ACTIVITY 7.7: RECOGNIZING TYPES OF QUESTIONS

Key	A	Closed question
	B	Open-ended question
	C	Leading question
	D	A disguised 'Why?' question

1	D	What makes you feel scared?
2	B	How are you feeling today?

3	A	What is your doctor's name?
4	C	Do you really enjoy drinking heavily?
5	B	When does your pain get worse?
6	A	Are you interested in seeing a volunteer from Alcoholics Anonymous?
7	D	What are your reasons for refusing your medication?
8	C	What kind of nurse do you think I am?
9	C	You really don't want any more pain medication, do you?
10	B	What did the doctor say?
11	A	Did that medication help with the nausea?
12	B	How do you like your breakfast tray to be arranged?
13	B	How did it go with physiotherapy today?
14	D	What makes you say that?
15	A	How old are your children?
16	B	How was the visit with your family last night?
17	A	Did you sleep well after having the sleeping tablet?
18	C	When are you going to stop bothering the other people/patients?
19	A	Are you worried about having sexual relations after your heart surgery?
20	C	Don't you think you had better try to stick to your diet this time?
21	B	How do you usually manage your diabetic diet?
22	C	Are you still hurting your baby by smoking while you are pregnant?
23	B	What would help you to be more comfortable?

ACTIVITY 7.9: CUES AND INFERENCES

1	Cue	Answered interview questions completely.
2	Inference	Uninterested in the interview.
3	Cue	Changed the topic when asked about her family.
4	Inference	An open person.
5	Cue	Sleeping quietly.
6	Cue	Shallow, rapid respirations.
7	Inference	Doesn't understand prescribed medications.
8	Cue	Keeps asking questions about diagnostic tests.
9	Cue	No eye contact during the interview.
10	Cue	Speech is pressured.
11	Cue	Puzzled expression on her face when I asked her about the surgery.
12	Inference	Doesn't know what to expect.
13	Cue	No visible signs of distress.

REFERENCES

Benjamin, A. (1969). *The Helping Interview*. Boston, MA: Houghton Mifflin.

Brown, S. J. (1994). Communication strategies used by an expert nurse. *Clinical Nursing Research*, 3(1), 43–56.

Brown, S. J. (1995). An interviewing style for nursing assessment. *Journal of Advanced Nursing*, 21, 340–2.

Burnard, P. (1989). *Teaching Interpersonal Skills: A Handbook of Experiential Learning Activities for Health Professionals*. London: Chapman and Hall.

Carnevali, D. (1983). *Nursing Care Planning: Diagnosis and Management*, third edition. Philadelphia, PA: J. B. Lippincott.

Hewison, A. L. (1995). Nurses' power in interactions with patients. *Journal of Advanced Nursing*, 21, 75–82.

Johnson, R. (1993). Nurse practitioner–patient discourse: uncovering the voice of nursing in primary care practice. *Scholarly Inquiry for Nursing Practice: An International Journal*, 7, 143–63.

Kristjanson, L. and Chalmers, K. (1990). Nurse–patient interactions in community-based practice: creating common ground. *Public Health Nursing*, 7(4), 215–23.

Macleod Clark, J. (1984). Verbal communication in nursing. In A. Faulkner (ed.), *Communication* (pp. 52–73). Edinburgh: Churchill Livingstone.

Shea, S. C. (1988). *Psychiatric Interviewing: The Art of Understanding*. Philadelphia, PA: W. B. Saunders.

Wilkinson, S. (1991). Factors which influence how nurses communicate with cancer patients. *Journal of Advanced Nursing*, 16, 677–88.

CHAPTER 8

COMFORTING, SUPPORTING AND ENABLING

INTRODUCTION

The material in the previous chapters has laid a foundation for establishing effective person/patient–nurse relationships. Through listening to people/patients' accounts, understanding people/patients' experiences and exploring people/patients' personal meanings of health and illness, nurses are able to interact with people/patients in ways that are helpful. Helpful interactions build relationships that are of assistance to people/patients and the person/patient–nurse relationship becomes a vehicle through which the nurse's actions come to life. The skills of listening, understanding and exploring are fundamental to the development of this relationship and their use must be continuous for the relationship's maintenance and further development.

Thus far, this book has alluded to how nurses take direct action in helping people/patients, but active intervention has not been fully explained. In fact, moving too quickly into action has been shown to be inappropriate in the absence of a relationship based on understanding. Focusing prematurely on action, intervention and outcome has the potential to stifle the nurse's understanding and appreciation of the person/patient's current experience.

There is inherent danger in taking action without first understanding the person/patient's unique orientation to the world. Interventions cannot be applied in a context-free manner, selected from a list of options as one selects a recipe from a cookbook. Such nonspecific, potentially hit and miss approaches can actually do more harm than good. For example, enabling people/patients to participate in their care by sharing information is most effective if nurses first determine how much information a person/patient wants and can use. Some people/patients want to know every minute detail about their nursing care, while others prefer to know only the bare essentials. It is inappropriate, even potentially harmful, to burden a person/patient with too much detailed information when the information is not wanted or cannot be put to some use.

This suggestion, initially to curtail direct intervention, may prove frustrating to some nurses because a felt need to do something often over-rides the need to understand the person/patient's experience from the person/patient's perspective. Time is a precious commodity in the clinical environment, and the time spent in coming to understand people/patients' experiences may be perceived as a luxury. Nevertheless, the time and effort expended in coming to understand the person/patient's frame of reference is well spent, because actions that direct and influence people/patients are then based on such understandings.

These actions include: comforting people/patients through interpersonal interaction; supporting people/patients in the use of resources; enabling them to participate in their health-care by sharing information; and encouraging people/patients to reframe their perspective through challenging and self-sharing.

CHAPTER OVERVIEW

This chapter presents skills that provide the means for nurses to take action beyond listening, exploring and understanding. These actions are psychosocial in nature, that is, they are interpersonally oriented and enacted through the nurse–person/patient relationship. Swanson's (1993) theory of nursing as informed caring is presented as a way of situating the skills in this chapter within the context of material in previous chapters. Ways of responding (first introduced in Chapter 5) are revisited in order to emphasize when psychosocial actions are appropriate. These psychosocial actions are grouped into three major areas: comforting, supporting and enabling. The primary comforting action is the skill of reassuring people/patients. Supporting actions, described next, promote people/patients' use of resources. Enabling focuses on actions that are aimed at encouraging people/patients to participate actively in their own care. The major enabling action described is sharing information and providing explanations to people/patients. The final skills of challenging and self-disclosure are two further examples of enabling actions.

PSYCHOSOCIAL ACTIONS THAT COMFORT, SUPPORT AND ENABLE

Often the nurse's actions are aimed at physical care and treatment of a disease, for example, administration of medication to provide physical relief from pain and technical competence is perceived by people/patients as caring (see Chapter 1). But caring actions are also psychosocial in nature. Psychosocial actions are aimed at promoting psychological ease and relief of distress, for example, through explanations that orient people/patients to what is happening around them.

Physical actions and psychosocial actions are inextricably linked in the caring environment. For example, hospitalized people/patients in Cameron's (1993) study indicated that focusing on physical care left them concerned about how they would be able to integrate illness into their lives, while focusing on psychosocial care resulted in worries about their physical care. Despite the artificiality of the separation of physical actions from psychosocial actions, this chapter focuses on psychosocial nursing actions that promote health and healing in people/patients and are accomplished through the person/patient–nurse relationship.

Table 8.1 Processes of informed caring and related interpersonal skills

Processes of informed caring (Swanson, 1993)	Interpersonal skills
Maintaining belief in people	Self-awareness (Chapter 3)
Appreciating personal meanings of health events	Understanding (Chapter 5)
Being with patients	Listening and exploring (Chapters 4 and 6)
Doing for patients	Comforting and supporting (Chapter 7)
Enabling patients	Encouraging participation by sharing information and challenging (Chapter 7)

Swanson's theory of 'informed caring' provides a useful model for situating the interpersonal skills necessary for psychosocial actions in the context of the skills outlined in previous chapters. Five processes of caring are explicated in the theory of 'informed caring' (Swanson, 1993). The first of these is a philosophical grounding of caring in an inherent belief in people and a conviction in personal meanings that are attached to health events (such a philosophy is enhanced through self-awareness, see Chapter 4). Once 'grounded' in this philosophical stance, nurses 'anchor' their caring through striving to understand the meaning that people/patients attach to health events. This second process is achieved by 'knowing the person/patient' (see Chapter 2), and is brought to life through the interpersonal skills of listening, understanding and exploring (see Chapters 5, 6 and 7). The third process in the theory of informed caring is enacted by nurses when they are fully present and available to people/patients. Referred to by Swanson (1993) as 'being with' people/patients, this process was reviewed in Chapter 5 in the form of attending and listening skills.

Once they are 'with' people/patients, nurses express their caring through actions that pertain to the final two processes in Swanson's theory, termed 'doing for' people/patients and 'enabling' people/patients to do for themselves. Although not rigid in the sense that the processes are passed through as stages and phases, there is a sequential manner to them. For example, 'doing for' requires nurses to understand what must be done, that is, to understand a person/patient's frame of reference before attempting to provide psychosocial help.

As seen in Table 8.1, the interpersonal skills for the first three processes of informed caring have been developed in previous chapters. This chapter focuses on the final two processes, 'doing for' and 'enabling'. Although the process of 'doing for' is predominantly expressed through physical care and skilled clinical performance of professional care, 'doing for' also includes comforting measures that are achieved through interacting with and relating to people/patients. Comforting measures such as reassurance are discussed in this chapter. Supporting actions are also considered in the process of 'doing for' people/patients. Swanson's (1993) process of 'enabling' includes having people/patients participate in their health care. Such participation is contingent on people/patients' knowledge and understanding of their health status and care. The interpersonal skills needed to inform and assist people/patients in obtaining this knowledge are also reviewed in this chapter.

INDICATIONS OF THE NEED FOR PSYCHOSOCIAL ACTION

When listening and understanding, nurses are guided by people/patients. When taking psychosocial action, nurses assume a more active role in guiding people/patients. This does not mean that a nurse takes charge and control of a person/patient's life, but rather intervenes in a way that encourages the person/patient to assume as much control as possible. For example, when an understanding is reached that a person/patient is facing a decision, the nurse takes action in order to help the person/patient make the decision, rather than taking over and making the decision for the person/patient. Actions that are psychosocial in nature are liberating, not restrictive, and they always work from within the person/patient's experience.

Taking action is based on indications that it is needed. The following list includes examples of person/patient situations that indicate a need to intervene directly.

Psychosocial action may be required when people/patients are:

- In need of more information
- Emotionally distressed, for example, feeling overwhelmed
- Facing a health-related decision
- Learning new skills
- Lacking in available resources
- Inadequately using existing resources
- Experiencing difficulties in coping, adjusting and adapting.

Person/patient outcomes

Psychosocial nursing actions of comforting, supporting and enabling are focused on outcomes and resources. When nurses employ these actions they do so with the deliberate intention of producing positive changes or reinforcing adaptive ones in people/patients. While the desired outcome may not always be directly observable and measurable, action is taken for a focused purpose. Some examples of desired outcomes include helping people/patients to:

- Adjust and adapt to changes in living imposed by illness
- Maintain self-esteem
- Find meaning in illness
- Feel secure and in control
- Contain and control emotional distress within manageable limits
- Make decisions about health care
- Access and use helpful resources.

Outcomes are based on the indication of need for action. For example, the indication that a person/patient is emotionally distressed calls for an outcome of containing and controlling that distress within manageable limits. Not only is it important for nurses to relate desired outcome to person/patient need, but more importantly nurses must work with people/patients in determining needs and outcomes from the people/patients' perspective.

Person/patient resources

Psychosocial actions are most effective when nurses work with people/patients' natural resources, their capabilities and means for coming to terms with health- and illness-related issues in their lives. Some actions work with the person/patient's existing resources, while others focus on the identification, development and use of new or unused resources. It is important for nurses to understand the person/patient's resources. Examples of resources include the person/patient's knowledge, will, desire, strength, and courage; also their family members and friends, other people/patients, self-help groups, and health services and providers (Carnevali 1983). Possible resources are endless for some people/patients and quite limited for others. Essential to the use of person/patient resources is the recognition and acknowledgement that nurses themselves are but one, usually temporary, resource in helping people/patients. Nurses must look to longer-term person/patient resources, basing their outlook on the belief that people/patients are themselves resourceful and capable.

WAYS OF RESPONDING REVISITED

The various ways of responding (presented in Chapter 6) include the action-oriented, influencing responses of advising and evaluating, reassuring and supporting, and analysing and interpreting. These responses were rejected as initial responses in favour of understanding responses. The major reason these action-oriented responses were deemed inappropriate early in the course of the relationship between person/patient and nurse is that the professional who employs them at this time is exerting too much control and influence on the person/patient. For example, an interpretation challenges people/patients to view their situations in a different light, which is based on the nurse's perceptions, rather than the person/patient's. There is a danger of alienating the person/patient if a nurse is too directive early in the course of the relationship.

The tendency for nurses to be directive in the face of person/patient problems was demonstrated in two recent studies (Motyka *et al.* 1997; Whyte *et al.* 1997). In these studies nurses were asked to write a verbal response to a person/patient complaint (tightness in the throat and difficulty swallowing). Of the 150 nurses who participated, the majority responded by directives such as 'Don't worry', 'Don't be upset' and 'I'll tell the doctor and you will be fine'. Only 2 per cent demonstrated an understanding response. When two groups of nurses were compared using the same research methods (Whyte *et al.* 1997), British nurses more frequently responded by collecting information about the person/patient complaint than did Polish nurses. Nevertheless, the majority of responses of nurses in both studies indicated that they operated from a position of authority and were directive in their responses. That is, the majority of responses indicated that the nurse assumed control rather than working with the person/patient to explore the meaning of the complaint further or to respond with understanding of the person/patient's discomfort.

Each way of responding is appropriate at various levels and stages in the development of the person/patient–nurse relationship. Nevertheless, the findings of the studies do indicate that nurses may tend to respond in habitual and automatic ways. The skills presented throughout this book, and especially those in this chapter, offer a range of possible alternatives. Nurses are encouraged to reflect and consider which type of response is appropriate at the time and under the circumstances. The importance of timing is highlighted as nurses consider what skills to use on which occasion. Early in the relationship the person/patient directs the interactions. As the relationship progresses, the nurse can exert more direct influence through direct action.

COMFORTING

Of the five ways of responding (see Chapter 6), a response that attempts to comfort and reassure is used most often by people who are trying to be of help (Johnson 2000). Nurses are no different in this respect. In the studies by Motyka *et al.* (1997) and Whyte *et al.* (1997), nurses most often tried to cheer people/patients with reassurance and consolation. Although participants' intentions were not investigated in these studies, the majority of their responses were most likely meant to comfort people/patients.

Caring and comforting

Comforting is associated with soothing distress, relieving pain and easing grief. To be comfortable is associated with being relaxed, contented and free from pain and anxiety. It is understandable that nurses attempt to comfort. In fact, Morse (1992) has urged nurses to re-focus care provision on the concept of comfort. She argues that caring focuses on the nurse, while comfort focuses on the person/patient. Caring is process-oriented and is the motivation for clinicians' actions. Comfort is outcome-oriented and is the aim of clinicians' actions. Caring is *why* nurses act; comforting is *how* they act (Morse 1992).

Morse's argument is compelling in the sense that it offers nurses a focus of care that can be described through practices that comfort people/patients. Caring is more nebulous in the sense that it offers little in the way of clear guidelines for clinical performance, especially for beginning nurses. Because comfort focuses on outcomes rather than process it offers a framework for nursing action.

People/patients' view of comforting

The meaning of comfort in the health care profession requires careful consideration, especially in relation to the person/patient's point of view. In a study exploring people/patients' views of comfort Cameron (1993) interviewed and observed a small sample (ten) of hospitalized people/patients. Results of the study indicate that people/patients are not passive in their view of comfort, that is, people/patients did not wait in hope of receiving comfort. Rather, they sought it out by, for example, gathering information about their condition and treatment from caregivers and other people/patients. These people/patients also vigilantly monitored nurses' responses to them in an effort to find reassurance that all was well. People/patients in this study also delved into themselves as a way of integrating their illness experience into the whole of their lives. These people/patients' views indicate that comfort is an active process that energizes. This view of comfort as enlivening, although part of its original meaning, contrasts to current conceptualization of comforting as soothing, easing or consoling (Cameron 1993).

In another study of comfort, people/patients gave an account of an illness in which they experienced agonizing pain, trauma or life-threatening conditions. In their analysis of the people/patients' accounts, Morse *et al.* (1994) concluded that comfort measures by nurses included taking control, reassuring, protecting, connecting, distracting (re-focusing), acknowledging, and supporting. Comfort measures enabled people/patients to retreat from discomfort and provided the opportunity for person/patient to regain strength and energy (Morse *et al.* 1994). The enlivening aspects of comfort echo Cameron's findings (1993).

In their analysis of person/patient biographies of illness Morse *et al.* (1992) describe a number of actions that promote comfort. These actions include pity (expressing regret), sympathy (conveying sorrow), compassion (sensitively sharing the distress of another), consolation (encouragement that things are not as bad as they could be), commiseration (sharing mutual situations), compassion (sharing feelings), and reflexive reassurance (appearing optimistic in order to counteract negative emotions). Each response has the potential to promote comfort because the response confirms negative emotions (pity), legitimizes the person/patient's response (sympathy), recognizes and shares feelings (compassion), reduces people/patients' distress (consolation), confirms universality of feelings (commiseration), and counteracts anxiety (reflexive reassurance) (Morse *et al.* 1992).

Each of these comforting responses focuses on the person/patient. More importantly, responses such as consolation and compassion interpersonally engage the person/patient by confirming their experience. In a similar vein, people/patients in Drew's (1986) study reported that they felt comforted and confident when they experienced confirming responses that were both cognitive and affective. When nurses' responses were confirming, they expressed a sense of concern for the person/patient, demonstrated through being unhurried, making eye contact and using a soothing tone of voice. Comfort and confirmation go hand in hand.

Nurses' expression of comforting

The measures described by people/patients in the studies cited in the previous section indicate that spontaneous (reflexive) responses promote engagement and involvement because they express identification with the person/patient's pain and distress. These responses are natural and naturally human, thus promoting a sense of connection between nurse and person/patient.

Sometimes nurses are taught to stifle these spontaneous responses in favour of 'professional' responses that are learnt (Morse *et al.* 1992). Traditionally, nurses are taught to provide comfort by therapeutic empathic responses (see Chapter 6). Therapeutic empathy de-emphasizes the emotional involvement of reflexive empathy. Emotional empathy, which is developed through experience, enables nurses to implicitly know what to do when people/patients are distressed (Morse *et al.* 1992). Informative reassurance, which provides explanation and information, is another learnt response. While intended to promote comfort, learnt responses are not as engaging as the spontaneous responses (Morse *et al.* 1992).

Results of studies that explicate comforting strategies (Bottoroff *et al.* 1995; Proctor *et al.* 1996) include actions of talking to people/patients in ways that help them to hold on, especially when they are in pain. Examples of 'holding on' strategies included supporting, praising and affirming the person/patient. Other comforting behaviours included providing information, explaining what is happening, being informal and friendly, and expressing concern. Offering choices in care is another way that nurses helped people/patients stay in control and feel comforted.

All the skills in this chapter could be subsumed under the umbrella of the comforting strategies that have been explicated through research; this reinforces the centrality of comforting in nursing. Nevertheless, for the purpose of simplicity and clarity, reassurance is the main skill that is fully developed as a comforting action. Supporting is another comforting action, and is described in a separate section. Other skills, such as informing and challenging are developed under the umbrella of enabling people/patients to participate in care.

Reassuring skills

Reassuring the person/patient is a common activity, often cited as a planned, purposeful intervention in care provision. But how is reassurance actually offered and provided by nurses? Under what circumstances is it indicated? How can reassurance be engaging and not dismissive of people/patients? Unless the answers to these questions are clearly thought through and understood, there is a danger that reassurance will be oversimplified as nothing more than a natural human response.

The responses analysed by Morse *et al.* (1992) as naturally comforting are spontaneous, that is, they are not learnt but are culturally conditioned. Sometimes cultural conditioning will result in a reassuring action that is not focused on the person/patient, but rather is protective of the nurse. This is false reassurance.

False reassurance

In everyday, social situations, reassurance is frequently offered in the form of trite, trivial clichés and platitudes, repeated so often that they have lost their meaning. Ready-made comments such as 'Everything will work out', 'Don't worry' and 'It will be all right' are uttered in an almost automatic, stereotypical manner. These types of 'reassuring' response were presented in Chapter 6 as examples of false reassurance. They do little to ease discomfort in the person being offered them. When reassurance is offered in this way, the effect is often opposite to its intention.

In saying to people/patients 'Everything will be all right', nurses may believe they have been truly reassuring; however, people/patients often feel dismissed by such an expression. Not only have nurses failed to meet people/patients in their world; they also have actually denied its existence or diminished its importance.

False reassurance distances the person/patient from the nurse, and may be used by nurses to distance themselves from unpleasant or difficult aspects of caring (Faulkner and Maguire 1984: 135). Telling a person/patient not to worry may make the nurse feel better but, as a general rule, unless the person/patient receives concrete reassuring evidence, this alone does little to calm the person/patient who is concerned and distressed.

Unless they are careful and thoughtful, nurses may inadvertently find themselves slipping into this automatic mode of falsely reassuring people/patients. Because years of socialization are difficult to change, it is likely that a platitude or cliché will 'slip out' before a nurse realizes it. When this happens, the realization that such responses are not truly reassuring, and even potentially alienating to people/patients, may produce a sense of failure in the nurse.

Nevertheless, a nurse who inadvertently utters a trite cliché can recover by following the cliché with a comment that indicates awareness and sensitivity. Here are some examples of how to recover:

- '(Everything will be all right), *but my saying so won't necessarily make it so.*'
- '(Don't worry). *That's easy for me to say, isn't it?*'
- '(Things have a way of working out), *but that thought may not help you to feel any better.*'
- '(Some good will come out of all of this). *That doesn't really help you, though, does it?*'

Recovering comments such as these demonstrate the nurse's awareness, and usually result in the interaction proceeding, rather than generating feelings of alienation and rejection in the person/patient. After recovering, the nurse is now free to proceed with a more realistic reassuring response.

Comforting reassurance

If effective reassurance is not about presenting such falsely reassuring responses, then what does it involve? To reassure is to restore confidence and to promote a sense of safety, control, hope, and certainty. Reassurance calms the anxious, abates the uneasiness of the worried and decreases concern in the uncertain. Reassurance is concrete and directly related to the person/patient situation, rather than global and non-specific, as clichés are. Realistic reassurance is novel, imaginative, unique, and most importantly, specific to the person/patient.

The desired outcome in providing reassurance is a restored sense of confidence and feelings of safety in the person/patient. To reassure literally means to assure again. In this sense reassurance is restorative. By supporting their inherent power and ability, effective reassurance enables people/patients to face situations with composure. Reassurance may not 'make everything all right' (sometimes this is not possible), but the person/patient who is reassured can face experiences with confidence, hope and courage.

Reassurance is often associated with person/patient coping (Fareed 1994). Like the previous analysis of caring and comforting, reassuring is what the nurse does, that is, it is nurse-focused, and coping is the desired person/patient outcome. Nevertheless, the provision of reassurance does not guarantee that the person/patient will feel more certain and confident, and therefore cope better. This lack of guarantee, however, should not stifle attempts to reassure people/patients.

People/patients' need for reassurance

As with all intervening skills, the recognition of the person/patient's need for reassurance, and an understanding of the person/patient's experience in relation to this need, precedes action. Nurses must understand and appreciate the concrete, specific nature of a person/patient's worry (Activity 8.1). The following situation serves as an illustration of the importance of assessing a person/patient's need for reassurance:

> James Carroll is scheduled for a mental health assessment. Over the past few months he has been quite low in mood, and is feeling unable to cope at home and work. He constantly feels tired and lethargic and now describes feelings of anxiety most of the time. Although his GP has prescribed medication it does not appear to be working and his symptoms have been getting worse. As the assessment commences he expresses his concerns by making statements such as 'I don't know how this is all going to turn out' and 'It's a bit of a worry'. The nurse caring for him avoids saying, 'Oh, don't worry, everything will be all right', appreciating the futility and potential harm of such a statement. Instead, the nurse explores what, specifically, is worrying Mr Carroll. Perhaps he fears what will happen during or after the assessment; he could be worried about how he will manage in the future; perhaps he is concerned that he may need to be admitted to hospital; perhaps he is worried that he might have to give up his job; perhaps he is worried that everyone will think he is 'mental'.

Perhaps . . . , perhaps . . . , the list is almost endless. Unless the nurse responding to him understands what exactly is worrying him, any attempts to reassure him may be misguided. Through the use of exploration and understanding skills, the nurse finds that it is the fear of loss of his functioning self and the impact of the illness on his work that is worrying him most. Now that the specific focus of his concern is identified, the nurse can reassure Mr Carroll with specific information about what he can expect to happen.

In the clinical environment there are common person/patient situations that indicate the need for reassurance. Awareness of these general situations, however, does not replace the necessity of exploring and understanding each person/patient's experience in relation to the need for reassurance.

The need for reassurance arises out of situations in which people/patients are apprehensive, doubtful, uncertain, worried, anxious, full of misgivings, or lacking confidence. In the health-care environment, there are myriad circumstances that result in people/patients experiencing such feelings and perceptions.

ACTIVITY 8.1

SITUATIONS REQUIRING REASSURANCE

 Process

1   Working individually, record a person/patient situation that you have experienced or can imagine that indicates the person/patient's need for reassurance. Ask yourself 'What made me think the person/patient needed reassurance?' Describe the situation as fully as possible.

2   Form groups of five to six participants and distribute the recorded situations randomly among the members.

3   Have each member review the situation and write a key word or phrase, from the recorded situation, that indicates the need for reassurance. Make a list of person/patient cues, from the recorded situation, that expressed the need for reassurance.

4   Record all key words and phrases, including those that are repetitive, on a sheet of paper visible to all participants.

5   On a separate sheet of paper, visible to all participants, record the identified person/patient cues.

Discussion

1   What themes are expressed in the key words and phrases?

2   How much variation is there in the list of person/patient cues?

3   What generalizations can be made about person/patient situations that indicate a need for reassurance?

Some examples include:

- Unclear/unknown medical diagnosis
- Facing unfamiliar situations
- Facing an uncertain outcome/future
- Facing painful procedures.

Uncertainty

The common theme in situations indicating a need for reassurance is uncertainty (Boyd and Munhall 1989). The need for reassurance arises out of situations that are unfamiliar, unknown, unsettling, threatening, and confusing. People/patients facing such situations often experience a loss of control, and need to have their

ACTIVITY 8.2

WAYS NURSES REASSURE PEOPLE/PATIENTS

 Process

1   Recall a time in your life when you were filled with uncertainty about something that was happening or about to happen to you.

2   Reflect on the situation and circumstances surrounding it.

3   What, if anything, would have allayed or did allay your uncertainty? Describe, on a piece of paper, how you were/might have been reassured.

4   Form groups of five to six participants and discuss both the described situations, and the ways of reassuring.

5   List the identified ways of reassuring.

6   Compare each small group's list, developed in Step 5.

7   Prepare a list that combines each small group's list.

Discussion

1   Of the identified ways of reassuring, which are appropriate within the nursing context?

2   How might a nurse reassure people/patients?

3   What hinders nurses in their attempts to reassure people/patients? What helps?

confidence restored (Teasdale 1989). They are in need of something on which, or someone on whom, they can rely to decrease their uncertainty. The intention of reassurance is therefore to decrease uncertainty and restore a sense of control.

Person/patient cues indicating uncertainty

Because of their uniqueness, people/patients will express uncertainty in a variety of ways. Return to the list of person/patient cues indicating a need for reassurance, developed in Activity 8.1. Some examples of person/patient cues indicating feelings of uncertainty, and therefore the potential need for reassurance, include:

■   Openly stating fears and anxieties
■   Asking numerous questions

▓ Continuous activity
▓ Being quiet and withdrawn
▓ Crying
▓ Numerous requests and demands.

The perceptive nurse will notice such cues, place them within the context of the person/patient's current situation, integrate them with an understanding of this person/patient's experience, and explore and validate the presence of uncertainty and need for reassurance. A general discussion of how to explore person/patient cues is found in Chapter 7. Having established the presence of a need for reassurance, nurses now can proceed to provide it in a variety of ways.

Nurses reassure people/patients in a variety of ways, not just through verbal responses. They provide reassurance to people/patients through their presence and manner, as well as through reassuring actions and verbal responses (Activity 8.2).

Reassuring presence of the nurse

People/patients are reassured by the knowledge that the nurse will be there, as the presence of another human being is reassuring in itself, especially during times of disquiet. Being present involves more than simply a physical presence; it involves the emotional presence of a nurse who is fully attending and listening. Hospitalized people/patients in Fareed's study (1996) described reassuring presence as 'being with [. . . me]' and 'being there [. . . for me]'. In fact, accessibility of the nurse was the key factor in these people/patients' sense of feeling reassured. Chapter 5 describes this presence, with specific reference to the comforting presence of the nurse whose entire focus is on the person/patient.

In addition, people/patients are reassured by knowing that the nurse will remain present, and will not abandon them, no matter how difficult, painful or overwhelming circumstances are for them. This vigilant, constant and reliable presence of the nurse promotes confidence within people/patients, thus providing reassurance.

Reassuring manner of the nurse

When a nurse conveys, primarily through nonverbal means, calmness and confidence, people/patients are reassured (Fareed 1996). This highlights the need for self-awareness (see Chapter 4), because nurses may unconsciously (nonverbal behaviour is largely unconscious) communicate a sense of uneasiness to the person/patient. A nurse's uneasiness may or may not have reference to the immediate person/patient, but it will compound the worry of an already worried person/patient. A nurse who appears unsure or uncertain can contribute to the person/patient's uneasiness and uncertainty.

The nurse's reassuring presence and manner maintain meaningful human contact between person/patient and nurse. Other nonverbal forms of communication, including touching, holding hands, massaging, and ministering, are examples of physically comforting, reassuring acts (Boyd and Munhall 1989; Fareed 1996). However, cultural and age variations in relation to the use of touch are important to understand.

Reassuring actions

In addition to the reassuring presence and manner of nurses, there are a number of actions that reassure people/patients (Activity 8.3). These include:

- Optimistic assertion (Teasdale 1989)
- Concrete and specific feedback
- Explanations and factual information.

These skills are considered facilitative because they encourage people/patients to reinterpret their situations in light of different or new information. They are especially helpful when a person/patient's current interpretation of a situation is threatening, for example, the new mother who believes that her blue feelings after birth are a sign that she is 'losing her mind'.

Optimistic assertion

An optimistic assertion is a pledge, promise or guarantee made with the intention of reassuring the person/patient (Teasdale 1989). Examples of optimistic assertions include:

- 'The analgesia that we will give you routinely after your surgery is quite effective. I think you'll find it really helps.'
- 'This wound is going to heal nicely, because you are a fit, healthy person.'
- 'I will visit your family every two weeks. Most families find this sufficient, but if you need to contact me in between visits you can reach me on this number.'

Notice how making an optimistic assertion is similar to sharing information (covered later in this chapter). While sharing information is related to optimistic assertion, it is not exactly the same. An optimistic assertion usually contains an interpretation, which the person/patient is asked to accept without analysis (Teasdale 1989). Information may be added to strengthen an optimistic assertion, but information itself does not provide an interpretation.

Optimistic assertions are similar to false reassurance, although they should not be empty promises or false guarantees. Termed reflexive reassurance by Morse *et al.* (1992), an optimistic assertion is encouragement to maintain an optimistic outlook, even in the face of dire circumstances. People/patients in Fareed's (1996) study felt reassured when they were encouraged to remain optimistic, even when nurses used clichés such as 'Don't worry' or 'I'm sure this will get better for you'.

The difference between false reassurance and an optimistic assertion is the nurse's focus. When a cliché or platitude is focused on protecting the nurse and hiding distress it is not reassuring. When it is focused on the person/patient, such a comment, genuinely and spontaneously stated, can result in comfort and reassurance.

ACTIVITY 8.3

REASSURING INTERVENTIONS

Process

1.   Return to Activity 8.1 and randomly redistribute the recorded person/patient situations to each participant.

2   Each participant reviews the person/patient situation and records how they would provide reassurance under the circumstances.

3   The recorded situations, along with the suggested way to reassure the person/patient, are once more randomly distributed to all participants.

4   Each situation and suggestion for reassurance is then read aloud by the participants. The types of reassurance suggested are recorded on a tally sheet, under the broad headings provided in the text.

Discussion

1   Which methods of providing reassurance were most preferred? Discuss the possible reasons for this.

2   Which methods of providing reassurance are easy to employ? Which are more difficult? Discuss reasons for this.

Concrete and specific feedback

Feedback about how the nurse perceives a situation can be reassuring to people/patients. In order to be helpful in providing reassurance, feedback needs to be concrete and specific to the person/patient. Simply saying to a person/patient, 'I think you are progressing just fine' is not concrete enough to fully reassure the person/patient. Examples of helpful feedback include:

■   'I can tell that you are getting a little stronger each day, because yesterday you could only walk to the edge of the bed. Today you made it to the shower on your own.'

■   'You have been through a lot with your father's illness. It's no wonder you are feeling a bit drained.'

■   'Last month you weren't sure what you were going to do about the tumour. This month, I see a different person.'

■   'When you first started the diet four weeks ago you seemed worried that you wouldn't be able to maintain it. Seeing that you have lost weight has made you much more determined to continue with the diet'.

Like optimistic assertion, feedback provides the person/patient with a new interpretation of the situation. This interpretation is based on the nurse's view of the situation, which is usually informed and knowledgeable. It is based on the nurse's view, but helpful feedback is neither a judgement nor an evaluation, nor again an analysis of the person/patient's situation.

In order that feedback be truly reassuring, it is essential that the nurse establishes first that the person/patient wants it and can use it. In addition, feedback, which focuses on the person/patient's strengths and resources, is more helpful than that which highlights weaknesses and shortcomings.

Providing explanations and factual information

Sharing information, especially about what is usual/expected under the circumstances, is reassuring to people/patients, particularly to those people/patients whose interpretation is based on faulty or misguided information. For example, a person/patient who is specified as nil by mouth, and receiving intravenous fluids, may fear that he or she will literally 'starve to death' due to lack of understanding. Explanations provide people/patients with an opportunity to re-evaluate their situation in light of new, more valid information.

Termed informative reassurance (Morse *et al.* 1992), explanations and factual information restore people/patients' sense of control over situations and reduce their uncertainty. Receiving factual information is a key factor in feeling reassured and gaining control (Fareed 1996); however, because informative reassurance is cognitive, it may not address people/patients' emotional fears (Morse *et al.* 1992).

SUPPORTING

To support is to provide a means of holding up something, in order to prevent it falling apart. Foundations support houses. Beams support ceilings. Their enduring presence provides the means to keep a structure intact and prevent its collapse.

In supporting people/patients, nurses 'stand in the wings' awaiting a call for assistance. Being supportive is an essential quality of nurses and it is needed whenever nurses relate to people/patients. The foundation skills of listening and understanding are the primary means of conveying a supportive attitude. Their use demonstrates that the nurse is available, accepting and encouraging. Nurses also express their support by upholding an inherent belief in people/patients' capabilities and resources, and through maintaining a sense of hope. In this regard, support encompasses a range of skills, because it is predominantly an attitude of being with and for the person/patient.

Types of support

There are a variety of ways in which nurses provide support to people/patients. First, there is informational support. Sharing information with people/patients is supportive because information assists people/patients in coming to terms with their health status, making decisions about health care and understanding what is usual and expected for a given situation. Another type of support comes in the form of direct aid and assistance. This type of support is the concrete, often observable, 'lending of a helping hand'. Helping a hospitalized person/patient out of bed is a clear example of this type of support. Another type of support is providing positive affirmation and encouragement to people/patients. This type of support is emotional in nature, and an example of it is the proverbial 'pat on the back'. It involves standing by and offering encouragement to the person/ patient. The last type is the most common usage of the term 'support'.

Wortman (1984) provides a useful schema in defining support. Support is conveyed to people/patients through:

- Expressions of positive regard and esteem
- Encouragement to express and acknowledgement of feelings and points of view
- Access to information
- Practical and tangible assistance
- A sense of belonging.

Most of what hospitalized people/patients describe as supportive is captured in this description of support (Edgman-Levitan 1993). The most important aspect of support for the people/patients in Edgman-Levitan's study were expressions of concern, acceptance, understanding, and hope. In addition, people/patients felt supported when they were offered useful information and realistic expectations.

From the preceding description of the types of support, it is apparent that nurses provide support to people/patients in a variety of ways. An effective relationship with a person/patient provides support. Most of the actions people/ patients find supportive are discussed in the previous chapters of this book, for example, Chapters 5 and 6. The previous section of this chapter on comforting and the following section on providing information are both examples of supportive nursing actions.

Nevertheless, nurses must also bear in mind that they are but one, often temporary, source of support for people/patients. Too much emphasis on nurses as providers of support can result in them feeling overwhelmed by people/ patients' needs.

Mobilizing person/patient resources

Another way for nurses to provide support for people/patients is through direct intervention to mobilize 'other' sources of support. This section focuses on such mobilization. The following example is an illustration of how nurses mobilize support for people/patients:

> Barbara Frenzell is in hospital following the stillbirth of a baby girl at full term. The pregnancy, her first, was planned, and both she and her husband eagerly anticipated the birth. The loss and disappointment following the stillbirth was devastating for Barbara. As expected under the circumstances, she was

extremely sad, upset and distraught. The nurses found her to be remote, non-communicative and inaccessible, although her emotional pain was visible to them. They understood Barbara's sadness but were especially concerned by her lack of responsiveness when interacting. Although every effort was made to interact with Barbara, the nurses began to feel helpless because they could not 'connect' with her. They recognized that their concern was greater than usual, and assessed the need for active intervention.

Of all the nurses caring for Barbara, Sue had established the most meaningful relationship with her. Although mostly unresponsive, Barbara spoke more with Sue than any of the other nurses. Through exploration Sue learnt that Barbara's husband, John, had refused to discuss the death of their daughter with her. John's attitude and approach was one of a 'stiff upper lip' style. He saw no reason to 'cry over spilt milk' and dwell on the negative; he just wanted their lives to return to normal as soon as possible. Sue noticed that when Barbara discussed John's reaction, she became a bit more communicative and animated. More than anything, Barbara wanted to talk to John about her feelings of despair and sadness. In this situation, one of Sue's supports, John, was not available to her. Sue decided to intervene to mobilize this support for Barbara.

The next time John came to visit, Sue made the effort to spend time with them both. Up to this point, the nurses had left the two of them alone during visiting time, out of respect for their needs for privacy. During the interaction with Barbara and John, Sue encouraged John to discuss his reactions to what had happened. When he stated that there was no reason to cry and feel sorry for himself, Sue suggested that, although he himself may not wish to cry, perhaps his approach was preventing Barbara from expressing how she felt. At this point, Barbara began to cry. John appeared a bit surprised, but made an effort to console her. Sue left the room, with Barbara and John in an embrace. The next day Barbara's general appearance and demeanour had changed. Although still quite sad, she was more talkative and open. Clearly, she felt better as a result of receiving support from her husband John.

This story illustrates, quite clearly, the importance of nurses perceiving support as more than something they supply directly. Through mobilizing support for Barbara, rather than focusing exclusively on the person/patient–nurse relationship, Sue provided intervention that was helpful and effective.

ENABLING PEOPLE/PATIENTS TO PARTICIPATE IN CARE

Person/patient participation has become a popular concept in nursing and health care provision (Cahill 1996) because it moves away from the notion of the person/patient as a passive recipient of care to the person/patient as an active agent in care. It shifts the role of nurse from provider of care to partner in care. Person/patient participation concurs with the modern view of the person/patient as a collaborator in care.

Person/patient participation varies from involving people/patients in care by considering their viewpoints to having people/patients acting as equal partners in decisions about care. Partnership implies a working association between two people, which is usually based on a contract (Cahill 1996). As such, both partners are knowledgeable about the work of the partnership. Involving people/patients in care, on the other hand, is more one-way, with the nurses being more knowledgeable, yet taking into consideration the person/patient's point of view. Whether at the level of partnership or involvement, there must be a relationship between person/patient and nurse in order for person/patient participation to occur (Cahill 1996).

Having people/patients participate in their health care is both an ethical ideal and a practical reality. From an ethical point of view, all people/patients should have a say in their care, that is, having a legitimate voice in care is a recognized person/patient right. From a practical standpoint, people/patients who participate in their health care are more likely to commit to that care because the care takes into account their particular circumstances. In this regard, health outcomes are more likely to be successful when people/patients have input into that care.

But having people/patients participate in their own care is not simply a matter of believing in an ideal or acknowledging a reality. Although nurses acknowledge the value of person/patient participation, they prefer people/patients to be passive and are challenged to determine whether and to what extent people/patients want to participate (Cahill 1998; Guadagnoli and Ward 1998).

Do people/patients want to be involved in their care? Research indicates that the answer to this question is both complex and variable. In most of the research on the topic, person/patient participation has been viewed as person/patient involvement in decision-making about health care. That is, participation is viewed as the extent to which people/patients are involved in health-care treatment decisions. Reviews of these studies reveal that people/patients want to participate to varying degrees *if* options exist and *when* they feel well informed (Cahill 1998; Guadagnoli and Ward 1998).

For example, hospitalized people/patients in Biley's (1992) study indicated that they wanted to participate in care if they felt well enough to do so, knew enough and were permitted to participate. In comparison, hospitalized people/patients in Waterworth and Luker's (1990) study were more interested in 'toeing the line' and fitting in with the nurses than they were with exercising their right to participate in health care. Another study that reveals insight into person/patient participation involved people/patients who were chronically ill and not hospitalized (Thorne and Robinson 1989). These people/patients involved themselves as 'team players' when they felt competent in managing their illness and when they trusted the health-care professionals. In the absence of trust and the presence of personal competence, these people/patients used their knowledge to manipulate the system to obtain necessary services, but did not engage with professionals.

The major theme in the literature on person/patient participation is the amount of information that people/patients have to participate. In the absence of information, people/patients did not feel capable of participating. Therefore, having people/patients participate in their care is contingent on them having knowledge about that care. Herein lies one of the major challenges to participation. Sharing information with people/patients is an important skill in meeting this challenge.

Sharing information

The skill of sharing information encompasses a range of actions from providing explanations, to giving instructions, to imparting knowledge, to formal teaching. When explaining to a person/patient the reasons for an extended delay in a scheduled procedure, the nurse is sharing information. When engaged in informing people/patients what they can expect to happen postoperatively, the nurse is sharing information. When teaching a person/patient how to care for a colostomy, the nurse is sharing information.

What nurses perceive as ordinary and everyday in the routine of health care delivery can seem foreign to people/patients. People/patients may have little previous knowledge and experience to draw on in trying to understand this sometimes strange, often frightening, world of health care. Clearly, nurses are in a prime position to help people/patients make sense of the environment, and their experiences in it, through the sharing of information.

Nurses play a key role in keeping people/patients informed, not only because of their sustained, continual presence but also because of their close proximity to the person/patient's specific experience. When sharing information, a nurse operates from within a person/patient's experience. It is the nurse who comes to know how much adjustment Mr Jones must make in order to follow a prescribed therapeutic diet. It is the nurse who appreciates the demands being placed on a new mother, who has recently arrived in the country and is isolated from her usual support systems. Empathy and understanding of the person/patient's experience enable nurses to share information that is subjective to the person/patient, and to appreciate what the person/patient wants to know in relation to health status and care.

Sharing information is more than merely providing information or imparting knowledge. In sharing, there is concern with how the information is received, understood and used. It is a two-way process. Providing information involves merely supplying information to people/patients and is a one-way process. In this sense, books, pamphlets, and videos provide information to people/patients. Sharing information, on the other hand, is interactive: it connects the people/patients' experience with the need for information; it concerns itself with how the information is received; and it views the person/patient as an active participant, not as a passive recipient.

As with all the skills of intervening, sharing information is grounded in the nurse's understanding of the person/patient. To some people/patients, remaining fully informed, down to the level of minute detail of their care, is extremely important to their sense of well-being. Other people/patients prefer not to know every detail and feel best when told only the bare essentials. Nevertheless, some information, for example, orienting information about the routine of the clinical setting, is necessary regardless of the person/patient's frame of reference and expressed desire to know.

Effects of sharing information

Having meaningful information about their health status and care helps people/patients gain a sense of control over sometimes uncontrollable, confusing or disturbing events. Frequently, information is shared when a person/patient is prepared for an anticipated health event. For example, knowing what can be expected following abdominal surgery assists people/patients in coming to terms with the usual postoperative course of events. Accurate information can do much to alleviate unnecessary anxiety stemming from false beliefs, misconceptions and even fantasies. People/patients facing decisions in relation to health care are able to determine the best course of action when they are fully informed. Explanations alleviate the anxiety of guessing what will happen next.

The skill of sharing information has been mentioned elsewhere in this chapter, in the sections on reassuring and supporting. In the case of reassuring, information is shared in order that people/patients remain aware of what is usual and expected in relation to their health status. In this regard, reassurance through sharing information is similar to informational support, a type of support mentioned in the section on supporting. In the next section of this chapter, sharing information is considered as a challenging skill because of its potential to trigger people/patients to reappraise their situations. This section contains a general overview and discussion of how best to employ the skill of sharing information.

A nurse's perspective on sharing information

Nurses sometimes show reluctance to embark on sharing information with people/patients, because the information to be shared is perceived as exclusively medical in nature. While it is inappropriate for one nurse to assume that of another health-care professional, for example a nurse assuming the role of doctor in presenting initial information about a medical diagnosis, nurses frequently serve as the interpreters of such information. People/patients frequently ask nurses questions that are medical in nature. Simply referring them to the appropriate doctor is often not enough. Nurses can assist people/patients to obtain relevant medical information by helping them to develop questions to be asked of the doctor and suggesting appropriate questions to ask. In this sense, nurses act as guides for people/patients.

Nevertheless, there is more to sharing information than helping people/patients to obtain and understand input that is medical in nature. People/patients also need assistance in understanding how their health status, including their medical diagnosis (when present and known), will affect their day-to-day living. They need to learn how to adjust and adapt to the demands that are placed on them by alterations in health status. When nurses share information about these aspects of health, they are functioning from a holistic perspective. By focusing on these aspects, nurses concern themselves more with people/patients' responses to their health status, rather than just their health status *per se*.

Examples of a holistic perspective on sharing information include helping people/patients to:

- Make sense of what is happening to them
- Learn new skills in caring for self
- Make adjustments and adaptations in relation to the demands placed on them by alterations in health status.

In short, nurses are in a position to share information about people/patients' daily living in relation to health status (Carnevali 1983).

The importance of sharing information is highlighted in this account:

> Harry had been on heart medication for two years. He was attending the hospital for his routine six-monthly check. After all of the investigations were carried out, the Sister from out-patients told Harry that the consultant wanted to admit him for a few days for further tests. Harry thought that this meant that they were going to alter his medication again. He had been through this process before and didn't feel anxious about it at all.
>
> When Harry was settled in the ward the junior doctor came to complete the assessment documentation. During the discussion the doctor said in a 'matter of fact' manner that Harry was being assessed for a heart transplant because his heart was in such a poor condition. Harry felt so shocked by this he felt he'd just walked into a brick wall. He couldn't think. He didn't know what to say. The doctor left Harry alone and said he would be back later.

None of the sharing of information elements had taken place. Although Harry has now successfully undergone the heart transplant surgery and recovered well, he talks about 'that moment' in the ward as being the worst time in his life.

Sharing information versus giving advice

It is easy to confuse giving advice with sharing information (this was mentioned briefly in Chapter 6). In sharing information, nurses offer a range of alternatives to people/patients. In giving advice, nurses present solutions to people/patients. There are times when people/patients expect advice and place nurses in the role of knowledgeable expert. Before assuming this role, however, nurses need to be clear that certain risks are inherent in advising.

When functioning within the nursing perspective, nurses share information in an attempt to help people/patients adjust and adapt to their daily living. By advising people/patients about what is 'best' to do, nurses assume they are experts about each person/patient's life. Clearly, the person/patient is the most qualified expert when it comes to managing their life. The risks of playing the expert when it involves another person's life are apparent – the advice can be unsuitable, unacceptable, inappropriate, or even dangerous.

It is better to present alternatives, through sharing information, and enable the person/patient to determine which course of action might be best. The following scenario highlights the process of presenting alternatives versus giving solutions:

> June Ford has been visiting the local mother and baby clinic on a regular basis since her first son, Ted, was born eleven months ago. During a recent visit she related that she is becoming increasingly distressed because Ted is still waking during the night to breastfeed. Although Ted feeds quickly during the night and settles back to sleep quite easily, June is distressed by her continually broken night's sleep.
>
> Eleanor, the health visitor in the centre, has been working with mothers and babies for twelve years. June asks Eleanor for advice about what to do, because she is becoming desperate for an unbroken night's sleep. Eleanor begins by explaining that Ted is of sufficient weight and age to go through the night

without a feed. She then proceeds to explain that June has various options. She could let Ted cry until he returns to sleep; she could use the 'controlled crying' method to get him back to sleep without a feed; June's husband could tend to Ted in the middle of the night; or she could continue to feed him, knowing that some day waking during the night will cease. Eleanor then continues, explaining how other mothers she knows have dealt with similar circumstances. Finally, she shares her own experiences learned through caring for her three children.

After presenting the options, Eleanor explains to June that only she can decide what is best for herself, Ted and the family. She finishes by stating that there are numerous theories about how to care for babies and a variety of possible approaches, but it really comes down to what June can live with. She then explores each of the options with June, to determine what June would like to try.

Obviously, Eleanor could have advised June about what she should do, rather than share information and let June decide. In doing so, however, she would have run the risk of suggesting a solution that is unacceptable or unworkable for June. Even if the advice is acceptable it may not work, so June would be left with no other options. Under these circumstances, June probably would not ask Eleanor again, and may even blame her for the failure of her recommendation. Most importantly, by giving advice Eleanor becomes responsible for the outcome. June could be left with feelings of inadequacy as a result. These are the risks of presenting solutions, rather than alternatives.

Giving advice is not the same as presenting factual, clinical information to people/patients, or explaining the potential consequences of certain health-related behaviours. Advice offers solutions when people/patients are facing situations that they can potentially manage. Instructing a person/patient to cough and deep breathe following surgery, in order to help prevent pulmonary complications, is an example of presenting information and instructions, although this could be construed as advice. There are times when nurses effectively offer advice to people/patients, but this should be undertaken with full awareness of the risks involved.

Approaches to sharing information

Sharing information begins with the nurse's recognition of the person/patient's need for it. While it could be said that all people/patients need certain information in order to cope with changes in health status, the specific need of each person/patient may be variable. This recognition and appreciation of the person/patient's unique requirements for information stems from the nurse's understanding.

While the person/patient's unique experiences provide a useful starting point for the use of any intervening skill, there are some general situations that indicate a specific need for information. These include:

- Facing new and unfamiliar situations
- Coping with demands of altered health status
- Developing new skills
- Being misinformed

- Requesting information and explanations
- Expressing the need for reassurance and informational support.

However, there is still a need for the nurse to gauge (a) readiness to learn, and (b) when to begin to share information.

(a) Readiness to learn

Timing is crucial when sharing information, and this is best expressed as capturing the person/patient's readiness to learn (Benner 1984: 79). If information is shared before a person/patient is ready it may fall on deaf ears or, worse, create undue anxiety in the person/patient. When it occurs too late, sharing information fails to achieve its desired outcome.

Capturing a person/patient's readiness to learn is a sophisticated process, which is described as an aspect of expert nursing practice (Benner 1984). The degree of sensitivity to person/patient cues that is required for this level of practice is developed through experience and involvement with numerous person/patient experiences. To beginning nurses, the concept of the 'right time' to share information may seem vague and elusive. Nevertheless, an acceptance and recognition that there is a 'right time' enables beginning nurses to make the effort to observe and notice person/patient cues that indicate readiness.

A good example occurs in the teaching of people/patients to care for a colostomy, a complex, sometimes overwhelming task for most people/patients. Because people/patients must first come to terms with the reality of a colostomy, they will not be ready to learn the details of caring for it and themselves until this happens. Cues indicating readiness include looking at the colostomy in more than just a fleeting manner; not reacting with disgust when looking at it; and asking questions of the nurse who is changing the colostomy bag. This is but one example of the importance of noticing when the person/patient seems ready to learn.

Obviously, capturing the person/patient's readiness means that nurses must be flexible enough to change their immediate plans, in order to accommodate this readiness.

(b) Beginning to share information

Once the need for information is established and the readiness to receive the information is noted, it is best to begin sharing information by establishing what the person/patient wants to know (Activity 8.4). Often people/patients will ask questions without prompting or probing, but it may be necessary for the nurse to use exploration skills (see Chapter 7) to establish what the person/patient wants to know first. Questions that are useful include:

- 'What questions are on your mind?'
- 'What would you like to know?'
- 'Where would you like me to begin explaining this?'

Through exploring what people/patients want to know, the nurse is requesting and encouraging the person/patient to ask the questions. It is important that these questions are answered at the depth and level at which they are asked. A simple question need not be met with a complicated, involved answer. Likewise, a complex question should not be brushed aside with a superficial answer. It is often a good idea to paraphrase (see Chapter 6) the person/patient's question prior to attempting to answer it.

After answering a person/patient's question, the nurse needs to check that the response satisfied the question. This is accomplished by following the response with another question, such as 'Does that answer your question?' The nurse may be surprised when the person/patient answers 'No'. Under this circumstance, it is obvious that the nurse needs to develop another response, or have the person/patient pose the question again, using different words.

From this point, the nurse now can move into further, more-focused exploration of what the person/patient already understands. A person who has experienced repeated hospitalizations may understand a great deal about ward routine. This exploration provides a good opportunity to correct any misinformation or misperceptions. The nurse can also use the person/patient's current level of understanding as a springboard for expansion and elaboration of further information. Notice how beginning in this manner encourages the person/patient to direct the flow of information. It also provides an opportunity for the nurse to further assess the person/patient's readiness to receive information.

Limiting the amount of information shared

When nurses are expanding into sharing new information, they need to appreciate that there are limits to how much information can be absorbed at one time. Too much information, presented at one time, can result in an overload of the person/patient's information-processing capacity. Presenting detailed, complex information all at once can create more confusion in the person/patient. For this reason, the general guideline of presenting no more than three new items at one time is recommended (Cormier *et al.* 1986).

Using appropriate language

Another important facet when sharing information is to use language that matches the person/patient's age, experience and cultural background. Nurses sometimes become so accustomed to the jargon of health care that they fail to appreciate that people/patients do not understand some of the language used. Terms such as 'IVs', 'nil by mouth', 'obs' and even 'bedrest' can create confusion in people/patients. For example, some people/patients think 'bedrest' literally means to have a rest in bed and liken it to an afternoon nap, thinking this is sufficient in maintaining bedrest. Not only should standard medical and nursing terms and jargon be fully explained to people/patients, but also their use should be kept to a minimum, if not avoided altogether.

Tailoring information to the person/patient

Of even greater importance, when sharing information, is the need to tailor explanations to the individual person/patient. Obviously, age and cultural

ACTIVITY 8.4

SHARING INFORMATION

 Process

1   Working in groups of five to six participants, develop a list of person/patient situations which indicate that the person/patient needs more information.

2   Each group member now writes a brief scenario based on one of the situations from the developed list. Include person/patient cues indicating a need for information.

3   Distribute the scenarios to each of the group members. Members are to take the scenario away from the session and gather the information required to fully inform the person/patient described in the scenario.

4   At the next class gathering, participants form into groups of three. Identify one member of the group as the person/patient, one as the nurse who will share information and the third person as an observer.

5   For each scenario, have the 'nurse' share information with the person/patient. The observer uses the following format:

Did the nurse:

(a)   Identify what the person/patient wants to know? Yes/No, How?

(b)   Clarify what the person/patient already understands? Yes/No, How?

(c)   Assess the accuracy of the person/patient's current information? Yes/No, How?

(d)   Determine the person/patient's readiness to receive information? Yes/No, How?

(e)   Limit the amount of information shared (about two items at a time)? Yes/No, How?

(f)   Use understandable language? Yes/No, How?

(g)   Present information clearly? Yes/No, How?

(h)   Assess the person/patient's comprehension? Yes/No, How?

(i)   Request feedback from the person/patient? Yes/No, How?

(j)   Discuss the person/patient's reaction to the information?

Discussion

1   What was easy about sharing information? What was hard?

2   What were some of the difficulties experienced in sharing information? Refer to questions on the observer guides that were answered 'No'.

3   How did the 'nurses' assess the 'person/patient's' current level of knowledge?

4   How did the 'nurses' determine the 'person/patient's' comprehension of the information?

5   What kind of wording and language was used in sharing the information?

variations need to be taken into account. But it is equally important to work from the person/patient's background and experience. For example, an engineer can easily relate the functioning of the heart to already-acquired knowledge of closed systems that work on pressure, pumps, one-way valves, and electrical conduction. Knowing a person/patient's background is necessary for this guideline to be enacted.

The need for reinforcement

It is often helpful to reinforce explanations and information verbally shared with prepared pamphlets, diagrams, models, and spontaneously written notes. Using an alternative means of expression such as these provides helpful reinforcement for people/patients. Summarizing (see Chapter 6) the shared information is another helpful means of reinforcing. Often people/patients' anxiety levels interfere with their ability to absorb information, and reinforcing will aid in the retention of presented information.

Additionally, there may be a need to reiterate information. Repetition provides reinforcement, although the need to repeat information may prove frustrating to the nurse. The person/patient may need to hear it more than once in order to incorporate the information and put it to some use.

Checking the person/patient's understanding

Sharing information is more than imparting knowledge, so the nurse sharing the information needs to check periodically that the person/patient understands the information. It is better to check frequently throughout an information-sharing interaction than to wait until it draws to a close. The skills of exploration (see Chapter 7) are employed for this purpose.

Expressing understanding when sharing information

Last, when nurses are sharing information, they need to be sensitive to the impact of the information on the person/patient. For the person/patient, there may be surprises and challenges in the information received. Observing person/patient cues that indicate their reactions, reflecting observed feelings and expressing empathy are all helpful skills to employ for this purpose. In the absence of person/patient cues, it may be necessary for nurses to explore people/patients' reactions to the information that is shared.

A final word on sharing information

Before embarking on sharing information, nurses must be reasonably confident with their own level of knowledge, related to the person/patient situation. This is not to say that nurses should 'know everything' there is to know about all person/patient situations, but there is little point in trying to share information when the basics of the situation are not understood. If this is the case, a cursory assessment of the person/patient's need for information could be undertaken; but there are limits. For example, a person/patient's misunderstanding might not be immediately corrected if the nurse lacks knowledge.

There are likely to be situations in which a person/patient's request for information is beyond what a nurse currently understands and knows. There is no real harm in nurses admitting that they do not know, as long as they are willing to find out for the person/patient, or refer the person/patient to an appropriate resource. When referral to another person, for example, the person/patient's doctor, is the most appropriate course of action, nurses can assist people/patients in framing questions to ask of this person.

Enabling participation through challenging

When challenging, nurses urge people/patients to reconsider their current perspectives and assist them in the development of new perspectives. A challenge encourages people/patients to evaluate their views, feelings and interpretations of a situation. This can be achieved by directly presenting a different interpretation, or by exploring alternative perspectives with the person/patient. Either way, a successful challenge enables people/patients to reframe their experiences in a new light and therefore participate in care with this new view.

Challenging is a skill that is high in terms of influencing people/patients. This is because the nurse is asking people/patients to call into question their experiences and to develop new perspectives on their experience. Challenging often forces people/patients to call on new or unused resources.

The challenging aspects of other skills

The section on reassuring skills makes reference to responses that encourage people/patients to reinterpret their experience. When enacted in this way, reassurance has a challenging edge to it. Sharing information can also be challenging, because the presentation of new information often results in the formation of new perspectives. Even exploration and empathy expression can be challenging. When nurses express empathy, reflect feelings and engage in exploration, the result may be that people/patients begin to challenge their own perspectives.

The nature of challenging

Effective challenging is beneficial because it influences people/patients to look at their situations in new and different ways. This reframing and reinterpretation may prove unsettling at first, and people/patients may experience anxiety as a result. For this reason, nurses are often uncomfortable with the notion of challenging a person/patient because it seems non-supportive to cast doubt on the person/patient's current perspective. Perhaps this is due to a lack of understanding of the nature and helpfulness of a challenge.

Challenging is not the same as disagreeing with or rejecting the person/patient's perspective, although it does rely on the nurse's judgement that another perspective may be more productive. For example, a person/patient may believe that having a myocardial infarction results automatically in permanent disability and dramatic alteration to previous functioning. An interpretation such as this can lead to feelings of depression and even despair. Such a person/patient is at risk of becoming a 'cardiac cripple'. By challenging this perspective, the nurse enables the person/patient to develop a more realistic view of the situation, post-infarction.

The conditions needed for effective challenging

As with all the psychosocial action skills, challenging is preceded by an understanding acknowledgement of the reality of the person/patient's current experience (see Chapter 6). Nurses 'earn the right' (Egan 1994) to challenge people/patients by first demonstrating understanding of their viewpoints and experiences. In this sense, understanding is a prerequisite to challenging.

Before embarking on challenging skills, a nurse must also consider the strength of the relationship with the person/patient. If little rapport, trust and understanding are developed, it is likely that a challenge will be ineffective. In fact, without trust, challenging may be counterproductive to the further development of the relationship. People/patients will accept a challenge from a nurse who has demonstrated interest, accessibility, reliability, and understanding. Challenging is more likely to be effective in longer-term rather than short-term relationships.

Other aspects to consider before embarking on a challenge relate to the vulnerability and fragility of the person/patient. Nurses must be reasonably certain that the person/patient being challenged has the strength, resilience and resources to develop and accept a new perspective. Minimally, the person/patient needs to be able to acknowledge that alternative views are possible.

The need to challenge

The need to challenge stems from the existence of person/patient perspectives that are unproductive, unsatisfying, poorly informed, unacceptable, and/or unnecessarily painful or distressing to the person/patient. The importance of that final phrase, *to the person/patient*, cannot be stressed enough. It is important that challenges are not presented as negative judgements, which give the impression that people/patients 'should not' think or feel the way they do. Although nurses rely on a judgement that a new perspective may be needed, they must operate from within the person/patient's value system in order to be most effective. A nurse cannot decide, without consultation, that the person/patient's perspective needs to be altered.

Tentativeness of the challenge

Challenges are best presented in a tentative manner, but not so tentative that nurses lack assertiveness in the process. A nurse wishing to challenge a person/patient can begin by suggesting that there may be another way of looking at the situation. This is an effective way to determine the person/patient's readiness to accept alternative perspectives.

Approaches to challenging

When people/patients indicate, often through subtle cues, that their current view is unproductive or difficult to maintain and acknowledge the possibility of alternative perspectives, nurses can proceed by:

- Exploring alternative perspectives
- Presenting their own interpretation and perspective
- Sharing factual information.

The first approach relies on the use of exploring skills (see Chapter 7). The second approach uses the skill of feedback, covered in the section on reassuring earlier in this chapter. The third approach is also covered in this chapter, under the heading of sharing information.

Exploring consequences

Another way to begin the challenge is to explore the consequences of the person/patient's present perspective. While this approach relies on the effective use of exploring skills (see Chapter 7), it is a focused exploration of the possible effects of the person/patient's current perspective, and delves into the potential risks and benefits of that perspective.

A nurse may be tempted to take the idea of consequences one step further and actually point them out to people/patients. This approach should be used sparingly (Ivey and Ivey 1998) because of its potential to degenerate into a judgemental, coercive activity that preaches warnings and punishment. Nurses need to be cautious about admonishing people/patients, because this can translate to 'blaming the victim'. If this happens, people/patients may form the impression that the nurse does not care to understand.

Assertiveness in challenging

The ability to be assertive (see Chapter 4) is necessary when challenging. Some examples of assertive, challenging responses include:

- 'I see your situation in a different light than you do.'
- 'I'm concerned that if you continue along these lines, you will just wither away.'
- 'You say you are doing everything to help yourself, but I can see some more things that you could do.'

When challenging, it is important to focus on the person/patient's strengths and resources, not just weaknesses and failures. In this regard, challenging is employed with an attitude of respect for the person/patient's inherent capabilities.

Reframing through self-disclosure

Self-disclosing is a skill whereby nurses share their own thoughts, feelings, perceptions, interpretations, and experiences in the interest of helping the person/patient (Activity 8.5). Self-disclosure is both a form of commiseration, which is a way of comforting people/patients (Morse *et al.* 1992), and a way of helping people/patients reframe their situations.

Reference to the use of this skill is made elsewhere in this book. In Chapter 7, it was presented as a means of opening areas for exploration. Using self-disclosure to prompt people/patients and encourage them to express themselves is one of the most common forms of this skill. Self-disclosure was also discussed in Chapter 6, as a way to clarify what people/patients have expressed. The skill of self-disclosure is included in this chapter because it can also be used to influence people/patients directly.

Sharing own experiences

One of the most frequent ways that self-disclosure is effective occurs when a nurse has experienced a situation that is similar to the person/patient's. For example, a nurse who has had the experience of a family member with cancer may share this experience with the family of a person/patient who is diagnosed with cancer. Under circumstances such as these, nurses share their experiences (commiseration) not only to demonstrate to the person/patient a personal understanding of the situation, but also to present an alternative perspective (reframing).

Self-disclosure also serves as a way to reassure people/patients that nurses are real people, with real lives. Being open enough to share their own accounts with people/patients demonstrates that nurses trust people/patients as much as they want people/patients to trust them. The genuineness and personal involvement that is demonstrated by self-disclosure has the potential to draw the nurse and person/patient closer together. But it also may frighten some people/patients, who do not desire this degree of intimacy, or who prefer nurses to remain distant.

ACTIVITY 8.5

SELF-DISCLOSURE

 Process

1   Discuss the following:

(a)   How much personal information about themselves should nurses share with people/patients?

(b)   Is there anything of a personal nature that nurses should not share with people/patients? If so, what?

(c)   Discuss the reasons for the answers to each of these questions.

Discussion

1   How much disagreement was there between participants in answering questions 1(a)–(c)?

2   Were there areas of agreement about what should and should not be shared with people/patients? What are they?

3   How do you account for the agreement and disagreement in the questions posed?

How much self should be shared?

This notion of sharing self with people/patients does challenge some notions of 'professionalism'. At times, professionalism is equated with distance, detachment and non-involvement with people/patients. This notion of professionalism is explored fully in Chapter 2. Self-disclosure raises questions about how much information about themselves nurses should share with people/patients.

A general rule of thumb can be applied in deciding how much self to share. The general rule stems from the nature of the relationship between person/patient and nurse. Although this relationship involves give and take, and, at times, is quite intimate, the nurse must remain oriented toward the person/patient. When self-disclosure is used to benefit the nurse, this orientation has shifted onto the nurse.

Pitfalls of self-disclosure

Self-disclosure does not mean that nurses should ask people/patients to bear some of the burden of their own personal difficulties and problems. This is one of the potential pitfalls of self-disclosure. Self-disclosing has the potential to shift the focus from the person/patient to the nurse and, as a result, the nurse dominates the interaction with discussions about self. In this case, the self-disclosure runs the risk of burdening the person/patient with the nurse's personal story. Obviously, if this happens questions are raised about how helpful this might be for the person/patient. It takes awareness to recognize when this is happening, and an aware nurse will shift the focus back onto the person/patient, perhaps by employing an exploration skill.

When sharing their own experiences with people/patients, nurses need to be careful not to use the self-disclosure as a subtle way of rejecting a person/patient's experience, in favour of the nurse's. Nor should self-disclosure be used in a competitive manner of 'let's see who has the best/worst story to tell'. Before disclosing themselves to people/patients, nurses should pass the disclosure through the following proverbial gate: 'Am I sharing this in order to benefit the person/patient or our relationship?' If the answer is 'yes', the gate opens for self-disclosure.

Person/patient requests for personal information

The above discussion of self-disclosure also raises the question of how nurses should respond when people/patients request information that is personal in nature. In this regard, the person/patient prompts the self-disclosure. Clearly, the decision about how much nurses share of themselves is a personal one, but there are also professional reasons to disclose or not to disclose. First, the context must be considered, including:

- The possible reasons why the person/patient requests the information
- The degree of personal depth in the request
- The potential consequences of answering or not answering the question.

Nurses are encouraged to reflect and explore how much or how little information about themselves they are willing to share with people/patients.

CHAPTER SUMMARY

The skills presented in this chapter focus on psychosocial actions of comfort, supporting and enabling. Nurses employ the skills of comforting in order to reassure people/patients. Effective reassurance releases person/patient anxiety so that energy can be used for dealing with the health event at hand. Effective support offers assistance and aid, again freeing the person/patient's energy to cope. Enabling people/patients to participate in care by sharing information and challenging helps people/patients to reframe their perspectives on their situation. All of these skills involve taking direct action to positively influence people/patients.

The power necessary for nurses to influence people/patients in these ways is not automatic; it is gained when the nurse has taken the time to understand the person/patient. Taking action is most effective when it works from within the person/patient's experience; therefore the continual need to listen, explore and understand has been emphasized throughout the chapter. Nurses are most effective when they use psychosocial actions with the view that people/patients are capable and resourceful. With this view, the skills in this chapter are used to mobilize, utilize and reinforce people/patients' capabilities and resources.

REFERENCES

Benner, P. (1984). *From Novice to Expert: Excellence and Power in Clinical Nursing Practice*. Menlo Park, CA: Addison-Wesley.

Biley, F. C. (1992). Some determinants that effect patient participation in decision-making about nursing care. *Journal of Advanced Nursing*, 17, 414–21.

Bottorff, J. L., Gogag, M. and Engelberg-Lotzkar, M. (1995). Comforting: exploring the work of cancer nurses. *Journal of Advanced Nursing*, 22, 1077–84.

Boyd, C. O. and Munhall, P. L. (1989). A qualitative investigation of reassurance. *Holistic Nursing Practice*, 4(1), 61–9.

Cahill, J. (1996). Patient participation: a concept analysis. *Journal of Advanced Nursing*, 24, 561–71.

Cahill, J. (1998). Patient participation: a review of the literature. *Journal of Clinical Nursing*, 7, 119–28.

Cameron, B. L. (1993). The nature of comfort to hospitalized medical surgical patients. *Journal of Advanced Nursing*, 18, 424–36.

Carnevali, D. (1983). *Nursing Care Planning: Diagnosis and Management*, third edition. Philadelphia, PA: Lippincott.

Cormier, L. S., Cormier, W. H. and Weisser, R. J. (1986). *Interviewing and Helping Skills for Health Professionals*. Boston, MA: Jones and Bartlett.

Drew, N. (1986). Exclusion and confirmation: a phenomenology of patients' experiences with caregivers. *Image: Journal of Nursing Scholarship*, 18(2), 39–43.

Edgman-Levitan, S. (1993). Providing effective emotional support. In M. Gerteis, S. Edgman-Levitan, J. Daley and T. L. Delbanco (eds), *Through the People/Patients' Eyes: Understanding and Promoting Patient-Centered Care* (pp. 154–77). San Francisco, CA: Jossey-Bass.

Egan, G. (1994). *The Skilled Helper*, fifth edition. Pacific Grove, CA: Brooks/Cole.

Fareed, A. (1994). A philosophical analysis of the concept of reassurance and its effect on coping. *Journal of Advanced Nursing*, 20, 870–3.

Fareed, A. (1996). The experience of reassurance: patients' perspectives. *Journal of Advanced Nursing*, 23, 272–9.

Faulkner, A. and Maguire, P. (1984). Teaching assessment skills. In A. Faulkner (ed.), *Communication* (pp. 130–44). Edinburgh: Churchill Livingstone.

Guadagnoli, E. and Ward, P. (1998). Patient participation in decision-making. *Social Science and Medicine*, 47, 329–39.

Ivey, A. E. and Ivey, M. (1998). *Intentional Interviewing and Counseling: Facilitating Person/Patient Development*, fourth edition. Pacific Grove, CA: Brooks/Cole.

Johnson, D. W. (2000). *Reaching Out: Interpersonal Effectiveness and Self Actualization*, seventh edition. Boston, MA: Allyn and Bacon.

Morse, J. M. (1992). Comfort: the refocusing of nursing care. *Clinical Nursing Research*, 1(1), 91–106.

Morse, J. M., Bottoroff, J. L., Anderson, G., O'Brien, B. and Solberg, S. (1992). Beyond empathy: expanding expressions of caring. *Journal of Advanced Nursing*, 17, 809–21.

Morse, J. M., Bottoroff, J. L. and Hutchinson, S. (1994). The phenomenology of comfort. *Journal of Advanced Nursing*, 20, 189–95.

Motyka, M., Motyka, H. and Wsolek, R. (1997). Elements of psychological support in nursing care. *Journal of Advanced Nursing*, 26, 909–12.

Proctor, A., Morse, J. M. and Khonsari, E. S. (1996). Sounds of comfort in the trauma center: how nurses talk to people/patients in pain. *Social Science and Medicine*, 42, 1669–80.

Swanson, K. M. (1993). Nursing as informed caring for the well-being of others. *Image: Journal of Nursing Scholarship*, 25(4), 352–7.

Teasdale, K. (1989). The concept of reassurance in nursing. *Journal of Advanced Nursing*, 14, 444–50.

Thorne, S. E. and Robinson, C. A. (1989) Guarded alliance: health care relationships in chronic illness. *Journal of Advanced Nursing*, 21, 153–7.

Whyte, L., Motyka, M., Motyka, H., Wsolek, R. and Tune, M. (1997). Polish and British nurses' responses to person/patient need. *Nursing Standard*, 11(38), 34–7.

Waterworth, S. and Luker, K. S. (1990). Reluctant collaborators: do patients want to be involved in decisions concerning care? *Journal of Advanced Nursing*, 15, 971–6.

Wortman, C. B. (1984). Social support and the cancer patient. *Cancer*, 53 (supplement), 2339–62b.

Part III

SKILLS IN CONTEXT

In Part I, we set out a theoretical framework (symbolic interactionism) for helping us to understand interpersonal relationships in nursing. We made a case for the nurse needing interpersonal skills in order to negotiate the relationship and the meaning of care. In Part II, we presented, and illustrated, the specific skills that underpin practice.

In Part III we locate interpersonal relationships in nursing in the wider culture of health, illness and care. Illness, in Western societies, is seen as a threat, a physical or mental crisis that interrupts the progress of life. To some extent, how illness is presented by health organizations, as something that can and should be avoided, affects the repertoire of 'illness responses' that people carry. Put simply, people have, sometimes unrealistic, expectations about their health and well being, often expecting a miracle cure from the professional system. Of course, this disempowers the person in relation to their care. However, illness simultaneously is a point of opportunity. It is a time to re-evaluate and negotiate how life is to be lived in the present and into the future. In Chapter 9, we look at how people can be 'ill well'. The nurse–person/patient relationship can provide a space for people to empower themselves in relation to their illness.

The theme of empowerment in illness is picked up in Chapter 10 where we look at the interpersonal relationship as the 'stage' on which empowerment may be enacted. Drawing on the ideas of Michel Foucault as well as symbolic interactionism, we examine what power and empowerment mean. We look at how specific 'situational variables' – age, gender, race, culture (and associated stereotypes) – need to be actively worked with. To illustrate the possibility of empowering interpersonal relationships we offer a philosophy/model and an example of empowering practice.

In Chapter 11 we look at how interprofessional working can be organized in order that nurses can be supported in delivering quality care. Without this sense of support nurses experience stress and disempowerment. Interprofessional working is a context in which nurses can be personally and professionally sustained. Successful interprofessional working allows the stresses and strains of the peculiar work of health professionals generally, and nurses in particular, to be contained.

CHAPTER 9

HEALTH, ILLNESS AND CRISIS: OPPORTUNITIES FOR EMPOWERMENT AND PERSONAL GROWTH

INTRODUCTION

During life, many, if not most, people experience illness. Some minor illnesses do not have a greatly disruptive effect on everyday life. However, when illness is significant enough to bring people in contact with health professionals such as nurses, it is a stressful event. Whether it is temporary or long-term, an illness places demands on people/patients to cope and requires the use of physical, personal and social resources. Through their interactions and relationships, nurses assist people/patients in meeting the challenges and demands often presented by an illness.

Appreciating and understanding the nature of the illness experience enables nurses to provide this assistance. Put simply, the disruption caused by illness involves transitions, for example, from well to ill, from independent to dependent. Often, being in a state of transition is experienced as disempowering. When interacting with people/patients, nurses' efforts are aimed at understanding the person/patient's experience of illness, which can be the first stage of re-empowering the person/patient (see Chapter 10).

Understanding the illness requires knowledge of the person/patient's physical condition, medical diagnosis and treatment (this is case knowledge, described in Chapter 1). Nevertheless, understanding illness is more than simply knowing about diseases; it entails knowing something about the person who experiences illness. This is knowledge of how the person is responding to the disease (patient and person knowledge, discussed in Chapter 1). In nursing practice the focus is on the relationship between illness and disease (Benner 1984). Disease is a medical diagnosis that explains symptoms of an illness. Illness is the experience of

237

disease, that is, how disease affects a person's life. Illness is also the whole personal experience of a disease, the 'story' of the person who is the patient. 'Illness is the human experience of loss or dysfunction whereas disease is the manifestation of aberration at a cellular, tissue, or organ level' (Benner and Wrubel 1989: 8).

Illness is the human response to disease; however, there can be illness in the absence of disease. Similarly a person can have a disease yet not experience illness. Whenever people/patients become ill there is a personal assessment of the meaning of the illness. Benner and Wrubel express this by stating that, 'Every illness has a story – plans are threatened, relationships are disturbed and symptoms become laden with meaning depending on what else is happening in the person's life' (1989: 9). 'When illness strikes, the illness and possible ways to cope with it are understood in light of personal background meanings, the situation and ongoing concerns in the patient's life' (Benner and Wrubel 1989: 88).

Illness and crisis

The written Chinese character for crisis combines signs of danger and opportunity. Similarly, illness can be seen as both a threat and opportunity. Nurses encounter illnesses that can become crises and crises that are not entirely based in illness in their daily practice. For example,

- Disability
- Dying
- Trauma from an accident
- Ageing
- Planned pregnancy
- Birth of a child
- A sick child
- Changes in lifestyle
- Social violence
- Natural disasters.

Not every illness or other event that is stressful and/or distressing results in crisis. Consider the following story:

> Sally Goldstein was returning home from work one rainy evening when she was involved in a low-speed, head-on automobile collision close to her home. Awaiting her arrival at home were her five children, ranging in age from three to twelve years and her husband. The accident left Sally's legs severely damaged and mangled. There was a chance that one of her legs would need to be amputated. Her family, friends and neighbours were shocked and devastated by the news of Sally's condition.
> But Sally's outlook was positive right from the beginning of what was to become a long journey back to functioning. She was grateful to be alive, and thankful that she had not sustained injuries to her brain or other internal organs. Although her physical pain was great, especially in the early days after the accident, she remained pleasant and cheerful. Even during the time when amputation of her leg was being considered, Sally maintained that if it eventuated she could find 'other ways of getting around' despite the fact that she may do so 'with only one leg'.

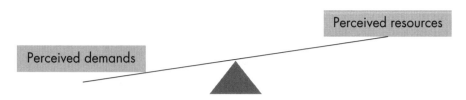

Figure 9.1 Crises develop when perceived demands outweigh perceived resources

Friends who visited her in hospital in the early days found her attitude uplifting and remarked that they left her bedside feeling better because Sally herself was in such good spirits. Some thought that it was only a matter of time before Sally would plunge into despair, sadness and anxiety about what was happening to her. Sally's outlook remained positive throughout the immediate and long-term recovery periods.

As soon as she was able, she contacted the driver of the other vehicle involved in the collision. She expressed her concern and reassured this young man, who was not physically injured in the accident, that it was just an unfortunate incident for which no one could be blamed. Sally's family and friends rallied around and took care of her family's household needs while she was in hospital. The day she was able to get out of bed and into a wheelchair, Sally began visiting the other patients who were on the hospital ward. She spent the remaining six weeks of her acute hospitalization visiting other patients, bringing encouragement and showing genuine interest in each of them.

Sally's heartiness and the way she approached her situation impressed the nurses who cared for her. She remained optimistic, pleasant and understanding even when she was suffering excruciating pain. Fortunately, Sally's leg did not require amputation but she did undergo a long period of rehabilitation during which time she learnt to walk again. Throughout the entire recovery period, Sally demonstrated an ability to cope, had available resources for her assistance, and was able to maintain a realistic and positive view of the situation.

Sally's story illustrates that it is not a stressful event itself that creates a crisis situation but rather how the event is perceived and approached. In Sally's situation, her perception that she was lucky to be alive balanced the potential devastation of her injuries. Because she did not feel defeated by her circumstances, she was able to meet the many demands imposed by them. She perceived herself as capable of handling the situation and she continued to focus on 'how lucky' she felt; a crisis did not develop for Sally. Another person could have been devastated by the extent of the injuries, and could have focused attention on what was lost instead of what remained.

Sally's coping skills in the situation related directly to her ability to remain realistically focused on her remaining ability to function, rather than dwelling on her temporary loss of full functioning. Her active concern and interest in other people, her own family and friends, and even the other people/patients on the hospital ward prevented her from becoming overly anxious about her own circumstances. She always had been an active, involved person and remained so, even though her injuries and hospitalization limited her.

The support systems available to Sally were numerous. She had friends who provided assistance to her family during her absence from home. Not only were these people willing and able to help, but Sally and her family recognized that they needed their help and accepted it without hesitation. Sally actively encouraged people to visit her while she was in hospital because she found these visits helpful in maintaining her positive outlook.

Sally did not experience a crisis despite the fact that she did experience a stressful event that placed enormous demands on her. The factors that equipped Sally to meet the demands of the situation were her perception of the event, her coping skills and her support systems.

Aguilera (1998) describes these three factors as balancing factors, because they are critical in determining whether available resources will meet the demands of a stressful event. When there is a realistic perception of a situation, when coping skills are effective in the situation, and when support systems are available, of use and accessed in the situation, the demands of a situation and the capabilities for meeting these demands are balanced. In the absence of these factors the scales of demands and resources are tipped toward the demands. The person becomes incapable of meeting these demands, and a crisis situation develops. The effects of these balancing factors are depicted in Figure 9.2 and discussed below.

How a person responds to a stressful event depends on how the event is interpreted, what meaning it has in the person's life and its perceived impact. Events have meaning in the context of the person's life. For example, had Sally been a professional dancer her view of the situation might have been quite different from what was presented in the story.

The impact and meaning of an event will influence whether or not the event will create anxiety and distress. Some people/patients view admission to hospital for routine surgery as a minor inconvenience. But a mother of small children who is unable to arrange adequate child care in her absence may view the same event as a major inconvenience and disruption of her daily life. For this mother, the event of hospitalization imposes demands for which there are no available resources and therefore it may trigger a crisis.

Aguilera (1998) emphasizes that the event must be perceived realistically because a distorted view of a situation creates mounting tension and anxiety. For example, if a new mother perceives that her lack of success in easily getting her premature baby to settle is a sign of inability to be an effective parent, her tension and anxiety will mount, and she may begin to feel helpless and hopeless as a result.

There is a danger in using the notion of 'realistic' perception, because nurses might be imposing their own values on the person/patient (see Chapter 4). What may appear distorted to the nurse may be realistic for the person/patient. The importance of understanding the person/patient's experience from her/his frame of reference (see Chapter 6) is reinforced in the context of crisis.

In addition to evaluating the event itself, people/patients in stressful situations also evaluate their personal coping capabilities in terms of whether they perceive themselves as able to meet the demands of the situation. Even when a person/patient has coping resources that may be effective in the situation, a failure to recognize these resources may stifle their use. Thus, the perception of

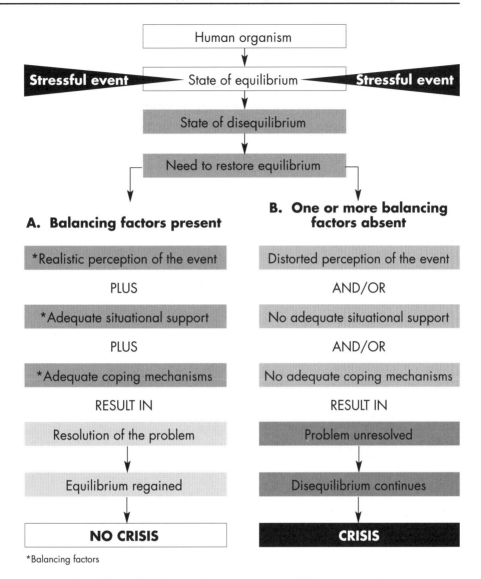

Figure 9.2 The effect of balancing factors in a stressful event (Aguilera 1998)

a stressful event refers to the meaning of the event as well as the perceived capabilities for responding to the event. Also included in the perception is the evaluation of available support systems. Support systems may be available but not tapped, because of a failure to perceive them or an inability to solicit help from other people.

Crises are generated by situations that place demands upon a person that exceed that person's available and usable coping resources and capabilities, thus depleting energy. A crisis is accompanied by extreme tension, high levels of anxiety and feelings of helplessness (Brownwell 1984). When a potential or actual crisis develops, nurses are often in a position to assist and guide people/patients through the experience by understanding the nature of crisis situations; recognizing those people/patients who are at risk of experiencing a crisis; and integrating this understanding and recognition into their interactions with people/patients. Through acknowledgement and comprehension of crisis situations, nurses are able to anticipate, even help to prevent the development of, a crisis and act to mitigate undesirable outcomes of a crisis. Such interventions are predominantly interpersonal: interactions and relationships with people/patients are the means through which they are enacted.

CHAPTER OVERVIEW

In the first part of the chapter we identify the nature and consequences of the transitions that people face on becoming ill. Next we set out some ideas of how people cope with transitions, framing this within a symbolic interactionist perspective. In the following sections, we look at illness/crisis as a threat and a challenge and we explore the ways in which illness/crisis can be an opportunity when the right conditions prevail. Using a narrative analysis (taking people's stories of illness as central) we show how the accounts that people construct around their illness experience are a means to reconstruct themselves. Finally, we focus on how nurses can respond to illness/crisis in a positive way in order to create opportunity for empowerment and growth from the illness/crisis situation.

TRANSITIONS

The people who are cared for by nurses are often experiencing life transitions because of the physical effects of illness. They are also making an adaptation to the experience of being unwell. The effects can be far-reaching. The people may be adults moving from being independent to being permanently or temporarily dependent on others. It may be a family coming to grips with a terminal diagnosis of one of its members. Others may be awaiting a medical diagnosis after experiencing symptoms of illness. All of these circumstances imply a transition, moving from one place, or way of being, to another. Because of its pervasiveness in health care, the process of transition is important for nurses to understand.

In its simplest definition, transition is passage from one place to another; in this regard transition simply refers to relocation. But in health care settings such passages are often more transformative. Transitions through health and illness are often transformative in the sense that lives are altered. Stress, anxiety, loss and grief may also mark health transitions, as people cope with life alterations such as being unwell, getting well again, becoming disabled and approaching death. More frequently than not, health transitions are perceived as negative events.

Nevertheless, transitions, even those related to health events, are not all negative. Transitions bring with them tremendous opportunity for positive growth. A transition, even one from health to illness, is inherently neither positive nor negative; often a transition is both. Consider the following story:

When Ted Johnston had a myocardial infarction (heart attack) at the age of 52, he was not surprised. Many years earlier he had witnessed his father suffer numerous myocardial infarctions that eventually left him debilitated and ultimately resulted in his death. Ted knew that there was a strong possibility that he might experience a fate similar to his father. Because of his family history, Ted had quit smoking and reduced both his cholesterol intake and his weight, ten years prior to his infarction. Ted received early warning signals in the form of angina three years prior to his infarction and the diagnosis of coronary artery disease was confirmed at that time. When Ted had the diagnosis confirmed, he began an exercise programme and visited a cardiologist regularly. None of these measures prevented his ultimate heart attack, but Ted knew that his efforts had helped to decrease both the severity and the effects of the infarction.

One aspect of Ted's life had not been altered in his efforts to reduce his risk of progressive coronary artery disease. It was his job. His work as a superintendent of a large production plant was stressful, and recent events in the industry had placed more demands than ever on Ted. When he had the heart attack, Ted realized that it was time to consider altering his current work activities. Just how he would or could do so was not immediately apparent, but the recognition that something had to be done either to reduce his work-related stress or cope with it in different ways became clear in Ted's mind as he lay in that hospital bed inside the coronary care unit.

Ted underwent coronary artery bypass surgery just four weeks after his infarction. His recovery from a medical and surgical viewpoint was uneventful, but the experience dramatically altered Ted's life. When he returned to work six months after the surgery, he did so on a part-time basis. No longer would he spend endless hours at work. Ted also altered his attitude toward work. No longer would he react with anger and frustration at what he perceived to be improper decision-making at upper management levels. He successfully changed both his attitude and reactions to work-related demands. While still functioning effectively on the job, he successfully altered his perception of his work environment and his response to it.

After two more years as superintendent, Ted was offered and accepted a newly created position in his company. This position was more relaxed and enabled him to have more flexibility and control over his work environment. After three years in this position, Ted took an early retirement package when it was offered.

Prior to his illness the idea of retirement had frightened Ted, because he could not imagine what he would do with his time if he was not at work. His illness changed all that. He took up more leisure activities in an effort to prepare for retirement, and as his final days at work approached, Ted was ready and able to leave it all behind, eagerly anticipating his new life as a retired worker. Many years later, Ted remains content in his retirement, relaxed and able to enjoy the slower pace of life that it brings. Ted sometimes reflects back to his illness and wonders what might have happened if he had not suffered the heart attack. He now realizes the learning that it triggered and is grateful that it caused him to reconsider his lifestyle and take action to alter what had become unhealthy work practices.

The account of Ted's life illustrates how a transition to illness can serve as a catalyst for learning and change. Ted met the challenge and opportunity presented by his illness, and the illness experience ultimately served him in a positive manner. In understanding the positive and negative aspects associated with transitions, it is important that nurses have a basic understanding of how people cope.

Coping with transitions

The link between coping and transitions is premised on the notion that transitions bring change and change brings anxiety and stress. There are at least two major ways that people cope with stress (Lazarus and Folkman 1984). They can attempt to change the situation or their perception of it, so that it does not continue to be so stressful; or they can attempt to change the way the stressful situation affects them, thus altering their response to it. The first of these attempts is known as 'problem-focused' or active coping. The second is known as 'emotion-focused' or passive coping. Active coping efforts are related to meeting the demands of the situation through direct actions. Such efforts include problem-solving; reframing the meaning of an event; seeking further information in preparation for an event; talking it over with a trusted person; finding alternative ways to meet needs and goals that are thwarted by the event; learning new skills; and altering goals or expectations.

Passive coping focuses on the emotional response to the problem at hand. Passive coping efforts are aimed at keeping uncomfortable feelings within manageable limits, and these include the use of defence mechanisms. Examples of this type of effort include avoiding the situation; minimizing the significance of the event; distancing techniques; focusing on the bright side; deriving positive value from negative events; meditating; turning to religion; laughing it off; and using physical exercise to decrease tension.

People need to be able to employ both types of coping effort. Passive coping efforts assist in maintaining emotional equilibrium by diffusing emotional responses and keeping anxiety under control. Active coping efforts enable people to change and grow through stressful experiences.

Coping effectiveness

Like transitions, coping methods are not inherently good or bad, and nurses must be able to view people/patients' coping efforts within the overall context of the situation. An evaluation of the effectiveness of coping efforts relies on the use of a variety of criteria, expressed in the following questions:

- Does the coping effort help to keep anxiety and distress within control?
- What are the long-term effects of the coping efforts?
- Does the coping effort help to maintain a sense of self-esteem?
- Is the coping effort helping to maintain interpersonal connections?
- Is there flexibility in the thinking about and the approach to the situation?

Effective coping is a sophisticated juggling act, which simultaneously maintains self-esteem and internal equilibrium, sustains interpersonal relationships, assists in securing adequate and relevant information, and promotes autonomy and freedom and flexibility of approach. These factors are important to take into account when nurses are considering the effectiveness of coping efforts (White 1974).

Some authors (Jacelon 1997; Wagnild and Young 1993) believe that the ability to cope with major life transitions (resilience) is a personality characteristic or trait within the person. Resilient people are capable of being injured and they bend under stress, but are equally capable of subsequent recovery (Garmezy 1993). Thus, for the trait theory of resilience, the following story is relevant:

> Sue Campdon wouldn't rest until she had an answer that made sense to her about what she felt in her breasts. Dissatisfied with what the doctors were telling her about her symptoms, she persisted in seeing more medical specialists. She did not believe that there 'was nothing wrong'. She told herself and her friends 'Just because the tests have come back negative doesn't mean I am fine. I know there is something wrong and I am not going to settle until somebody does something.' Sue knew she could not afford to take any chances. Her family, especially her three children, needed her.
>
> She was not at all surprised by the diagnosis of cancer when finally a specialist agreed to do a breast biopsy. While the diagnosis and subsequent mastectomy were extremely distressing, at least some action was being taken. She felt strong because she knew what she was fighting. And fight she did. Through every course of radiotherapy and chemotherapy Sue remained incredibly optimistic. She reassured her friends and family members when they expressed worry or fear. In fact Sue's fortitude was an inspiration to everybody. When secondary sites of the cancer were found she was a bit disheartened, but not discouraged. She courageously endured three years of cancer therapy and never lost the beaming smile on her face. Her major frustration was a low level of energy and the need to curtail her usual activities. Sleeping during the day was not her style, but she did adjust to the change of pace in her life. Her friends and family members stepped in to assist with her daily responsibilities of caring for her children.
>
> Despite ongoing treatment the cancer gradually invaded all of Sue's body. When it became clear that no more active treatment was indicated, some of her friends and family members fell apart. Nevertheless, Sue did not. She remained an inspiration to all. Her cheerfulness was unending. Even though her 'fight' with the cancer was over, she did not feel or act defeated. She enjoyed every day that she had with her family. Sue was thankful for and cherished every moment until the end of her life. When she died peacefully and in comfort in her home, her friends and family members were grief-stricken. But they also knew that their lives had been enriched by Sue and her phenomenal strength and human spirit.

However, Jacelon (1997) also sees resilience as a learnt process. As a process, resilience is a response to stress in which a person directs energy to minimize the impact of stressful events through novel approaches to problem solving and reframing their perception (active coping). Taking resilience as a learnt process is more consistent with a symbolic interactionist perspective. Problem solving and reframing involve the manipulation of symbols. Having the capacity for abstract thought means that people can interpret and reinterpret symbols. They can engage in inner conversations in order to impose meaning on unclear or previously unencountered situation (see Chapter 1 for a more comprehensive explanation of symbolic interactionism).

The ability to manipulate symbols and think in an abstract way underpins another feature of 'coping'. Aaron Antonovsky (1987) developed a theory about how people stay healthy in order to counteract the tendency in health care to focus on why people get sick. Antonovsky emphasized the resources that people use to cope successfully with the stresses of life. These resources combine and converge to form what he refers to as a sense of coherence, an orientation towards life's challenges that averts tension and assists in managing life stress and transitions.

A sense of coherence (Antonovsky 1987, 1996) is marked by three attributes: an ability to understand situations that happen in life (*comprehensibility*), an abiding trust that things will work out because there are resources available to meet the demands of life's various situations (*manageability*), and the motivation to invest time and effort in life's challenges (*meaningfulness*). For example, people who have a strong sense of coherence perceive life's challenges as having some structure and clarity as opposed to the perception that life is a series of random events. This is what is meant by comprehensibility. Manageability, the second attribute, is the extent to which a person perceives that resources to cope successfully are available. The sense that resources are available is gained through the encounter with the care system. The final characteristic, meaningfulness, is the extent to which a person believes it is worth putting time and effort into coping with life stresses (Antonovsky 1987; Wolff and Ratner 1999).

Antonovsky's theory has received attention in the nursing literature (for example, Sullivan, 1993). Recent nursing studies indicate that a sense of coherence is related to remaining healthy and socially connected (Wolff and Ratner 1999); maintaining hope in the face of a diagnosis of cancer (Post-White *et al.* 1996); and returning to work following liver transplant (Newton 1999). The positive nature of the theory, with its emphasis on health, is concordant with a nursing perspective of health care because nurses assist people/patients in dealing with the whole of a health event, not simply managing a disease.

Both resilience and a sense of coherence have a common thread, that of the presence of a social network that provides support to the person. Symbolic interactionism places the social network central to defining 'self'. Social support involves connection with and mutual obligation to other people. People who experience social support feel cared for, loved and esteemed (Cobb 1976). Social support is based on the assumption that people need to have supportive relationships with other people in order to manage the demands of daily living and cope with life transitions (Norbeck 1988). These relationships serve to fulfil social needs for affection, approval, belonging, security and identity (Thoits 1982).

Social support is positively related to health and recovery from illness (Ell 1996). That is, family and friends offer needed assistance and emotional support in illness, thus helping in recovery. Likewise, there is a correlation between being strongly connected through a social network and remaining healthy (Ell 1996). People who have a strong, supportive social network remain healthier than people who are socially isolated and lacking in a social network.

Apart from the provision of tangible aid, for example, physical assistance with getting around, just how does support from other people assist with coping? There are two main hypotheses (Keeling *et al.* 1996), both of which marry up with a symbolic interactionist world view. The first is that having people around who care for and are about a person helps that person's self-esteem and sense of security. In addition, other people may encourage healthy behaviour, such as regular exercise. Another way that other people provide support is by helping with the perception and appraisal of a situation, that is, looking at the world with different eyes. Whether by providing information or offering a different perspective, other people often help with seeing a situation in a new and different light. All of these instances of social support have a positive effect on coping and being healthy.

The concept of social support is sometimes presented as all positive, expressed through catch phrases such as 'your friends are your best medicine'. Nevertheless, this is a simplistic notion of social connections because people in a social network can place demands on each other as well as offer assistance. Friends and family can create stress as well as alleviate it. Also, support that is offered must match what is needed (Hupcey 1998). There is no use in a friend offering help that actually hinders, for example, offering advice that is neither wanted nor useful.

Therefore social support is a complex, multi-dimensional concept, which means there are many aspects to it. One aspect is that social support encompasses an acknowledgement of the importance of social relationships. Other aspects include descriptions of social networks and the interrelationships between the people in that network (for example, an extended family). In addition, there are functional aspects of social relationships, the perceived availability of support and actual support that is received (Keeling *et al.* 1996). Because of its complexity, social support has many definitions (Hupcey, 1998; Keeling *et al.* 1996). At their most basic level, social connections between people are part of a healthy life.

ILLNESS AS THREAT AND CHALLENGE

How people/patients respond to illness depends to a large degree on their perception of it. While it might be easier for nurses to consider a person/patient's responses in the light of what they know about the clinical condition of the person/patient, they also need to understand how the person/patient is perceiving and experiencing the illness. Nurses need to read the cues that people/patients offer in order to begin the process of collaboratively constructing a definition of the meaning of the illness experience and possible interventions. There are four important perceptions that nurses may 'read' in the person/patient's presentation: (i) illness as threat; (ii) illness as best denied; (iii) illness as challenge; (iv) illness as threat and challenge.

(i) Illness as threat

Often there is a perception of threat or danger in illness, especially when it begins or exacerbates: a threat that the person's life may no longer be the same; a threat that there may be an inability to proceed with life as anticipated and planned; and a threat in the sense that the body once relied on to perform and work effectively is no longer able to do so. This sense of threat is often accompanied by anxiety and fear, and if these feelings become too strong or pose too much of a disruption, they are met with efforts to keep them under control.

Of primary importance in coping with illness is the ability to maintain emotional balance. People/patients must be able to keep distressing feelings within manageable limits, in order to cope with other demands of illness. If feelings of anxiety and fear become overwhelming, then people/patients become disorganized or almost paralysed. Passive coping efforts, such as minimizing, denying, rationalizing and ignoring, are all examples of how feelings of anxiety are kept in check.

In Chapter 6 there is reference to the importance of recognizing when patients are trying to control their emotions and appreciating the importance of not focusing on feelings during these times. The reasons for this are reinforced in this section, and nurses who understand the importance of timing their responses will be able to refrain from discussing feelings with people/patients who are coping by containing and controlling their emotional responses.

(ii) Illness as best denied

Denial is frequently used as a means of containing anxiety within manageable limits. Denial can take many forms, ranging from denial of feelings about an illness to denial of the existence of a disease even when it has been diagnosed and explained to a patient. It is an effective way for people/patients to manage the perceived consequences of an illness. Denial is often used whenever these consequences are dire for the patient, for example, when life goals are under threat.

There is often an automatic tendency to confront and challenge denial, because it is perceived by nurses as an ineffective way of handling an illness. Before challenging denial, nurses need to understand and appreciate the benefits of it.

Denial serves as a buffer for a disturbing and disruptive reality by allowing a temporary respite from this reality. Because people/patients will let reality (*their* reality) seep into their awareness at a rate that is manageable for them, the degree of denial is in keeping with this rate. This rate may be different from the nurse's desired rate. Whenever nurses are tempted to challenge a patient's denial, it is essential that the person/patient's readiness to accept the challenge be assessed. The nurse wishing to challenge denial must ask, 'Is this for the *person/patient*, or for *me*?' and co-ordinate with the person/patient.

(iii) Illness as challenge

Illness, either temporary or permanent, may also be viewed by people/patients as a challenge. Illness poses many challenges: to adapt, adjust, or learn new ways of achieving life goals; to alter these goals in light of present realities; and to develop new skills and resources. When viewed as challenge, the demands of illness are met with a sense of 'fighting spirit'. This approach is characteristic of people/patients who meet the demands of illness head on and come to grips with adjustments and adaptations by facing the situation and 'getting on with it'.

(iv) Illness as both threat and challenge

Most people/patients perceive both threat and challenge through the course of an illness, especially when it is chronic in nature. In doing so, they vacillate between confronting the reality of the illness and retreating from it.

Some people/patients may have a characteristic style of coping that is not effective in the situation at hand. For example, when symptoms are experienced yet no definitive diagnosis can be made, or is delayed through extensive testing, some people/patients with a preferred repertoire for attacking situations may not cope effectively because they are essentially trying to come to grips with an unknown. As long as there is effort made to determine the cause of symptoms, people/patients in this situation would be better off temporarily forgetting or denying the possibilities. Focusing on 'what if' scenarios could lead to increased distress and anxiety.

Consider the following story:

> Leanne was 43 years old when she was diagnosed as having a brain tumour. Her symptoms during the three years prior to diagnosis had been annoying, puzzling and, at times, alarming to her. But, despite these symptoms, she did not see herself as ill. It was her gradual loss of hearing in her left ear and the subsequent referral to a neurologist that finally resulted in tests that confirmed the presence of the tumour. Initially she was shocked and frightened but somewhat relieved when a biopsy showed that the tumour was benign.
>
> Nevertheless, she was informed that she would need to undergo a lengthy and complicated surgical procedure for the removal of the tumour. She began to prepare herself for this. She was accustomed to leading an active and involved life, filled with a job she enjoyed, friends and family, and extensive travel. From what the surgeon explained, Leanne realized that her life would change dramatically in the immediate months following the surgery. Although the long-term prospects for full recovery were hopeful, Leanne also realized that there were no guarantees. She understood the implications of her surgery and knew her future was filled with uncertainty.
>
> Leanne's friends and family were amazed by the way she was facing the situation. Naturally, she had periods of distress, anxiety, sadness, and even anger. But most of the time she thought about and discussed her impending surgery with an informed awareness of what it would entail. She understood and accepted that her recovery would take time and require effort to re-learn some daily functions that she previously took for granted.
>
> In the weeks leading up to the surgery, however, Leanne found that she focused less and less on what was about to happen. Instead she busied herself by sewing fancy nightgowns so she would at least 'look nice' while in hospital. There was really no more for her to do but wait and try not to dwell on her worries.

Leanne's story illustrates how a combination of efforts is used to cope with an illness. Initially she focused on 'attacking' the problem by having all the necessary tests and gathering information that would help her to understand the surgery. Once plans for surgery were under way, she coped with the waiting period by focusing her energies elsewhere. Worrying seemed of little value to Leanne at this time, so she coped by 'not thinking too much about' the surgery. Critically, Leanne was able to negotiate the meaning of each situation with significant others involved. For example, she was able to discuss with doctors what the surgery would mean at the appropriate point and to let friends and family know what her needs would be post-op.

As well as general perceptions of illness, people/patients have situated experiences that are specific to the stage of the illness. There are some person/patient situations that nurses commonly encounter in their everyday practice:

- A disease is suspected yet unknown or unclear, the person/patient feels unwell and is ill but no identifiable cause is known
- The person/patient's condition is one in which full recovery is anticipated, although the person/patient may be ill and incapacitated for a period of time
- Although recovery is likely, the person/patient experiences complications that delay recovery and create the possibility of a long-term illness
- An acute condition is present for which the person/patient will need to make dramatic adjustments and alterations to daily living and lifestyle
- The person/patient's condition is one that is likely to proceed on a progressive downhill course, leaving her/him increasingly incapacitated and ill
- The person/patient develops a chronic condition that is usually characterized by periods of illness and periods of wellness
- There is a life-threatening condition that brings uncertainty both immediately and in the future
- The person/patient's condition is one in which death is likely to occur in the near future.

In relation to the specific situation the nurse may seek signals as to whether the person/patient is experiencing: (a) uncertainty; (b) vulnerability.

(a) Uncertainty

Whenever there is an alteration in people/patients' health status, they are dealing with uncertainty. What is wrong? Will recovery occur? What type of medical intervention will be required? Can the demands of such intervention be met? Will there be a permanent alteration to lifestyle? Will there be pain and suffering? Uncertainty is accompanied by emotional distress and anxiety, and affects both the quality of a person/patient's life and the adjustment to illness (Mast 1995).

In understanding the experience of illness, nurses are often sensitive to the uncertainty that is part of the experience. In symbolic interactionist terms, the nurse is able to take the role of the other and so gain some level of understanding. In fact, for adults, uncertainty is considered to be the greatest single psychological stress in acute illness (Mishel 1997). Perhaps the widespread existence of uncertainty in the illness experience is the reason that nurses so frequently offer false reassurance by directing people/patients not to worry (see Chapter 8).

Factors thought to contribute to uncertainty in illness include severity of illness, specificity of diagnosis, personality of the person/patient, degree of social support, and trust and confidence in health-care providers (Mast 1995). Of these possible contributors to uncertainty in illness, research has correlated the lack of a specific diagnosis to increasing uncertainty. Research into remaining possible causes of uncertainty is inconclusive, although the provision of relevant information by health-care professionals has been shown to decrease uncertainty.

Furthermore, support from family and friends eases the anxiety that accompanies uncertainty (Mishel 1997).

People/patients who are uncertain are more likely to use passive, emotion-focused coping, although the active-coping activity of seeking information is often spurred by uncertainty (Mast 1995). Like illness, uncertainty can be perceived as both threat and opportunity. Those people/patients who perceive uncertainty as danger are likely to use emotion-focused coping, while those who see uncertainty as opportunity will use problem-focused coping (Mishel 1997).

(b) Vulnerability

When people/patients are experiencing illness of any nature they are likely to feel vulnerable. Vulnerability is a subjective experience in which people/patients perceive that their capabilities are inadequate to cope with the situation (Clark and Driever 1983). It is based on an interpretation that the demands of a situation exceed personal capabilities for meeting these demands. Coming into contact with nurses can compound people/patients' vulnerability. The very fact that they perceive their situation as one that requires the use of health-care resources (for example, nurses) indicates that they may evaluate their own capabilities for dealing with the situation as inadequate. The potential dependence and disempowerment resulting from the need for health care may further increase feelings of vulnerability. On the other hand, the fact that people/patients have mobilized health-care resources may indicate a sense of competence and resilience. They may still perceive themselves as capable of handling the situation but recognize the need for professional assistance.

ILLNESS AND CRISIS AS OPPORTUNITY

Illnesses and crises offer opportunities for growth because successful resolution enables people to extend themselves beyond their current capabilities. Because crises occur when there is inability to cope, successful resolution results in new or different coping methods, resources and supports being developed. The outcome of a crisis may result in regeneration and rejuvenation. Focusing exclusively on stressful events and crises as negative experiences blinds nurses to the potentially positive aspects of them. While the negative side of crisis must be understood and appreciated, an awareness of the positive aspects enables nurses to maintain hope and a 'vision of possibility' for the person/patient who is experiencing actual or potential crises. For example, Cutcliffe and Barker (2002) have pointed out that being engaged with suicidal patients and inspiring hope can help them to move into the future from their existential crisis.

The way an event is perceived in terms of its importance, realism and relevance affects how it is handled. In order to cope effectively, people/patients must be able to construct an interpretation of an event so that meaningful action can be taken. Support from others helps people/patients to evaluate their situation realistically, to challenge and alter their existing perspectives, to maintain their self-esteem by reinforcing a belief that they are able to manage, and to establish emotional balance by absorbing the impact of strong feelings. Other people's involvement can also serve as a temporary distraction from the patient's distress. Cultural and religious rituals, beliefs and practices, largely social in nature, can also provide support during stressful events.

To be effective in balancing a stressful event, support from other people must be available, usable and suitable for the context. A hospitalized person/patient's relative who cannot cope with the sights and sounds of a hospital will be of little value in the situation. In this sense, the effectiveness of the support needs to be evaluated in light of the current context. Supportive people must be suitable for the context and available in the situation. A supportive person who lives in another county or country may not be able to provide support regardless of how helpful this person may be. The following story illustrates what happens when balancing factors are absent or ineffective in preventing a stressful event from becoming a crisis. Contrast this account to that of Sally Goldstein, presented earlier.

> Joanne and Harold Gray had been married 50 years when Harold suffered a heart attack. The heart attack was minor from a medical viewpoint and physical recovery was expected. Harold's hospitalization and convalescence were following the usual pattern of recuperation, without complications. The nurses in the coronary care unit recognized that although Harold was progressing toward recovery, Joanne remained extremely anxious. Each time she visited Harold she asked the same questions over and over again. Her questions centred on the theme of Harold's recovery and she expressed fears that he was not going to be 'all right'. She kept focusing on a fear that Harold might die.
>
> No matter how many times the nurses attempted to reassure Joanne, through offering factual, encouraging information about Harold's continued improvement, she remained visibly anxious. In fact her anxiety seemed to be escalating as Harold recovered. With each visit she appeared more distraught. One day as she was leaving the hospital, Joanne's anxiety mounted to near panic. She began to cry uncontrollably and reached a state where her behaviour became disorganized. She was making random attempts to cope with the situation and her verbalization reflected that she was having difficulty keeping her thoughts on one track. Joanne needed immediate attention.
>
> Victor, one of the nurses caring for Harold, took Joanne to a quiet area of the ward. He listened to Joanne in an effort to understand what was happening. It took some time to piece together the story that Joanne related. Victor learnt that Joanne and Harold had both been survivors of a train crash that occurred many years ago when they were young. They lived through the ordeal but lost family and friends in the accident. The event brought them close together, bonding them in a common experience that would remain significant for the rest of their lives.
>
> Joanne's major worry now was that Harold would die. She believed the nurses were just telling her everything was all right because they did not want to worry her. She had not been sleeping or eating well since Harold was in hospital because 'they always did these things together'. Harold and Joanne's only son was out of town on a business trip that had been delayed because of Harold's illness, but could not be postponed any longer. Many of Joanne and Harold's friends had either died or moved away after retirement.

Joanne's perception of the situation was that Harold would die, despite what she was hearing from the nursing and medical staff. Her major way of coping previously was to talk things over with Harold, an avenue that was not available to her under the circumstances. Joanne's son, a potential source of support, was unavailable to her at the moment. The lack of balancing factors – realistic perception of the event, adequate and usable coping skills, and available situational supports – resulted in Joanne's experiencing a state of crisis.

Another way to think of Joanne's perception is as a narrative of her life, past, present and future, which constrains how she can react to her current circumstances. 'The concept of "narrative" does not hold an established theoretical place in any sociological school or tradition' (Williams 1984: 177). Narratives tend to have certain features: a linear form, with a beginning, middle and end; they presuppose a teller and a listener; they are rich in the feelings, understanding and concerns of the tellers. We all have many narratives available to us, influenced by many sources at different levels; societal stories, for instance about the entitlement of 'the sick' to care, psychological theory that has entered the public domain, for instance, the psychoanalyst's couch; family/lay beliefs about health and illness, for instance, 'feed a cold, starve a fever'. Similarly, professionals hold a range of theories and ideas about people who come to them for help. The theories are often concerned with the causes of the problem and its solution.

Critically, narratives are important because they are enacted. For example, a biological explanation is one possible account of psychiatric experience. It may have some currency for both the psychiatric professional and the person seeking help if she/he has benefited from psychotropic medication in the past. As such it may be a helpful narrative in that it is a shared account of the likely course of the 'illness', the treatment outcome, and so on. An alternative account might be that the psychiatric distress is a way of communicating some dissatisfaction with the person's circumstances of living, encouraging the psychiatric nurse to help the person find external solutions to the problems. In Joanne's case, her narrative about Harold dying and the consequences was at odds with the preferred professional narrative. The lack of understanding of the respective accounts was preventing Joanne from coping with the crisis.

Recently, there has been a growing interest in narrative medicine (see the series of papers in the *British Medical Journal* in 1999, edited by Trisha Greenhalgh), based on a concern that objectivity has limits in clinical method. Patients are individuals whose illness behaviour is necessarily 'contextual and idiosyncratic' (Greenhalgh 1999: 324). People vary their narratives according to the context of their telling, and towards a meaning about an event generated through dialogue. In listening carefully to the narratives of the person/patient, the clinical symptoms and signs can be reinterpreted by the attentive doctor towards a formulation that is meaningful for both parties. As Launer (1999) suggests there is the opportunity to generate a different story of what is happening for the person/patient that both respects the person's expertise enshrined in her/his biographic narrative but which also offers new possibilities by joining up with the narratives of the doctor's experience. Person/patient and doctor can strive for a new 'meaning as use' (Wittgenstein 1953) about the illness. In relation to Joanne, revealing her narrative about the illness experience would have been an opportunity to help her both to deal with her distress in the here and now and to re-visit and resolve the distress about the past that she was still burdened with. In this way, the crisis can be seen as an opportunity for growth for both Joanne and Harold.

WORKING WITH CRISIS, ILLNESS AND LOSS AND GRIEF

In the following section we look at some of the practical issues and skills that nurses can use in working with crisis, illness, and loss and grief. Most of these will be familiar to readers who have read Part II of this book. Implicit to the processes described is a symbolic interactionist framework. Being able to work practically means that opportunity for person/patient empowerment and personal growth is maximized.

Working with crisis

In responding to crisis situations, nurses must be able to recognize when crises are occurring in people/patients' lives. Awareness of situations that have a potential to create crises is the first step in recognition. But there is a danger that nurses will believe that *any* person/patient experiencing a stressful event will also be experiencing a crisis. Noticing a person/patient's distress, however significant, in itself does not mean that the person/patient is experiencing a crisis. A view that a stressful event is a crisis is based on the person/patient's perspective of the situation. Nurses need to explore the situation with the person/patient in order to reach this level of understanding.

The balancing factors (described above) that prevent a stressful event from becoming a crisis are useful focal points in directing such exploration. In this regard, assessing the meaning of a stressful event takes the form of focused exploration (see Chapter 7). The potential for crisis can be assessed through answering the following questions, which are based on the balancing factors:

- What is the person/patient's perception of the event?
- What is the impact of the event on the person/patient's life?
- How much tension and anxiety is the person/patient experiencing?
- What does the person/patient usually do to manage stressful situations?
- Will these usual ways of coping meet the demands of this situation?
- How is the person/patient attempting to manage this situation?
- How effective are these attempts in meeting the demands of the situation?
- How capable does the person/patient feel in meeting the demands of the situation?
- How effectively is the person/patient keeping anxiety within manageable limits?
- What supports are usually helpful to the person/patient?
- How effective are these supports for *this* situation?
- Is the person/patient able to mobilize these supports?
- Are these supports available *at* the moment?

An understanding of each of these areas must be achieved in order for nurses to assess whether the person/patient is experiencing a crisis and what actions may be of assistance when they intervene to assist the person/patient in managing the situation.

Intervening in a crisis

When intervening in a crisis situation, either potential or actual in nature, nurses should focus their efforts on strengthening or altering the balancing factors. Any of the intervention skills presented in Chapter 8 can be employed and placed within the context of potential crisis situations. Such interventions include:

■   Assisting and enabling the person/patient to develop different and new perspectives, and altering current perspectives through the use of enabling skills
■   Strengthening coping skills through comforting and supporting skills
■   Assisting in the development of new coping skills through encouragement to try different approaches by offering information and advice
■   Mobilizing and providing support.

When intervening in a crisis it is best to remain focused on the immediate situation and limit interventions to those actions that directly relate to it (Aguilera, 1998). The offer of suggestions and advice about how to manage the situation is often needed in crisis intervention because when people/patients are experiencing a crisis they are open to suggestions. In doing so, nurses must take care to provide advice that is based on an understanding of the person/patient's experience, culture, age, lifestyle, and values. They should follow the guidelines below:

(a) Remain calm

Because crisis situations create tension and anxiety, it is important that nurses remain calm and confident when they interact with people/patients in crisis. Anxiety is often interpersonally contagious, that is, nurses who are interacting with anxious people/patients may themselves begin to feel anxious and unsettled as they interpret signs and put themselves in the position of the other person. Likewise, a calm and comforting manner (see Chapter 8) is also contagious, and people/patients will feel relaxed in the presence of a nurse who is able to remain calm.

(b) Maintain hope

Throughout interactions with people/patients in crisis, it is also important that nurses maintain a sense of hope that the crisis can be resolved. Hope serves to mobilize reserve energy (Brammer 1988) and counteracts feelings of despair. Nurses who demonstrate confidence in people/patients' capabilities to cope with and manage the situation promote hope. This belief in people/patients also demonstrates respect.

During an illness, no matter how serious or minor, a sense of hope must be promoted and maintained. Hope that the situation will improve and that efforts to cope will meet with success is vital to people/patients' perseverance. In the absence of hope people/patients often give up, perceiving that their efforts to cope are in vain. This frequently occurs for brief periods during recuperation from a long-term illness or when illness is chronic. If it becomes pervasive, people/patients may fail to put any effort into recovering or adjusting.

While it is important that nurses maintain a sense of hope, this should not take the form of presenting false reassurance, minimizing the significance of people/patients' distress, or promoting a false sense of well-being through deception. At times nurses may think that deceiving people/patients is in the person/patient's best interest. Conversely, deceit signals a lack of respect for the person/patient's abilities to cope and undermines any trust the person/patient may be feeling in the nurse. While it may be tempting to offer false hope, such actions are usually counterproductive to the establishment of an effective relationship and the resolution of a crisis.

Helping people/patients cope with illness

In coping with crisis or illness, people/patients call upon needed resources. Nurses are potential resources if they are involved, interested and concerned. But nurses can only be resources when they have taken time to understand the situation from the person/patient's perspective.

Nurses help people/patients cope with illness by assisting them in many ways; for example, nurses help people/patients to contain uncomfortable feelings, generate a sense of hope and redefine the situation in solvable terms. Perhaps most significant is the way in which nurses assist people/patients in maintaining or regaining their sense of self-esteem.

Illness often threatens this sense, for example, when there is loss of physical functioning or an alteration in body image. Acknowledging and understanding people/patients' experiences is one of the most effective ways that nurses can maintain people/patients' self-esteem. However, there may be specific needs associated with specific illnesses. Illnesses can be acute, critical, chronic, or terminal. When interacting with people/patients, nurses need to consider the nature of the illness, not in an attempt to classify people but rather to anticipate which themes might be most relevant to the experience. Nurses must still rely on their own recognition of people/patients' situations and also develop understanding of how individual people/patients are experiencing an illness.

(a) Acute illness

The term *acute illness* in this context refers to situations in which people/patients are experiencing symptoms significant enough to bring them into a health-care setting. A medical diagnosis of a specific disease may or may not be known, but regardless of this there is a personal impact on the person/patient's life. Nurses need to be sensitive to this impact and how the person/patient is responding to the situation.

When people/patients come into contact with nurses because they are experiencing an acute illness *and* the cause of this illness is unknown or unclear, there is a great deal of uncertainty. People/patients are usually concerned and worried about the situation and may ask numerous questions. In responding to these questions, nurses need to be sensitive to the fact that they are often asked out of uncertainty. While it might be easy to dismiss questions with, 'Let's wait and see', such a response invalidates the person/patient's concern. While it might not be possible for nurses to reassure people/patients with factual information, it is possible to reassure people/patients that their worries are understandable.

Not all people/patients in this situation will ask questions. Some will worry in silence. When this happens it is often helpful for nurses to take the lead in exploring the person/patient's potential uncertainty. Focused exploration or a self-disclosing statement (see Chapter 8) reflecting the likelihood of uncertainty can be employed for this purpose, as long as nurses evaluate the person/patient's degree of comfort with discussing feelings and assess the level of trust in the relationship.

If medical tests are being conducted to determine the presence or absence of a disease, nurses can inform people/patients about what they can expect to experience during such tests. Some people/patients will want to know everything about a procedure, while others will be happy to undergo a procedure with very little information.

Chapter 2 highlights the need for nurses to ascertain how much information a person/patient wants before actually sharing it. Sensitivity to the individual person/patient and understanding of the world from the person/patient's frame of reference are necessary if the information that is shared is to have relevance to the person/patient.

It is a good idea to ask people/patients how they would like test results communicated to them. Some people/patients may prefer to have family and friends present while others may prefer to hear the news, good or bad, on their own. Nurses are in the best position to understand the significance of the results in terms of their potential impact on the person/patient's life. This is part of understanding the experience of illness.

When the person/patient's condition is understood from a medical viewpoint, nurses can then focus their interpersonal efforts on understanding how the illness and consequent medical treatment may affect the patient as a person. All of the skills presented in Chapters 5–8 offer guidance on how to approach situations such as this.

(b) Critical illness

When an illness is *critical*, it is most often life-threatening as well. During these types of experience people/patients are often living in 'dream world' and may even 'lose' a period in their life in the sense that, after recovery, they cannot recollect what happened. During critical illness the traditional ways of verbally communicating may be shut off, for example, because of mechanical ventilation, thus increasing the challenge for nurses to connect with people/patients on an interpersonal level.

In understanding the experience of critical illness it is important that nurses recognize the significance of people who know the person/patient on a personal level. Family and friends are often the link between the person/patient and the nurse, so their presence and participation during the illness can be vital. Without the information that family and friends can provide, interpersonal connections with people/patients become extremely difficult, if not impossible.

The sophisticated technology and equipment in the critical-care environment are often unfamiliar to people/patients and their friends and families. The importance of providing explanations about equipment, procedures and nursing care cannot be underestimated. But again, care should be exercised by nurses to limit such explanations to a level that people/patients and families and friends can absorb, and to an extent that they desire.

(c) Recovering from an acute or critical illness

During recovery from an acute or critical illness people/patients often want to relive their experiences and discuss them with nurses, who they perceive have an intimate understanding of the significance of illness. Feelings are often expressed because the risk of losing control over emotions is reduced. The immediate danger has passed and uncertainty is lessened. For these reasons, reflecting feelings (see Chapter 6) is often effective during this time.

Frequently, people/patients are not prepared for the amount of time it takes to regain their strength and former ways of functioning following an acute or critical illness. An explanation from nurses that this is to be expected is reassuring, demonstrates understanding of the person/patient's situation and provides anticipatory guidance in the recovery experience.

(d) Chronic illness

Chronic illnesses can be progressively deteriorating, or they can be characterized by periods of stability and instability with little or no deterioration. Chronicity places demands on people/patients to learn new skills, alter their lifestyles, and make adjustments and adaptations as they learn new ways of functioning. In caring for people/patients whose illness is chronic, nurses need to focus their efforts on helping people/patients to develop resources in meeting these demands. Nurses can minimize people/patients' sense of vulnerability through 'anticipatory guidance' that builds new worlds before old ones are destroyed (Birchfield 1985).

Assisting people/patients whose illness is chronic involves helping them learn to live with their condition. In doing so, nurses must be aware that there is often loss in the learning. They must be prepared to listen with understanding as people/patients whose lives have been changed as a result of their illness mourn the losses that accompany these changes. They are often in a grief process of letting go as they learn to move on.

In relating to people/patients, nurses need to understand the up-and-down nature of most chronic conditions. They must be able to remain with people/patients as they cope with losses as well as gains. It is far easier to share the triumph of success in coping with chronic illness than it is to listen with understanding to the pain that accompanies an exacerbation of the illness or a setback in recovery.

With chronic illness there is often an opportunity for nurses and people/patients to come to know each other over a long period of time and, therefore, the possibility that relationships will progress beyond the therapeutic level of involvement (see Chapter 2), developing into a connected relationship. Through this level of relationship, people/patients and nurses come to understand each other as people. The pain of loss and the joy of successful adaptation that accompanies living with chronic illness is often shared on a personal level between person/patient and nurse.

(e) Living with dying

The ability to form a meaningful relationship with people/patients whose prospects for the future are slim requires a special kind of nursing knowledge and experience. Helping people/patients to live with dying is a specialized area of nursing practice, but it is likely that most nurses will at some time come into contact with people/patients who are acutely aware of their own death.

Many people enter nursing with thoughts of helping people cope with and recover from illness, so the thought of helping people die may be somewhat alien. There is a risk that people/patients who are dying experience abandonment because nurses find it difficult to come to grips with the reality of death. This 'denial of death', as it is often referred to, is a reflection of societal values that revere youth, health and vitality, and look to technological advances that will 'win the battle over death'.

The reality that death is an inevitable part of life is one that nurses will find difficult to deny. While nurses may know that death is a part of life, they may not want to be reminded of this fact by coming face-to-face with a person/patient who is living with dying. Not all nurses have the attributes that equip them to relate effectively to patients whose death is imminent. One of the essential attributes is comfort with the thought of death. The most significant aspect of interpersonally relating to people/patients who are living with dying is that of simply being there, unafraid and unencumbered by fears about death.

Acceptance of death and an awareness of their own thoughts, feelings and values related to dying is essential for nurses who want to connect with people/patients in this situation. Like self-awareness in general (see Chapter 4), if these thoughts, feelings and values are left unexamined and unrecognized, they may interfere with nurses' ability to establish interpersonal contact. A discomfort with thoughts of death may result in inadvertent rejection of people/patients.

A popular conception of how to deal with people/patients who are living with dying is that they pass through various stages as they adjust to their impending death. While such stage theory provides a useful way of understanding how people/patients cope with dying, there is a risk that people/patients will be forced to conform to the theory. For example, once people/patients have experienced denial, nurses may relate to them with an expectation that now is the time to begin the bargaining, the next phase of dying. Rigid adherence to this type of theory forces people/patients to conform to nurses' expectations or may lead to consternation on the part of nurses if people/patients do not conform to the theory.

It is more effective for nurses to listen and understand what these people/patients are experiencing, and to be fully present as other human beings who are willing to be there during the period of 'waiting for death'. Listening and understanding helps to decrease the potential loneliness of this experience.

When nurses do become comfortable with the thought of death there is another risk that they will want, indeed expect, people/patients to discuss dying with them. People/patients who are living with dying do not want to think and focus exclusively on their death, but rather be recognized as still *alive*. People/patients express the need to be cared for in an atmosphere of normality, rather than one that is focused on the fact that they are dying (Arblaster *et al.* 1990). It is not that these people/patients want nurses to deny or ignore that they are dying, but rather they prefer that nurses do not actively direct their conversations to the subject of dying.

When people/patients *do* want to discuss their experience of dying, nurses need to be responsive to such discussions. This requires that nurses follow the person/patient's lead, that is, they should respond to the person/patient with comfort and ease, rather than direct their interactions to the subject of dying.

Helping people/patients with loss and grief

Losses are often experienced during illness. There may be loss of ability to function, loss of ability to achieve life goals, loss of hope, loss of contact and connection with significant people, or loss of flexibility and freedom to determine life goals. Coping with loss is a process of letting go, often accompanied by feelings of sadness, anxiety and sometimes guilt. People/patients who are facing or experiencing loss are frequently consumed by this process and therefore are unable to focus their thoughts.

Most often there is emotional pain as people/patients come to grips with a loss. There is a tendency to focus on the deprivation created by the loss. People/patients whose loss is acute often feel immersed in the experience. When this natural process of healing is allowed to happen, what often follows is a new sense of gain in meeting the demands of the illness.

Grief is a natural reaction to loss. It, too, is a process of letting go, mourning, reflecting, reliving memories, and eventually summoning resources to proceed with life, despite the fact that it may never be the same. Through the experience of grief, people learn to let go and adjust, and eventually adapt to changed life conditions. Grief is a process of closing a chapter of life and gathering energy to begin the next chapter. While there may be energy to begin new phases of life, unveiling the closed chapter is still possible. But this is done as a way of recollecting how it was, of choosing to remember, rather than remaining in the acute pain of loss and grief.

Nurses who understand and appreciate that grieving is a natural process of healing are able to facilitate its spontaneous progression. Through understanding, nurses are able to accept people/patients' expression of feelings, their reliving and reflecting, as an expected and usual progression towards healing.

A central consideration when interacting with people/patients who are grieving is *not* to impede the process through trying to make it all right, ignoring the suffering or dismissing the emotional pain. One of the greatest challenges to nurses is staying with the grieving patient, both emotionally and interpersonally. Remaining with people/patients who are in the depths of despair during a loss is often an emotionally draining experience for nurses. When the loss is real and can no longer be denied or minimized, nurses recognize that they cannot magically alter the situation and bring back what has been lost. Because of this harsh reality nurses often feel helpless and sometimes out of control. In an effort to regain control, false reassurances are sometimes uttered. 'It will be all right', 'Please don't be so upset', or 'You will learn to live again' may *sound* helpful on the surface, but do little to acknowledge the pain that is experienced in loss.

It is better for nurses to come to grips, on a personal and professional level, with the reality of the pain of loss. Accepting that loss is an aspect of nursing that cannot be denied or avoided minimizes the risk of treating it as something that can be intellectually 'problem-solved'. In dealing with people/patients who are experiencing or facing loss, nurses must be able to assist them with reviving memories of what has been lost. Nurses must be comfortable in allowing people/patients' feelings to emerge and be expressed. When the experience of loss is shared with and understood by nurses, people/patients feel consoled and nurtured.

We conclude this section with a final word on helping people/patients with crisis and illness. There is another aspect that nurses need to be aware of when interacting with patients who are experiencing crisis or illness: they should *expect* patients to be self-absorbed with their situation. Crisis situations create tunnel vision that often prevents people who are experiencing them from seeing beyond the immediate circumstances. They are looking inward, trying to make sense of the situation. When helping people/patients in crisis, nurses can assist by broadening the person/patient's perspective and encouraging alternative perspectives. Nevertheless, what may seem obvious to the nurse may be difficult for the person/patient to perceive.

Likewise, because illness can be a lonely experience, people who are ill are often concerned only with themselves. The degree of self-absorption is related to the seriousness of the illness and the amount of pain and suffering that is being experienced. Nurses can help to ease the loneliness of the experience by being available, willing to listen and concerned enough to understand. But they should not expect that people/patients would have the same degree of concern for them.

CHAPTER SUMMARY

Illness, crisis, dying, and death are part of everyday life. They inevitably mean transitions for the person/patient and her/his family, for example, from healthy to ill, independent to dependent, father/mother/brother/sister to carer. However, there is the potential to define these situations in different ways – as threats, challenges and even opportunities. Nurses have the privilege of being in a position to work with the symbols of illness, crisis, dying, and death; with the cues that people in transition offer. Collaboratively, nurses, people/patients and family members can create descriptions and coping strategies to allow the person/patient to feel empowered in relation to the illness experience and able to grow personally. Of course, nurses need to have practical skills in understanding the experience of illness and crisis in order to be able to offer a space in which such construction can occur. The skills of assessing and working with crisis – being calm, fully present and maintaining hope – are critical. But nurses must be sensitive also to the nature of the illness, whether acute, critical, recovering, chronic, or living with dying, loss and grief, while hearing the individual narrative clearly.

REFERENCES

Aguilera, D. C. (1998). *Crisis Intervention: Theory and Methodology*, eighth edition. St Louis, MS: Mosby.

Antonovsky, A. (1987). *Unraveling the Mystery of Health: How People Manage Stress and Stay Well*. San Francisco, CA: Jossey-Bass.

Antonovsky, A. (1996). The sense of coherence: an historical and future perspective. *Israel Journal of Medical Sciences*, 32, 170–8.

Arblaster, G., Brooks, D., Hudson, R. and Petty, M. (1990). Terminally ill patients' expectations of nurses. *The Australian Journal of Advanced Nursing*, 7(3): 34–43.

Benner, P. (1984). *From Novice to Expert: Excellence and Power in Clinical Nursing Practice*. Menlo Park, CA: Addison-Wesley.

Benner, P. and Wrubel, J. (1989). *The Primacy of Caring: Stress and Coping in Health and Illness*. Menlo Park, CA: Addison-Wesley.

Birchfield, M. E. (1985). *Stages of Illness: Guidelines for Nursing Care*. Bowie, MD: Brady Communications.

Brammer, L. M. (1988). *The Helping Relationship*, fourth edition. Englewood Cliffs, NJ: Prentice-Hall.

Brownwell, M. J. (1984). The concept of crisis: its utility for nursing. *Advances in Nursing Science*, 6(4), 10–21.

Clark, H. F. and Driever, M. J. (1983). Vulnerability: the development of a construct for nursing. In P. L. Chinn (ed.), *Advances in Nursing Theory Development* (pp. 207–20). Rockville, MD: Aspen.

Cobb, S. (1976). Social support as a moderator of life stress. *Psychosomatic Medicine*, 38, 300–13.

Cutcliffe, J. R. and Barker, P. (2002). Considering the care of the suicidal client and the case for 'engagement and inspiring hope' or observations. *Journal of Psychiatric and Mental Health Nursing*, 9, 611–21.

Ell, K. (1996). Social networks, social support and coping with serious illness: the family connection. *Social Science and Medicine*, 42, 173–83.

Garmezy, N. (1993). Children in poverty: resilience despite risk. *Psychiatry*, 56, 127–36.

Greenhalgh, T. (1999). Narrative based medicine in an evidence based world. *British Medical Journal*, 318, 323–5.

Hupcey, J. E. (1998). Clarifying the social support theory–research linkages. *Journal of Advanced Nursing*, 27, 1231–41.

Jacelon, C. S. (1997). The trait and process of resilience. *Journal of Advanced Nursing*, 25, 123–9.

Keeling, D. I., Price, P. E., Jones, E. and Harding, K. G. (1996). Social support: some pragmatic implications for health care professionals. *Journal of Advanced Nursing*, 23, 76–81.

Launer, J. (1999) A narrative approach to mental health in general practice. *British Medical Journal*, 318, 117–19.

Lazarus, R. S. and Folkman, S. (1984). *Stress, Appraisal and Coping*. New York: Springer-Verlag.

Mast, M. E. (1995). Adult uncertainty in illness: a critical review of research. *Scholarly Inquiry for Nursing Practice: An International Journal*, 9, 3–24.

Mishel, M. H. (1997). Uncertainty in acute illness. *Annual Review of Nursing Research*, 15, 57–80.

Newton, S. E. (1999). Relationship of hardiness and a sense of coherence to post-liver transplant return to work. *Holistic Nursing Practice*, 13(3), 71–9.

Norbeck, J. S. (1988). Social support. *Annual Review of Nursing Research*, 6, 85–109.

Post-White, J., Ceronsky, C., Kreitzer, M. J., Nickelson, K., Drew, D., Mackey, K. W., Koopmeiners, L. and Gutknecht, S. (1996). Hope, spirituality, sense of coherence, and quality of life in patients with cancer. *Oncology Nursing Forum*, 23, 1571–9.

Sullivan, G. C. (1993). Towards clarification of convergent concepts: sense of coherence, will to meaning, locus of control, learned helplessness and hardiness. *Journal of Advanced Nursing*, 18, 1772–8.

Thoits, P. A. (1982). Conceptual, methodological and theoretical problems in studying social support as a buffer against life stress. *Journal of Health and Social Behavior*, 23, 145–259.

Wagnild, G. and Young, H. M. (1993). Development and psychometric evaluation of the resilience scale. *Journal of Nursing Measurement*, 1, 165–78.

White, R. W. (1974). Strategies of adaptation: an attempt at systematic description. In G. V. Coelho, D. A. Hamburg and J. E. Adams (eds), *Coping and Adaptation* (pp. 47–68). New York: Basic Books.

Williams, G. (1984). The genesis of chronic illness: narrative reconstruction, *Sociology of Health and Illness*, 6, 175–200.

Wittgenstein, L. (1953) *Philosophical Investigations*. Trans. G. E. M. Anscombe. Oxford: Blackwell.

Wolff, A. C. and Ratner, P. A. (1999). Stress, social support and sense of coherence. *Western Journal of Nursing Research*, 21(2), 182–97.

CHAPTER 10

EMPOWERING INTERPERSONAL RELATIONSHIPS

INTRODUCTION: THE PROBLEM OF POWER

In life generally, and in nursing encounters, we tend to behave as if power is a 'thing', something that can be possessed, lost or found, given or taken; as if there is only a certain amount of power to go around. Currently, in the UK, there is much discussion in the nursing literature about the need to empower patients. The concern is driven by government policy that requires patients to be involved at all levels of the care system. For example, patients have greater rights and responsibilities in relation to individual treatment (Department of Health 2001a). At a trust level, they are to have a voice in clinical governance (DoH 1999) and setting benchmarks (DoH 2001b) and through the establishment of Patient Advice and Liaison services (DoH 2000). More widely, they are to contribute to the development of health care strategies (DoH 2001c, d).

But there is a paradox of empowerment (Baistow 1994), if power is conceived of as a thing. Empowerment seems to involve professionals giving back power to patients (see Ryles 1999 for a review of work that takes this position). Price and Mullarkey (1996) define empowerment as 'The process of [*the nurse*[1]] helping the client achieve a position or equality of power within the nurse/client relationship . . .' (p. 17). As the act of giving back power is itself a powerful act, a paradox is evident. Another example of the failure of empowerment concerns consulting service users about services. As Ron Coleman (2000) describes, when service user involvement in planning is initiated, 'tame' user representatives are invited who do not upset the hierarchical status quo. Such paradoxes occur because, more often than not, power is unexamined and people use terms like empowerment and collaborative care unreflectively without recourse to theories of power (Ryles 1999).

Drawing on the theoretical work of Michel Foucault, we argue that power is not simply a commodity, but that it is present only in its enactment, in the

---

[1] Our addition.

interpersonal space between people. In symbolic interactionist terms, power is negotiated in the call–response–call cycle that occurs when people interact.

CHAPTER OVERVIEW

The following discussion aims to encourage the reader to think about power and empowerment in a more sophisticated way that might invite more emancipatory practice. First, the ideas of Michel Foucault, in relation to power/knowledge and surveillance and resistance are outlined. We go on to set out a philosophy and model of empowerment based on the work of Barker *et al.* (2000). Next we discuss the issue of disempowering stereotypes, before turning to a nursing model (Tidal Model, Barker 2000) that offers nurses a different way to practice. Working in a more empowering way requires special skills and we outline these, with reference to Part II of the book. Finally, we give a case example of empowerment in practice.

FOUCAULT'S IDEAS ABOUT POWER

A Foucauldian perspective offers a more liberating understanding of power and empowerment than that based on dividing people into classes, for example the divisions of nurse, doctor, patient, etc., where one class wields power over others. Overturning class hierarchies requires revolution. Using a Foucauldian perspective, especially his position on knowledge/power, surveillance and resistance, invites reflection about how power is enacted in everyday encounters, potentially leading to a re-visioning of nurse–person/patient relationships.

(a) Knowledge/power

Foucault did not believe that power is a commodity or that it resides with certain groups in society. Power is only visible in its enactment between people, in their social practices. For Foucault, knowledge and power are inextricably linked. Any 'version (knowledge[2]) of an event brings with it the potential for social practices, for acting in one way rather than another, and for marginalizing alternative ways of acting' (Burr 1995: 64). Foucault (1979, 1982) noted that the growth in the social sciences provided a more extensive knowledge base for health professionals. As such knowledge increasingly came to be seen as legitimate, serious speech acts (Foucault 1972) were more readily available. Serious speech acts are statements that have their base in knowledge that is accepted by society. Such speech has effects on how people act. 'Therefore the power to act in particular ways, to claim resources, to control or be controlled depends on the "knowledges" currently prevailing in a society' (Burr 1995: 64).

   In relation to biomedicine, Foucault (1976) notes that the knowledge held by doctors about the human body, health and illness, supplies the substance by which medical dominance is established and maintained. Thus, when nurses adopt the knowledge base of medicine, it is unlikely that they will relate to the patient as a

---

[2] My addition in brackets.

person. For example, one kind of knowledge that is available to both doctors and nurses is diagnostic knowledge. Foucault notes the growth of professional power was accompanied by a need to classify and categorize people and their behaviours. There was a need to distinguish between the normal and abnormal. Diagnosis (as a serious speech act) is seen by professionals as helpful, in that it helps to distinguish 'what is not'. Speaking of psychiatry, Jenner (2000) argues that diagnostic categories are meaningful in so far as they allow differentiation of things and allow intellectual content. 'Special words' allow professionals a way of talking about their world of practice. It is convenient shorthand to describe a person as hypertensive, 'schizophrenic' or HIV Positive.

However, this may be disempowering for people/patients. Andrews *et al.* (1996) note that family therapy team members have traditionally kept the process (knowledge) of their work secret from the family members. As 'staff talk' takes place in the private domain, it is an opportunity to say what the staff 'really' think about the family, their diagnosis; special words reflecting special knowledge. However, this tends to be critical, objectifying talk. Thus, implicit in professional diagnostic language is a notion of 'us and them' (Birch 1995). This is implicit power, which becomes explicit in the enactment of diagnosis and treatment. In relation to psychiatry, Birch (1991) points out that medical discourses lead to self-sustaining disabling cycles; a cycle of disqualification, where 'sufferers' and families lose their sense of expertise and defer to the opinion of psychiatric experts; a cycle of victimhood, where 'sufferers' see little hope for a socially fulfilling life; a cycle of fatalism in which the 'sufferer' and her/his social network wait for the next relapse. Thus, how professionals use knowledge has huge repercussions for how the person is treated and how s/he views her/himself, for example, as powerless and out of control, and for how relatives view and respond to the person, for example, as sick and irresponsible. From a symbolic interactionist perspective, the exchange of symbols, diagnosis from the professional in exchange for signs and symptoms from the patient, leads to a definition of the situation that is limited in its possibilities. It does not allow for a negotiation of power because the diagnosis is imposed and is more meaningful for the professional than the patient. In order to arrive at a more democratic and fair position in relation to patients, nurses might reflexively consider how their past and current professional knowledge, personal experience, class, gender, race, ethnicity, and age, create barriers in relation to hearing the expertise of people/patients. In so doing, they may be able to re-connect with the person and establish a different order of interpersonal relationship.

Jackson and Stevenson (2000) have studied the positions that psychiatric nurses can adopt in relation to their people/patients, and the social distance, kinds of knowledge and power these entail. Respondents in the study (people from different psychiatric disciplines, service users and their families) all thought that nurses do, and/or ought to:

- Veer towards being the person/patient's friend (rather than being a detached professional)
- Have the most intimate knowledge about the person/patient (rather than objective case knowledge, but see the section on 'Surveillance and resistance' below)

- Engage with the patient in 'ordinary' conversation (rather than using excluding talk – jargon or professional terminology)
- Become powerful in a non-coercive way, through caring with the patient/person (rather than caring for her/him).

(b) Surveillance and resistance

In relation to health care, Fraser (1995) notes that the professional knows the patient by what they say. People are willing respondents, because to be the focus of inquiry is attractive. From a symbolic interactionist perspective, being asked and answering questions is part of the expectation set that patients bring to the care encounter. But like a collected butterfly impaled on a pin, the patient becomes subject of the professional gaze, interrogated in order that knowledge of the individual is amassed. This knowledge allows the individual 'to be constructed as good or bad, ill or well, moral or immoral, worthy or unworthy . . .' (Fraser 1995: 159). These are implicitly powerful discourses. Once so constructed, the person is obliged to live by this construction. For example, in psychiatry, professionals may engage in an assessment of risk. This can involve the patient answering a broad range of personal questions, which are then the source of an assessment made by the professional. The assessment of risk is acknowledged as problematic, because of the number of variables that need to be taken into account, because of the fluctuations in intention, etc. Yet, professionals frequently behave as if they have captured a picture of the individual. If a high level of risk is perceived, the person is subject to intense surveillance, medication and/or other invasive treatment.

However, there are always different discourses available in relation to a state of affairs, and so there is always the possibility of resistance to the prevailing discourse (or knowledge or 'common' sense). 'For Foucault, power and resistance are two sides of the same coin. The power implicit in one discourse is only apparent from the resistance implicit in another' (Burr 1995: 64). This is a very different view of power from those that see power as being *over* others – the ability to compel others to do something they do not want to do. In a Foucauldian analysis, repression or coercion is demonstrative of a lack of power, a time when the power of discourse breaks down. For Foucault, 'Power is tolerable only on condition that it masks a substantial part of itself. Its success is proportional to its ability to hide its own mechanisms' (Foucault 1976: 86). For example, Bloor and McIntosh (1990) found that Glaswegian mothers resisted the overt surveillance undertaken by health visitors. They did not do this openly, but found covert means to engage in non-co-operation: 'Ye just agree wi' her [health visitor] and do yer own things, 'cause she's no here every day to check' (p. 174). From a symbolic interactionist perspective, mothers and health visitors have not satisfactorily agreed upon the meaning of the situation and there is a divergence in their understandings and consequent practices. Conversely, there is always an opportunity for different understandings to merge. As Crawford *et al.* (1995: 1143) put it:

> Clinical practice is the intersection where meanings of the world converge. The health worker (theories), the client (stories and narratives) and culture (myths, rituals and themes) all converge in the linguistic interaction. Acknowledging

this enables the health care worker not to pathologize or psychologize problems, which might better be conceptualized in political or social [*or personal*[3]] terms.

In this circumstance, it seems more feasible for newly evolved meanings to form the basis of care. For example, in a US study, Meiers and Tomlinson (2003) noted that nurses and family members in a paediatric intensive care unit co-constructed meaning together which then informed the nurses' care giving.

A PHILOSOPHY AND MODEL OF EMPOWERMENT

Empowerment has become a buzzword in relation to being with patients. However, the rhetoric has not been matched with a careful analysis of empowerment, leading to the paradox of empowerment described above. There are other paradoxes that are inherent to nurses trying to empower patients outlined by Elliott and Turrell (1996: 46):

- Advocating 'active' patients while allowing for patient individuality
- Acknowledging patients' right to decide but accepting the practical constraints about their freedom to choose
- Ensuring informed choice without creating information overload
- Providing individualized care without invading patients' privacy
- Anticipating 'normal' patient behaviour in an abnormal (hospital) environment
- Expecting patient behaviour to conform to specific cultural or social norms but accepting individual freedom to adhere to other norms in a pluralistic society.

Despite these challenges, some progress has been made towards empowering interactions. A study by Barker *et al.* (2000) engaged key stakeholders (people/ patients, service-user consultants and CPNs) in an (implicitly) symbolic interactionist research project. The aim was to establish (through the process of grounded theory [Glaser and Strauss 1967] research) a shared meaning concerning a philosophy of empowerment and a model for enacting empowering interactions in psychiatry. The research identified the following underpinning philosophical values:

- Improvement of the person's situation and lifestyle is possible
- Building on strengths is better than focusing on problems
- Collaboration is the key
- Participation is the way
- Self-determination is the ultimate goal and enhancement of the person's capacities will be the result.

A key aim of the empowering relationship is to negotiate, from the outset, power sharing and to, gradually, shift the balance of power towards the person (Barker *et al.* 2000: 8).

---

[3] Our addition.

Barker *et al.*'s (2000) research also led to a model of empowering interactions. In the model, the person is seen as the core, to which all the empowering processes are joined up. The empowering processes are as follows:

1 Being respectful. The empowering CPN recognizes that respecting the person's knowledge and expertise [is essential]. She begins her approach to the person with the implicit assumption that everything about the person is worthy of respect. . . .

2 Putting the person in the driving seat (or client-driven responsiveness). The empowering CPN recognizes that to feel empowered the person needs to have a clear sense of control over the proceedings of the interaction . . . it is essential for the clients to retain control of the purpose, pace and direction of the work.

3 Seeking permission and valuing people's experiences and contributions. By constantly seeking permission to explore any aspect of their experience and encouraging people's contributions, the empowering CPN promotes informed consent within the relationship and an active role for the person.

4 Being curious. The empowering CPN recognizes the importance of expressing genuine interest in the person, her/his life story and aspirations.

5 Learning the language. In the empowering relationship, the disempowering effects of language and labelling on the individual are recognized. Instead, the CPN and person try to negotiate some common ground upon which both may share an appreciation of the preferred use of language and meaning.

6 Taking stock or review and evaluation. The empowering CPN recognizes the importance of summing up the discussion, checking the accuracy of their interpretation and evaluating the usefulness of the whole meeting.

7 Designing the future. The empowering CPN recognizes that the person's life moves on, albeit invisibly. . . . the CPN helps the person to determine what needs to be done next and how. (Barker *et al.* 2000: 8–11)

Taken together, the empowering interactions philosophy and model provide nurses with a different repertoire to bring to the interpersonal encounter, which, in turn, offers the opportunity for a new response from the person/patient. The model was developed for use in acute psychiatry, but its principles would seem to be applicable across specialities and across the life span. However, it is clear that the application of the principles will involve sensitivity to age, gender, and racial and cultural stereotypes.

DISEMPOWERING STEREOTYPES

There are many ways in which empowering interactions and relationships can be prevented. An important consideration is how stereotypes get in the way of seeing the person and so in the way of establishing meaningful partnerships. The following case scenario illustrates this:

A nine-year-old Lebanese boy, Amal, was admitted to a surgical children's ward post surgery for a ruptured appendix. Amal was very ill for the first three days, receiving a continuous morphine infusion for pain. As the days passed, Amal 'should' have been improving; he remained highly anxious and refused to talk to anyone other than his mother, whom he would not allow to leave his side. His mother was continually at the nurses' station asking for something for his pain and the nursing staff developed strategies to administer what they considered inappropriate amounts of analgesia. At the shift handover, nurses began to talk about this 'over-anxious child and his over-anxious mother'. There was a sense that this was typical from people from 'that part of the world'. On day seven, however, a large quantity of pus was drained from behind the suture line. Within 24 hours Amal was up playing with the other children and the next night his mother was able to sleep at home.

In the following section we look at how ageist and cultural stereotypes prevent communication and the establishment of an empowering interpersonal relationship and shared meaning about a care episode.

(a) Age and ageism

Nurses encounter people of all ages in their professional lives. They need to be able to adapt their practice accordingly. For example, communication with younger people needs to take account of the level of sophistication the person has in relation to language and concepts used. At the other end of the human life cycle, older adults who have a more extensive life experience may challenge nurses. Difficulties in interacting may be due to generational differences (Kimmel 1980). For example, young people tend to be oriented towards the future, whereas older people tend to spend more time thinking about the past. This is not surprising since most of a young person's life is in the future and most of the older person's life is in the past. Values and attitudes to life tend to be shaped by the major economic and other world events through which people have lived. Often, however, there are particular stereotypes concerning youth and age that are negative, for example, ideas that young people are not able to take responsibility for their health and are more likely to engage in risky behaviour, ideas that older people are less able to change or are less capable in relation to remembering or contributing to society. These attitudes are embedded in ageist societies. If nurses want to take empowerment seriously, it is important to respect the expertise of the person (young or old) in relation to their world. Taking a symbolic interactionist perspective, selfhood is constantly being re-invented as the person monitors other people's reactions to her/him. The 'other' provides a 'looking glass self' (Cooley 1902) that contains information about the person. Thus, the reflection of negative attitudes to the younger or older person can create a negative sense of self that means the person feels unworthy or inadequate, and most definitely not empowered to be a partner in care.

(b) Culture

Culture is the total system of beliefs, values and practices in a society or social group. It provides the framework for that particular society's way of life; it influences the way social life is regulated; it guides interactions between the members of a social group; and it influences the way they understand and make sense of the world. Differences in cultural understanding commonly lie outside conscious awareness. For example, Western medicine tends to see health and illness in biomedical terms. On the other hand, indigenous peoples of Australia believe that disharmony and discontinuity cause ill-health and healing seeks to reintegrate people with one another and with the environment (Short *et al.* 1998: 156). There is the potential for one cultural understanding to dominate the other. Without cultural awareness, there is the possibility of the nurse misreading cues from the person. For example, Martin and Belcher (1986) found that North Americans tend to believe that screaming is a common response when people experience intense pain, while South Africans believe that people in severe pain are more likely to be quiet and withdrawn. So, the interpretation of the person/ patient's presentation can be inaccurate and this, in turn, communicates a lack of understanding. If the person/patient feels misunderstood, they are unlikely to have a sense of empowerment. To interact effectively with members of different cultural groups, it is necessary to be more culturally aware and less ethnocentric. Ethnocentrism is a tendency to see the world as having one standard, that of one's own cultural group, and to judge other cultural groups in relation to it. In becoming more culturally aware, nurses develop an understanding and acceptance of the differences that exist between different groups of people and are more willing to investigate the practices and rituals that are associated with different cultural groups. Some of the more fundamental of these practices include the care of the body after death, religious rituals, beliefs associated with food, and childbirth customs.

However, cultural awareness is not enough. Cultural safety is a term that embodies empowerment. Nurses have a duty to provide care that is physically and psychologically safe, but their duty extends to providing culturally safe care (Polaschek 1998; Ramsden 1993). Cultural safety is more than simply learning about cultural practices and beliefs; it is an ethical standard that recognizes the position of cultural groups and how they are perceived. Likewise, unsafe practice is any action that demeans or diminishes cultural identity and well-being (Polaschek 1998). Imposing a biomedical perspective on illness while dismissing beliefs that do not fit a biomedical model is an example of culturally unsafe practice. Cultural safety is more than a recognition of the uniqueness of cultural identity and the need for equity in health care. Cultural safety includes recognition of social structures that disempower cultural groups, for example, the hierarchy of care systems based in scientific knowledge described above.

Barnes and Bowl (2001) rightly state that the important question concerns how power is used and not what it is. In common with Foucault, they see power as potentially creative, in that it can be used to make opportunities in relation to helping people live their lives. The Tidal Model of psychiatric and mental health nursing (© Barker 2000) is based on empowering interactions and illustrates the nuts and bolts of empowering practice, whether in psychiatry or more broadly in nursing care. It is culturally sensitive and it minimizes the possibility of basing care on stereotypes because it requires the nurse place the person/patient's story central in assessment and care planning. It embodies cultural safety because it uses the person's own language and definition of the problem situation, and does not use diagnostic structures that disempower cultural groups, for example, by associating being black with being schizophrenic (Fernando 2000).

THE TIDAL MODEL

As mentioned above, The Tidal Model (TM, © Barker 2000) is based on empowering interactions, but it draws also on Peplau's (1952) theory of interpersonal relations, and the Newcastle Need for Nursing Study (Jackson and Stevenson 2000). The TM has three different, but related, dimensions of care: the 'world', 'self' and 'others'. In the 'world' dimension, the focus is on the person's need to be understood. Irrespective of whether the person is in physical or mental distress, s/he needs to have the experience validated by other people. In assessing the person, the nurse accesses what the problem is and what effect it has on the person's life. The aspects of the person's story that the person considers significant are documented in her/his own words. In the 'self' dimension, the focus is upon the person's need for physical and emotional security. The nurse's line of inquiry concerns what has to happen or be in place for the person to feel safe and supported. In the 'others' dimension, there is an emphasis on finding the right kind of support from a wide range of people and services, in order that the person can function at the best possible level. Box 1 outlines the critical features of the TM.

Box 1 Critical features of the Tidal Model (adapted from Stevenson and Fletcher (2001: 34) to be generalizable to nursing across specialities)

- Active collaboration with the individual and family, where appropriate to plan and deliver care
- Empowerment of the person by locating the narrative experience (McIntyre 1981) of illness and health at the heart of the care plan (Newnes *et al.* 2000)
- Integration of nursing with the service provided by other members of the multidisciplinary team
- Resolution of problems of living and promotion of health through narrative-based interventions, which complement physical interventions

---

In the following section, we suggest some practical skills for working in a more empowering way with people/patients.

SKILLS OF EMPOWERING INTERPERSONAL RELATIONSHIPS

The shared meaning of what might be therapeutic arises through the process of the interpersonal relationship. As Barker (© 2000: 20) rightly points out, the most realistic intervention is one that is consonant with the needs, worldview, and values and motivation of the person concerned. Therefore, the most important skills are those that can help empowering interactions to occur that elicit information about these areas. By focusing as follows (adapted from © Barker 2000) and using the identified skills, the nurse may help the conversation to flow.

1   *Why this and why now?*   The nurse needs to know what the major presenting problem is (see Chapter 7). However, the context in which the problem came into existence and the current situation are also important. The nurse uses curious questioning skills – 'What's brought you here to the clinic?' – and active listening to make sure s/he has a feel for what the person is experiencing and what must be done as soon as possible to relieve distress and begin to resolve the problem. Sometimes, the process of listening to and hearing requires some creativity, sometimes because of differences in intellectual functioning or age-related differences. For example, Alderman (2000) reports the work of John Killick, who was a writer in residence with Westminster Health Care and worked in nursing and residential homes. After a year, he was asked to work in a dementia unit with 30 people with different kinds and stages of dementia. He openly described himself as terrified. However, he spent time with the people/patients and encouraged them to talk of their life experiences. He noted that people 'often respond to him in quasi-poetic language, which he then develops into poems for them. Many of these conversations reveal awareness of the future, the passage of time and social change and a reluctance to trouble others' (Alderman 2000: 18). Killick noted that it was crucial to 'shut up and listen' (see Chapter 6) and amazed nursing staff by typing up a life story that the home staff had not managed to access in the six months the man had been resident.

   With children, it may be necessary to use different modes of communication. For example, to ask a young child to draw a picture of the problem which can then be the focus of a conversation.

2   *What works?*   The person has a personal expertise about the problem. They may (because of expectations about 'the professional front) not think that they have a contribution to make. They may say 'Well, you're the expert, what do you think?' However, the nurse does not offer standardized therapeutic techniques that have some general value. S/he tries to discover what has worked for the person in the past ('When you last had the pain, what did you find was useful in reducing it?'), or what might work for the person in the future, given the person's history, personality and general life circumstances ('Given that you have nobody at home who can look after you during the day, do you think that you might want to spend some time with a relative or attend a day centre?'). The nurse may outline some treatment possibilities but is careful to explain these thoroughly, especially if the person has difficulty in understanding (see Chapter 6).

3   *What is the person's personal theory?*   Unless the nurse understands the person's personal theory regarding the illness, then s/he may offer the person an intervention that is simply not 'fitting' (see Chapter 9). The nurse may ask questions such as 'When you think about the breastfeeding, why do you think the baby seems reluctant to suck?' The nurse does not offer the professionalized explanation as in any way superior, but listens carefully to what the personal theory is. The personal theory may vary across the lifespan or because of religious or cultural reasons. It is important that the nurse does not place a value judgement on the person's theory but explores where it has come from, how it affects the person's responses in the present

and how it may work or not work with any particular treatment. Nor should the nurse simply try to replace the person's explanation with her own preferred version. For example, children often perceive that those that are caring for them do not tell the truth (Ross and Ross 1984). For the 'truth' to be heard by children, it needs to be couched in terms that can be absorbed and in a form that is compatible with the particular child's developmental age, as they will have different kinds of explanation at different stages, for example, concrete explanations such as 'You just get it' through to psychophysiological, for example, ' When you're all stressed out, that makes your immune system not work properly'.

4   *How to limit restrictions?*   The nurse tries to allow the person the space in which to conduct her/his own care as well as being there to offer help. The nurse does not own the interpersonal relationship, and is giving the person responsibility for it and bringing about change. Consequently, the nurse has to feel able to answer difficult questions ('Will it hurt?') with as much honesty as possible but with a sense of caring and at an appropriate level also. It would be useless to explain to a two-year-old the links between intravenous therapy and the circulatory system and movement of a part of the body. But s/he might be able to accept a magical explanation, for example, 'The new blood will make you pink and strong enough to play with the other children'.

From the above, it is clear how the interpersonal skills outlined in the previous chapters will contribute to empowering relationships with people/patients. However, the case study below further demonstrates how empowering relationships and caring with the person are enacted.

A CASE STUDY IN EMPOWERING INTERACTIONS

The case study reports the work of Reed and colleagues who developed a unique way of working with people who are admitted to an acute in-patient psychiatric ward (Reed *et al.* 1998). When a person is admitted to hospital, s/he has much anxiety and confusion in relation to the change that is occurring. Disempowerment is almost inevitable. Often family members are upset and do not know what to do for the best. Staff are not always able to keep the boundary between hospital and community open (Scott 1973), and the person is stripped of the context in which s/he has been living. Reed developed social network meetings, which were offered to people/patients and their significant others (including family, friends, ward staff, and other involved professionals) shortly after admission. Members of a local systemic therapy team who had expertise in co-ordinating a group discussion facilitated the meetings. The meetings had multiple functions, all of which are consistent with the empowering interactions model outlined above:

- To tell the story or previously untold stories of events leading up to the admission
- As a forum to express emotions

- To express fears about the severity of the problems and about their involvement with psychiatry
- As an opportunity for the family to inform and educate the staff about the family's culture
- To explore myths about mental illness and psychiatry
- For finding out from staff about the ward and the service generally [for example, staff roles, how decisions are taken in the unit, etc.]
- To ask questions, express concerns or dissatisfactions regarding aspects of the service
- As a forum for making plans
- As a safe place to raise difficult topics between family members
- To discuss actual or potential issues of stigma or discrimination that the service user/family might encounter as a consequence of the admission
- For the discussion of practical arrangements.

(Reed *et al.* pp. 52–3)

Because the meetings were inclusive of family members, it was sometimes necessary to have an interpreter present to help any attendees who did not have English as their first language. Indeed, this was the situation in the reception meeting reported below. It is important to use a trained health interpreter.

A reception meeting was organized for Ms X, a Bangladeshi woman in her early twenties and her family. Ms X had been admitted to hospital once before and had stayed a short while before going back to the family home. She had been described as a 'difficult patient', as she had not engaged with the nursing staff. There was no sense that being in hospital had made a difference to her 'condition', which was thought to be some kind of psychosis. She had refused routine admission procedures (medical examination and nursing assessment) on both admissions. Ms X declined the invitation to attend the meeting but was happy for her parents to come along and a community worker who was involved with her. An interpreter was invited, as the parents were not able to express themselves in English.

In the meeting, Ms X's parents were asked to tell their story about what had led up to the admission, what had been helpful or unhelpful in the past, for their ideas about what was happening for their daughter now that she was in hospital, and what would have to happen to make the stay useful for both her and her family. It transpired that Ms X had refused medical examination because of cultural and religious beliefs about her body being seen by a male doctor. She could not be in a one-to-one with a male member of nursing staff for assessment. Her parents thought that this would tarnish her. Once the cultural difference was exposed, it was easily arranged with the member of ward staff that a female doctor would be asked to make an examination, and it was arranged that if a male member of nursing staff needed to approach Ms X he would be chaperoned by a female nurse. These simple measures allowed care to proceed on a different basis on the second admission, with Ms X more in the driving seat.

CHAPTER SUMMARY

In order to allow the person, as well as the patient, to express her/himself it is important for power to be negotiated within the interpersonal relationship.

However, power is not a commodity to be given or taken. As Foucault points out, power is visible only in its enactment. Having privileged knowledge (discourses) affects how people act. Professional use special (serious) speech acts that position people as patients. However, alternative positions are available. Barker *et al.*'s (2000) philosophy/model of empowerment puts the person's needs, strengths and potential central and encourages collaborative, participatory care. It circumvents the damage that disempowering stereotypes create. The Tidal Model of psychiatric and mental health nursing (© Barker 2000) and a clinical case study illustrate how empowering interactions are possible in the real world of caring.

REFERENCES

Alderman, C. (2000). The art of listening. *Nursing Standard*, 14(20), 18.

Andrews, J., Birch, J., Reed, A., Spriddell, G. and Stevenson, C. (1996). The construction of authority: context and power in family meetings. *Changes*, 14, 282–8.

Baistow, K. (1994). Liberation and regulation? Some paradoxes of empowerment. *Critical Social Policy*, 14(3), 34–69.

Barker, P. J. (2000). *The Tidal Model: Theory and Practice*. Newcastle: University of Newcastle.

Barker, P. J., Stevenson, C. and Leamy, M. (2000). The philosophy of empowerment. *Mental Health Nursing*, 20(9), 812.

Barnes, M. and Bowl, R. (2001). *Taking Over the Asylum: Empowerment and Mental Health*. UK: Palgrove.

Birch, J. (1991). Borderlines. *Journal of Family Therapy*, 18, 285–8.

Birch, J. (1995). Chasing the rainbow's end, and why it matters: a coda to Pocock, Frosh and Larner. *Journal of Family Therapy*, 17, 219–28.

Bloor, M. and McIntosh, J. (1990). Surveillance and concealment: a comparison of techniques of client resistance in therapeutic communities and health visiting. In S. Cunningham-Burley and N. P. McKeganey (eds), *Readings in Medical Sociology*. London: Routledge.

Burr, V. (1995). *An Introduction to Social Constructionism*. London: Routledge.

Coleman, R. (2000). In P. J. Barker and C. Stevenson (eds), *The Construction of Power and Authority in Psychiatry*. Oxford: Butterworth Heineman.

Cooley, C. H. (1902). *Human Nature and Social Order*. New York: Scribners.

Crawford, P., Nolan, P. and Brown, B. (1995). Linguistic entrapment: medico-nursing biographies as fictions. *Journal of Advanced Nursing*, 22(6), 1141–8.

Department of Health (1999). *Clinical Governance. Quality and the New NHS*. Health Service Circular 1999/065.

Department of Health (2000). *The NHS Plan*. London: DoH.

Department of Health (2001a). *The Patients' Charter and You: A Charter for England*. London: DoH.

Department of Health (2001b). *The Essence of Care: Patient Focused Benchmarking for Healthcare Practitioners*. London: DoH.

Department of Health (2001c). *Building a Safer NHS for Patients*. London: DoH.

Department of Health (2001d). *Involving Patients and the Public in Healthcare: A Discussion Document*. London: DoH.

Elliott, M. and Turrell, A. (1996). Understanding the conflicts of patient empowerment. *Nursing Standard*, 19(45), 45–7.

Fernando, S. (2000). Imperialism, racism and psychiatry. In P. J. Barker and C. Stevenson (eds), *The Construction of Power and Authority in Psychiatry*. Oxford: Butterworth Heineman.

Foucault, M. (1972). *The Archaeology of Knowledge and the Discourse on Language*. New York: Harper.

Foucault, M. (1976). *Birth of the Clinic*. London: Tavistock.

Foucault, M. (1979). *Discipline and Punish*. Harmondsworth: Penguin.

Foucault, M. (1982). Afterword. In H. L. Dreyfus and P. Rabinow (eds), *Beyond Structuralism and Hermeneutics*. Brighton: Harvester.

Fraser, M. (1995). The nurse as social scientist: the use of Michel Foucault's analytic. *Social Sciences in Health: International Journal of Research & Practice*. 1(3), 158–63.

Glaser, B. and Strauss, A. (1967). *The Discovery of Grounded Theory*. Chicago: Aldine.

Jackson, S. and Stevenson, C. (2000). What do people need psychiatric and mental health nurses for? *Journal of Advanced Nursing*, 31, 378–88.

Jenner, A. (2000). Deconstructing over half a century of increasing involvement with psychiatry. In P. J. Barker and C. Stevenson (eds), *The Construction of Power and Authority in Psychiatry*. Oxford: Butterworth Heineman.

Kimmel, D. C. (1980). *Adulthood and Ageing*. New York: John Wiley.

Martin, B. A. and Belcher, J. V. (1986). Influence of cultural background on nurses' attitudes and care of the oncology patient. *Cancer Nursing*, 9(5), 230–7.

Meiers, S. J. and Tomlinson, P. S. (2003). Family–nurse co-construction of meaning: a central phenomenon of family caring. *Scandanavian Journal of Caring Sciences*, 17(2), 193–201.

Polaschek, N. R. (1998). Cultural safety: a new concept in nursing people of different ethnicities. *Journal of Advanced Nursing*, 27, 452–7.

Price, V. and Mullarkey, K. (1996). Use and misuse of power in the psycho-therapeutic relationship. *Mental Health Nursing*, 16(1), 16–17.

Ramsden, I. (1993). Kawa Whakaruruhau: cultural safety in nursing education in Aotearoa (New Zealand). *Nursing Praxis*, 8(3), 4–10.

Reed, A., Stevenson, C. and Wilson, M. (1998) Social network meetings ease trauma of psychiatric admission. *Nursing Times*, 94(42), 52–3.

Ross, D. M. and Ross, S. A. (1984). The importance of type of question, psychological climate and subject set in interviewing children about pain. *Pain*, 19, 71–9.

Ryles, S. M. (1999). A concept analysis of empowerment: its relationship to mental health nursing. *Journal of Advanced Nursing*, 2, 600–7.

Scott, R. D. (1973). The treatment barrier: Part 1. *British Journal of Medical Psychology*, 46, 45–55.

Short, S., Sharman, E. and Speedy, S. (1998). *Sociology for Nurses: An Australian Introduction*. Melbourne: Macmillan Education Australia.

CHAPTER 11

INTER-PROFESSIONAL WORKING: BEATING STRESS AND EMPOWERING PROFESSIONALS

INTRODUCTION

The central premise of this book is that good relationships between people/ patients and nurses are at the heart of good nursing care. This is because inter-personal relationships are the location where meaning in the situations of health, illness, crisis and care are negotiated. Various contextual factors that need to be taken into consideration in the formation of these relationships have been described in previous chapters. These factors are embedded within the nurse (for example, self-awareness, professional attributes), within the person/patient (for example, the desire to be informed, expectation of the nurse) and within the health event at hand (for example, the nature of an illness and the responses to it).

Nevertheless, there are considerations that extend beyond the specifics of the individual nurse, the person/patient and the situation. Of equal consideration is the environment of the health-care setting in which person/patient and nurse come together. For example, if person/patient care is organized so that a person/patient and a nurse rarely see each other on more than one occasion, then the depth of involvement and mutual understanding is restricted by limited opportunity to get to know each other. This chapter focuses on another important consideration: promotion of a supportive inter-professional working environment that promotes person/patient-centred care.

For many years the Department of Health (1989, 1998, 2000) has stressed the need for closer collaboration and inter-professional[1] working between health and

---

[1] Inter-professional within this context means where professionals learn from and about each other to improve collaboration and the quality of care.

social care professionals in the delivery of effective person/patient care. From a symbolic interactionist perspective, it makes sense for professionals to interrelate. For example, it allows feedback to individual practitioners about the care that they have been involved in; it provides a space in which the professional can experiment with different ways in which s/he can present her/himself within a care episode, for example, as a counsellor or as a psychotherapist; it is a means of constructing a sense of self, as a set of personal and professional attributes becomes defined and re-defined. Indeed, the last point is very important. As professional boundaries are being realigned, it is possible that individuals become disconnected from their practice, lose a sense of self and feel de-skilled, disempowered and stressed. As we argue later, inter-professional working can help to address these difficulties. Despite these obvious advantages, studies such as Reeves *et al.* (1999) and Annandale *et al.* (1999) showed that difficulties are still being encountered relating to inter-professional co-ordination and communication.

Each professional body, for example, the Nursing and Midwifery Council, the General Medical Council, Allied Health Professional Governing Bodies, has identified benchmarks that each award holder must demonstrate they have met in order to achieve their professional qualification. The QAA (2001) identified the benchmarks referring to collaboration for health care, some of which are listed below:

- Participate effectively in inter-professional and multi-agency approaches to health and social care, where appropriate
- Work, where appropriate, with other health- and social-care professionals and support staff and patients/clients/carers to maximize health outcomes
- Communicate effectively with patients/clients/carers and other relevant parties when providing care
- Assist other health care professionals in maximizing health outcomes
- Contribute to the well-being and safety of all people in the workplace
- Recognize the place and contribution of his/her assessment within the total health care profile/package, through effective communication with other members of the health-care team.

These are only a sample of the benchmarks that identify the need for effective inter-professional working and collaboration between health-care professionals.

The political agenda is changing the face of the NHS and the workforce within it. Health-care providers, including the nurse, are now expected to develop new roles, to extend their practice to take on the roles of other professionals in the promotion of a more seamless care provision for the person/patient. Today we see nurses developing their roles as Nurse Consultants, Specialist Practitioners, Clinical Specialists, Nurse Champions, Nurse Prescribers, to name but a few. All of these roles involve blurring the professional boundary for the nurse working in a more effective collaborative health-care system. The implications of taking on such roles include coping with change, developing the required knowledge from nursing and other professionals to underpin the new roles, as well as remaining the autonomous and accountable professional nurse in the decision-making process of care provision.

Not only are the roles of staff changing within health-care provision, but also the role and the expectations of the person/patient have changed in regard to health care provision. The introduction of the Patient's Charter (1992) encouraged people to become more aware of their rights and have more input into decisions on their care provision. The passive participant in care is now often an active participant in the health-care decision-making process, keen on contributing more to the definition of the health situation. However, the staff are more accustomed to leading the process and at times the individual and her/his family's priorities for health care are in conflict with the professionals providing the care. Dealing with the conflict of care provision engenders a highly emotive stressful situation for the health-care provider.

The need for supportive inter-professional relationships in the work environment is dealt with in this book as it can be seen from the previous section interpersonal involvement with people/patients can be professionally and personally demanding for the carers involved. The changing roles of the nurse may tax the nurse's internal coping resources as they are brought close to their own human vulnerability as well as that of the person/patient's vulnerability, suffering, pain, fragility, anxiety, and death. These realities, potential sources of stress in nursing practice, are not easily denied or avoided when there is interpersonal connection between nurse, person/patient and other care providers. Emotional detachment, one possible way of coping with the reality of nursing practice, is not possible under such circumstances. Alternative methods for coping must be accessed.

Peer support is now a recognized and encouraged method of dealing with the stress of nursing and working within the health-care setting. Support from others is not a coping mechanism *per se*, but rather a fruitful resource that reduces stress and enhances effective coping. Supportive relationships with colleagues are not automatic; they require active cultivation in order to develop and grow.

CHAPTER OVERVIEW

This chapter first explores the need for social support in nursing by reviewing general aspects of nursing practice that contribute to work-related stress and disempowerment. The changing roles of the profession and the interpersonal involvement with patients/persons is highlighted as specific facets of this stress. The need for social support in occupational stress is briefly reviewed with specific reference to colleagues as a basis for such support. The relationship between colleague interaction and work-related stress is reviewed in the next section. Potential constraints in the formation of a supportive interpersonal work environment are explored on three levels: personal, professional and organizational. Enhancement of a supportive inter-professional work environment in nursing is a natural follow-on to this discussion, and the final section of the chapter includes recommendations for the development of this environment.

STRESS AND NURSING

The provision of nursing care is both physically and emotionally demanding, and stress in nursing is acknowledged and accepted as part and parcel of the profession. The number of articles about stress that appear in the nursing literature attests to this fact. Stress and disempowerment are logically linked. Disempowerment is experienced when people lose their citizenship rights (sometimes through unemployment, poverty and poor housing), through active discrimination, through assumed incompetence or less competence, through feelings of lack of self-worth and hopelessness (Barnes and Bowl 2001). It is clear that nurses are in positions where they are particularly vulnerable to these factors, as demonstrated above and below. It is unclear whether disempowerment causes stress, stress causes disempowerment, or whether they feed each other. However, the reduction of stress and empowerment are likely to go hand in hand.

Workload, too much to do in too little time with too few resources, and dealing with death and dying rank high on the list of factors contributing to stress in nursing (Dunn *et al.* 1994; Gentry and Parkes 1982; Gray-Toft and Anderson 1981; Hipwell *et al.* 1989; Kushnir *et al.* 1997; Ness 1982; Snape and Cavanagh 1993; Tyler *et al.* 1991). Nurses often face people who are distressed, vulnerable and in need of assistance and support. Even when not directly caring for ill people, as in the case of health promotion, nurses must still provide assistance and support in fostering others to change health patterns. Health care is provided on a 24-hour-a-day, 365-days-a-year basis, and nurses often provide and/or organize the bulk of this care. Hours are often long and shift work can be energy-depleting. Nurses in the community are often stretched to provide nursing care for increasing numbers of patients/persons who are now cared for in the home environment.

Health-care organizations impose additional demands, such as new roles, limited resources and an over-developed bureaucratic hierarchy. In these organizations, nurses are often accountable to multiple authorities, such as employers, doctors' orders, professional standards, and government bodies. An individual nurse also has personal expectations and standards of care that may conflict with the demands of the bureaucracy. Small wonder that nurses describe themselves as disempowered. As Davidson (1997) puts it, (psychiatric) nurses do not have a well-defined theoretical position to help them define their territory. They have low prestige within the medical hierarchy, and as a result, seem to experience a sense of disempowerment. According to Ryle (1999) attempts to establish a 'power base', such as the movement to 'new nursing' (Salvage 1988, 1990, 1992) often rely on establishing élite practice, which serves to distance the nurse and person/patient from one another. Of course, the creation of distance is contrary to ideas conveyed in this book about the centrality of the interpersonal relationship in caring and comforting, even allowing that these relationships can be a source of stress, as shown below.

Thus, stress and disempowerment in nursing is generated from a multiplicity of sources – personal, professional and organizational. Irvine and Evans (1996) have integrated findings from a number of research studies to investigate the relationship between job satisfaction and nurses leaving their jobs (job turnover). In their meta-analysis they found that individual differences in nurses were not as pronounced as work-environment variables in determining the cause of dissatisfaction with work and turnover in nursing. Rather than focusing on characteristics of individual nurses, it is more fruitful to consider organizational realities such as colleague support and collaboration when considering job stress.

Interpersonal involvement

The added dimension of close interpersonal involvement with people/patients could be viewed as yet another demand placed on nurses. Interpersonal closeness with people/patients may challenge and even threaten the nurse's sense of competence and control because there are often no clear answers to people/patients' expressed concerns or expectations, no procedure or protocol to consult. Nurses may experience a sense of loss if people/patients die or fail to recover. Coming close to human suffering and pain brings into conscious awareness the nurse's own vulnerability as a human being.

Furthermore, interpersonal involvement with people/patients, as a professional value, may come into conflict with bureaucratic values such as tangible productivity and cost-effectiveness. Spending time talking with people/patients is still viewed by some nurses as 'wasting time' or an activity that is done after the 'real' work is completed. A good nurse is a busy nurse and nurses who are spending time relating with people/patients simply do not appear busy! All of this may add to the perceived work-related stress of nurses who try to put into effect the interpersonal skills described in this book.

The experience of stress

Each of the factors mentioned, or any combination of them, can produce stress in nursing. Stress is a complex phenomenon that encompasses more than simply the factors that provide its stimulus (stressors). Stress is a transactional process involving a complex interplay between perceived demands of the environment and the perceived resources for meeting these demands (Lazarus and Folkman, 1984). It results from a perception that a demand is potentially harmful, will result in personal loss, is threatening or challenging *and* that resources for meeting the demand are inadequate, unavailable, unusable, or inappropriate in the situation. A lack of balance between the perceived demands and the perceived availability of resources results in feelings of vulnerability (see Chapter 9). Therefore, it is not an event itself (stressor), or the personal resources and coping capabilities alone that create stress, but rather their dynamic combination that produces a stressful experience.

Personal appraisal (perception) is critical in this process because it determines whether the demand is interpreted as harmful or threatening, and whether internal and external resources for coping are seen to be accessible and adequate (see Chapter 10). These perceptions relate to questions such as: 'What is the situation?', 'What can I do to manage it?', 'Who or what can I call on to manage it?' For example, a nurse working in a critical care area may be required to wean a person/patient off a mechanical ventilator (demand). An experienced critical-care nurse, who has weaned many people/patients from ventilators, may perceive this situation as relatively benign (no stress). On the other hand, a nurse who has recently completed an advanced course in critical-care nursing may view the same situation as a challenge and call on available coping resources such as knowledge and problem-solving. A newly registered nurse, with little or no experience and education in critical care, may appraise the same situation as a threat for which there are no capabilities or resources. The same event results in three different responses according to how it is perceived.

The need for support

Asking nurses to become interpersonally involved with people/patients without addressing the need for resources to cope with this is unrealistic at best and irresponsible at worst. The perceived demands placed on nurses that occur as a result of interpersonal involvement need to be met through the cultivation of a supportive inter-professional working environment that functions as a resource for coping with such demands. Other nurses and professionals involved in the person/patient care are central players in this environment because support from colleagues not only helps to decrease the perceived stress but also functions as a resource for coping.

This support comes in a variety of forms. The proverbial pat on the back, which offers personal encouragement, affirmation and validation, is the most frequent interpretation of how support for others is demonstrated. Nevertheless, there are other manifestations, such as tangible aid and assistance, and informational support in the form of feedback, suggestions and advice. A final type of support, particularly relevant to the work environment, is situation-specific support (Norbeck *et al.* 1981). This form of support emanates from another person who has experienced or is experiencing a similar situation, one who understands the complexity and nuances of the situation, one who has 'been there, done that'. This situation-specific support encompasses all the other types of support mentioned, as illustrated in the following story:

> Tom, a first-year nursing student, faints during his initial visit to the operating theatre. Mary, a veteran theatre nurse, assists Tom in recovering from the fainting episode and escorts him to the staff tea room [tangible support]. After he recovers, she says to him, 'I bet this is embarrassing for you, and you probably wish you could crawl into a hole [emotional support]. I'll let you in on a little secret. The same thing has happened to me. I do have one question, have you eaten breakfast?'
> 'No,' Tom replies hesitantly.
> 'I knew it,' Mary responds. 'Look, let me give you a bit of advice. It's a good idea to eat breakfast before you come on duty, especially in theatre. It may help prevent this from happening again.' [informational support]

Mary's support is both emotional and informational; she reassures Tom and shares information that is useful to him. Her awareness of Tom's situation emerges from her understanding of this event, in this context, at this time. Her support is situation-specific.

The importance of supporting colleagues within the health care environment has been documented in many reports such as the Clunis Report (1994) and the Clothier Report (1994). The Falling Shadow report (1995) suggested that 'even the most skilled and experienced amongst us can benefit from reflecting on our practice under the guidance of a skilled practitioner whom we trust' (p. 140).

From a symbolic-interactionist perspective this makes sense. When a nurse finds her/himself struggling or stuck with an episode of care, it is likely that s/he has not managed to negotiate a meaningful definition of the situation with the person/patient. By seeking support and guidance there is a chance to re-visit and analyse the situation, and generate ideas that might free up the conversation/ interaction with the person/patient allowing care to be negotiated.

Clinical supervision is often used in the caring environment to provide this situational support. Reflecting on the situation and exploring why it happened with other colleagues enables the nurse to use the experience of others as a basis for developing strategies to cope with the situation should it arise again. Although the above example demonstrated how an experienced theatre nurse supported the student nurse, the support could have been given by a doctor, an operational department practitioner, an anaesthetist, in fact anyone in the team who had experienced fainting on their first encounter in the theatre environment.

INTER-PROFESSIONAL WORKING AND WORK-RELATED STRESS

The relationship between inter-professional working and stress in nursing is complex because each individual functions both as a resource for handling or modifying this stress *and* as a source of stress. Each professional has her/his own aims for the person/patient care and at times this will conflict or support the professional considerations of others in the team. Supportive inter-professional relationships and interactions have potentially positive effects; inter-professional relationships and interactions that lack support can add to work stress, creating negative effects not only for the nurse or professional involved but for the person/patient who is receiving the care.

Supportive inter-professional relationships and interactions need to be developed by the professionals involved. Inter-professional working is a fairly new concept in health care provision. Many times this is interrelated with multi-professional working.

Multi-professional working has been evident in the caring environment for decades. It is still commonly seen in the health care setting today, particularly within the adult-care environment. This is where professionals work side by side but stay isolated within their professional boundary – the doctor gives the order and the other professionals carry these out, for example, when a person/patient is admitted with breathing difficulties after clinical assessment, it is traditionally the doctor who orders the drugs, the X-rays, the physiotherapy assessment and so forth. The nurse then co-ordinates the team roles and ensures all information is related back to the doctor for his/her next decision on the person/patient's care. Each professional decision for the person/patient is made in isolation. The person/person is not normally involved in the decision-making process. Team meetings are sometimes held to discuss the person/patient's progress, but ultimately it is again the doctor who makes the decision on the the next plan of action for the person/patient. In this type of environment, challenging the doctor's orders is seldom heard of.

Today the face of nursing is changing. Nursing knowledge, nursing models and philosophies are expanding, giving nurses a stronger theoretical base that should support them in positioning themselves in relation to delivering care (Davidson 1997). Nurses are gaining status from receiving pre- and post-registration education within a university setting. The requirement to provide evidence-based care, the legal and ethical responsibilities of the nurse, give nursing direction. However, these changes implicitly require nurses to question and challenge their own and others' practices every day of their working life. This can cause nurses great stress, particularly if they wish to challenge the decision of another professional or the person/patient.

Inter-professional working is more apparent within the child, learning disabilities and mental health care environment. Care is more frequently carried out in the community settings where inter-professional working is often evident. The Christopher Clunis Report (1994) and the Clothier Report (1994) highlighted the importance of inter-professional working and collaboration, clearly recommending and encouraging the development of inter-professional working strategies to enhance person/patient care by reducing the potential gaps in care and providing a more seamless approach. Within inter-professional working teams it is the team leader who takes ultimate responsibility for the planning of the clients' care. The team leader can be anyone involved in providing the person/patient's care – they could be a nurse, a psychologist, a care worker, a doctor, a physiotherapist, a clinical nurse specialist, . . . the list goes on. Working across professional boundaries is more readily carried out by the team members involved. Frequent inter-professional team meetings are held to discuss alternative care-management strategies and often a collaborative decision on the person/patient's care pathway is made. The teams hold briefing and de-briefing sessions regularly to provide support for all members of the team. The professional knowledge within the team is shared, for example, in the mental health care team it may be the psychologist who provides the care worker with some information or skills to support them in the delivery of client care. Clinical supervision was first introduced in mental health care provision, where in general the mixture of the teams in the community necessitates one professional to supervise another from a different professional background. The development and continuation of this has supported the inter-professional working relationships within this health care environment.

The move from a multi-disciplinary approach to an inter-disciplinary approach to care provision requires co-operation among the professionals who recognize the uniqueness of each individual member, where each member of the team is considered to be a colleague who adds value and experience to enhance the quality of care the person/patient experiences.

Many of the activities in this book are there to enhance the person/patient's care through developing an attitude of openness, receptivity to ideas, valuing and respect for others, and a willingness to share and take responsibility through empowerment of self and others – not only valuing your colleagues' contributions to care provision but also by valuing the person/patient's contribution, encouraging and supporting them to have an equal say in their care provision. This is an ideal that is inherent in the governmental philosophy of care provision, which is expressed in documents such as the Patients' Charter (1992) now superseded by *Your Guide to the NHS* (2001) and reinforced once again recently in the *NHS Plan* (2000).

For the remainder of the discussion in this chapter, when a colleague is mentioned we are referring to any member of the team that is involved in the provision of person/patient care.

Positive effects

What beneficial effects on work-related stress would be evident if colleague support was fully enacted in the work environment? Colleague support has the potential to alter positively the experience of stress in three identifiable ways. First, support from colleagues can have the direct effect of reducing or preventing stress itself. Second, colleague support can buffer the negative effects of stress. And third, it can function as a resource for coping.

Direct effects

Social support functions to lower the amount of perceived stress by encouraging a reappraisal of the situation. The actual perception of a situation as threatening or harmful can be altered by fellow-worker feedback and input. Take the example of death and dying, a commonly cited source of stress in nursing practice. While the presence of supportive nursing-staff relationships cannot change the harsh reality of death, it can mitigate some of the stressful aspects of such a loss. Death is frequently viewed as stress-producing because it often threatens nurses' sense of professional competence (see the definition of disempowerment above). An appraisal of death as a natural and expected part of life lessens the likelihood that death will be viewed as a failure. The realization that nurses are not personally responsible for a person/patient death from cancer, for example, is achievable through open, honest interaction with other nurses, during which the situation is re-defined. The reappraisal of the situation is a direct effect of social support on stress because it actually lowers the level of perceived stress (MacNeil and Weisz 1987; Mossholder *et al.* 1982; Norbeck 1985; Gray-Toft and Anderson 1983).

Buffering effects

Another result of colleague support on work-related stress is its mediating or buffering effect: colleague support reduces negative effects and consequences of stress. In exploring the relationship between social support and stress-related indices in nursing, it was found that colleague support helps to reduce negative factors such as role ambiguity (Gray-Toft and Anderson 1985); burnout (Cronin-Stubbs and Rooks 1985; Firth *et al.* 1986; Lee and Henderson 1996); accident and error rates among nurses (Gentry and Parkes 1982); and job dissatisfaction (Decker 1985) – all factors in the experience of disempowerment. A New South Wales study (Battersby *et al.* 1990) indicates that 'friendly nurses' are a major factor in determining whether nurses stay at or leave a particular hospital. The reported strength of the buffering effect of colleague support on work-related stress is less than the reported strength of its direct effects (LaRocco *et al.* 1980;

Norbeck 1985). That is, colleague support helps more with emotion-focused passive coping than problem-focused active coping.

Colleague support as a coping resource

Stress in the nursing work environment cannot always be reduced or moderated, and coping efforts are activated whenever stress is present (Lazarus and Folkman, 1984). The use of colleague support as a resource or avenue for coping is another way that social support in the work environment affects the stress process. Nurses report 'talking it out' as a frequently employed coping strategy (Cross and Kelly 1983; Oskins 1979), and adaptive coping is correlated to being able to admit feelings of stress to oneself and others (Chiriboga *et al.* 1983). Supportive colleague interactions offer ideal opportunities for this open expression of stress.

The example of death is again a useful one because of the potential to view this event as a threat or loss. Reflecting with colleagues provides a forum to discuss reactions and responses to people/patient deaths. Sharing thoughts and feelings related to grief is an essential aspect of coping with death. Other team members/colleagues are the most appropriate people with whom to share these reactions because they have the greatest potential to offer situation-specific support in dealing with death.

Negative effects

The view of colleagues as supportive is encouraging, even uplifting, but runs the risk of sounding naive and unrealistic without an acknowledgement that colleagues can also contribute to work-related stress in nursing practice.

Effective inter-professional working relationships with colleagues are a necessity in health-care provision because of the need for collaboration and team effort in most work situations. The interdependence created by this need to pull together has the potential to strain inter-professional relationships when nurses do not demonstrate that they operate from a similar value system. This aspect of colleague relationships is shown in a study of caring practices in nursing, in which it was highlighted that 'Fellow staff nurses on the unit are often the greatest source of comfort and support to an emotionally burdened nurse, yet one's colleagues can also provide a real source of frustration and disappointment when their actions are seen to indicate a lack of caring for the patients' (Forrest 1989: 818). This statement exemplifies conflicting expectations and value systems between nurses. In the absence of interdependence, this type of conflict would not be as evident. 'Supportive behaviours have a greater impact on employees who work on interdependent teams than those who work in relatively autonomous jobs' (LaRocco *et al.* 1980: 214).

Strained relationships and open conflict add stress to any working environment, but it is an absence of support rather than the presence of conflict that creates stress in inter-professional relationships in the health care environment. More often than not, it is support that is missing in colleague relationships that contributes to stress in nursing. Lack of support from supervisors, lack of feedback, lack of understanding in response to mistakes, and lack of colleague cohesion were all reported as factors that positively correlate to stress in nursing

(Dunn *et al.* 1994; Hipwell *et al.* 1989; Humphrey 1988; Linder-Pelz 1985; Ness 1982; Nichols *et al.* 1981; West and Rushton 1986). Nurses create stress for other nurses largely by failing to provide support when it is needed.

The following story, told by a recently registered nurse, highlights this lack of support:

> It's as if I'm not myself when I'm at work. I don't mean with the patients. I mean with my other colleagues. There were all these problems with the charge nurse when I first started. He wasn't liked by any of the other staff on the unit and he gave the new team members a really hard time, especially when we made mistakes.
>
> One time, I made an error in preparing a drug for a patient but, fortunately, the mistake was caught before I actually gave it to the patient. The charge nurse really reacted badly to this, and made me fill out all these incident reports. The nurse manager was notified and there was all this discussion about the new team members and what their role was. You would have thought nobody had ever made a mistake before. After all, it was bad enough that I almost hurt a patient and I dread even the thought of this ever happening.
>
> At any rate, at no time did I receive any understanding and support from the charge nurse. Some other members of the team confided to me that they thought he (the charge nurse) had over-reacted and the situation was blown out of all proportion. Mostly, they were thankful that it was me and not them.
>
> Other colleagues also used the situation as a means of complaining about the charge nurse and there was constant griping and backbiting going on about this incident and other things occurring on the ward. But nobody was really being honest and open about their reactions. I suppose that's why, in the end, I just kept quiet. I couldn't really trust anybody.
>
> On the one hand, nobody seemed to like or respect the charge nurse and, on the other hand, not one of my other colleagues openly supported me when the drug error happened. It is as if we are supposed to care about patients but it doesn't really matter how we treat each other.

This situation illustrates the potentially disastrous effects of an environment that is lacking support for other team members. Lack of support compounded the stress already being experienced by this new member of staff. The sad irony is that work-related stress on nurses is exacerbated when colleague support is absent, and colleague support is lacking when it is needed most – during times of increased stress. What is most disturbing is that colleague relationships add to stress, not necessarily by creating overt conflict, but by failing to provide needed support.

Most references to this lack of support in the above example specifies nursing managers and charge nurses, while less emphasis is placed on other team members' support. This is curious and could indicate that those with legitimate authority are expected to provide support, and there is perceived stress when it is not forthcoming. It could be that this is the case because most health-care organizations emphasize a hierarchical structure. Studies that have specifically explored supervisor support have indicated that support from those further up the hierarchy reduced stress-related factors such as role ambiguity (Gray-Toft and Anderson 1985), emotional exhaustion, depersonalization, and thoughts of leaving (Firth *et al.* 1986); job dissatisfaction and propensity to leave (Decker 1985). In addition, support from charge nurses' superiors (next up in the hierarchy) increased the support charge nurses demonstrated to the nursing staff on their wards (Firth *et al.* 1986). Supervisor support enhanced peer support by creating openness in work-group relationships (Gray-Toft and Anderson 1985). This suggests a domino effect of supportive interactions between nurses that would ideally filter to people/patients. When nurses are supported and nourished they are better able to support and nourish others. When nurses feel empowered themselves they feel more able to engage in empowering interactions with people/patients.

Added to the complexity of the relationship between stress in nursing and colleague interaction is the fact that poor colleague relationships is a sign of stress and burnout, and therefore could be an outcome of stress rather than a cause of it. The question that remains is whether poor colleague relationships are a cause of stress or its outcome (Bergagliotti and Trygstad, 1987). Either way, there is clearly a reciprocal relationship between colleague interaction and stress.

CONSTRAINTS IN DEVELOPING COLLEAGUE SUPPORT

The lack of colleague support raises questions about why and how this happens in a caring profession. Nurses risk losing their credibility as caring persons when caring for other members of the team is not apparent and active in their work environment. Nurses should be able to demonstrate support for colleagues and cultivate a nourishing work environment, but there are a variety of factors that inhibit these activities. Although these factors are not present in every work environment, identification of the constraints that do exist in their work environment is an initial step that nurses can take in dismantling them as barriers and decreasing their negative impact.

Lack of time

The most obvious of these constraints, and the one most likely to be cited by nurses, is a lack of time to demonstrate concern for other colleagues (Kavanagh 1989). When nurses are already over-burdened with the sheer demands of the workload, how could there possibly be time to help and support their peers? The limitation of time is often very real, but sometimes the perception of 'never any time' goes unchecked and unchallenged; for example, nurses frequently do find the time (or make the time?) to complain to each other about such things as working conditions, short staffing or manager insensitivity.

The time spent on complaining could be used to provide support to other nurses. Perhaps listening to a colleague's complaints is supportive – to a certain extent. Acknowledging another's perceptions through attentive listening can be helpful in and of itself. Frequently, however, complaints are used as springboards for the escalation of further complaints. The usefulness of this behaviour as a coping resource is questionable, as the outcome often lends itself to more feelings of discontent and an increase in stress levels. Listening to complaints for the purpose of clarifying real issues and seeking ways to address them is one helpful and supportive alternative.

The other constraint related to time is the perception that supporting others takes extra time. The validity of this in the work setting is questionable. The time it takes to offer words of understanding to a colleague is less than the time it takes to understand a stranger. Other team members already know their working colleagues, and the the person/patient care environment and work context is familiar. Empathy is easy to demonstrate under these circumstances because colleagues have shared experiences and meanings.

Repression of own needs

Even if adequate time is available, nurses may still fail to provide open support for each other because the recognition that nurses have needs challenges the image of selfless dedication to others. Nurses often repress their own needs and feelings, while focusing their efforts on the needs of others, in what is described as the 'burden of helping'. The strength of this self-sacrificing image is waning in modern nursing but runs the risk of being replaced by a detached and distanced professionalism, whereby the nurse projects an image of one who is in control, impenetrable and dispassionate. Both of these images result in a denial of nurses' own needs, feelings and human reactions.

Difficulty in disclosing

Is there really an outright denial that nurses do have needs and feelings, or is it just that these needs and feelings are not disclosed, especially to other nurses? An open, honest acknowledgement of feelings, such as uncertainty, sadness or confusion, is often avoided out of fear that it is a sign of personal weakness and an inability to cope. This prevents nurses from seeking and offering advice and comfort with colleagues, thus closing off all other coping options except denial.

Larson (1987) uncovered difficult thoughts and feelings nurses have about their work that are kept hidden from colleagues, because of discomfort in discussing them. These secrets include concerns such as: distancing oneself and then feeling guilty for having done so; fears of inadequacy and incompetence; angry reactions; feeling over-burdened by too many demands; wishing for a person/patient's death or feeling relief when a person/patient dies; and the desire to receive as well as give. These are understandable, even expected, reactions to the work nurses do, so there is no great surprise that these concerns exist.

It is unfortunate that such thoughts and feelings are actively concealed from colleagues, because other team members are in an ideal position to offer understanding, reassurance and guidance about these secret concerns. Presumably, they are kept secret because discussion of such feelings is considered unacceptable and unprofessional. After all, nurses cannot really admit to feeling inadequate because they are supposed to know what to do.

Overcoming fears of disclosing

More than likely, other nurses are experiencing or have experienced similar feelings and reactions, but this conspiracy of silence prevents these experiences from being shared. Keeping feelings hidden, especially fears, places nurses in the position of worrying alone and perpetuates the fallacy that, 'I am the only one who feels this way' or 'There must be something wrong with me'. There is comfort in knowing one is not alone, not the only one with fears, worries and negative reactions.

Other nurses provide a special and unique insider perspective that can challenge unrealistic fears and expectations and also allows coping options to be explored and developed. For example, if fears of incompetence and inadequacy stem from lack of knowledge, then this could be addressed through an informal sharing of knowledge or more formalized staff-development programmes. It is far better for nurses to acknowledge their feelings and reactions in a safe, accepting, supportive environment than to maintain a façade of immunity and control.

Organizational realities

Another constraint in the development of colleague support is the phenomenon of oppressed-group behaviour that has been observed in nursing (Roberts 1983). The constraints outlined in the previous section assume that colleague support is available but not forthcoming because it is not actively solicited, offered and used, while oppressed-group behaviour actually stifles the development of support between nurses. As such, it is far more insidious because it creates a disruptive climate within nursing groups and pits nurses against each other, thus destroying camaraderie and group cohesiveness. Understanding the dynamics of groups that are oppressed is essential if this negative phenomenon is to be reversed in the health-care environment.

Nurses often perceive themselves as powerless against a system that dominates them, shouldering great responsibility in health care organizations without a commensurate degree of authority. The dominant culture reveres technology and devalues caring (Benner and Wrubel 1989) and places curing as superior to caring. This oppression results in feelings of inferiority and creates the myth that the dominant group's value system and culture is 'right' and superior (Roberts 1983). In oppression there is an internalization of the dominant group's view of the world and a tendency within the oppressed group toward self-blame and rejection of their own values and culture as inferior. This leads to the development of a collective poor self-esteem within the group.

There are frustrations and complaints about the oppressor and the oppression, yet no direct action is taken. Instead, the anger that builds as a result of oppression is released on members of the group rather than on the oppressor, because there is less risk of consequences in fighting each other than there is in fighting the dominant group. Oppressed groups remain submissive to those who dominate them. The lateral violence within the group keeps the group divided, prevents cohesion and maintains the status quo (Roberts 1983). The only real challenges are those that occur within the group.

Blaming and scapegoating other nurses are evidence of the behaviour of oppression in nursing work environments (DeFeo 1987; Lartin 1988). As long as blame can be found, and it usually is found within the oppressed group, real issues are not addressed because the culprit, another nurse, has been targeted, and there is no need to delve further into what is behind the cause of problem.

Reversing the behaviour of oppression requires recognition that the culture and value system of the oppressed group is legitimate and worthy. Currently, the discipline of nursing is rediscovering its identity as that of *caring*, and this cultural re-awakening is a sign that the oppression in nursing is being addressed. The concept of the value of caring and caring practices holds great promise in helping nurses to celebrate their professional culture. It would naturally follow that nurses would also begin to demonstrate caring for their colleagues as part of this cultural re-awakening, not only because caring for each other would be highly regarded in a caring profession, but also because the professional self-esteem of nurses would be improved and heightened.

This caring culture places demands on the health-care system in which nurses work because 'caring as a concept is dependent on adequate time being available so that people/patients and nurses can interact' (Weaver 1990: 452) and the current system does not provide ample time for nurses and patients to connect (Fry 1988). These demands place stress on the system by upsetting the status quo, and nurses need to support each other in meeting these demands and coping with the stress they create. A recognition and valuing of the culture of nursing leads to the type of collegiality that is required if nurse–nurse support is to be fully developed and used. The inspirational words of Margretta Styles sum it up: 'Collegiality is as sacred as a vow; it is a solemn promise whereby we bind ourselves to those who share our cause, our convictions, our identity, our destiny' (Styles 1982: 143).

Other organizational issues that prevent effective colleague support need to be addressed (Kavanagh 1989). Limited reward systems that promote competition between nurses, over-dependence on the administrative hierarchy and even the method of patient care delivery (McMahon 1990), all affect colleague relationships and cannot be ignored. There is a risk in asking nurses to be supportive of each other if the organizational culture does not value this. Time and resources to facilitate support between nurses need to be accessed (Kavanagh 1989).

DEVELOPMENT OF COLLEAGUE SUPPORT

Creation of a climate of colleague support does not mean that nurses should spend most of their time focusing on the needs of other team members and counselling their colleagues; nor does it imply that nurses should express every emotion they experience. It means paving a way by which nurses can actively share their concerns and emotions generated by the job, and be heard and understood by their colleagues. To make this environment most effective in developing inter-professional relationships and collaborative working, the individuals involved in the team need to develop an awareness of each professional's role and consider the barriers they may have as individuals to other team members. Too often, professionals within disciplines are focused on their own 'work' of their particular practice and have limited awareness of the scope of practice of other providers or team members. This, according to Forbes and Fitzsimons (1993), develops a rivalry between the professions related to territorial concerns, traditional role concepts and lack of understanding of the complexities and contributions of the varied team members in the provision of care.

All of the skills described in Chapters 5–8 of this book would support the individual to effectively reduce some of that rivalry and the barriers to enable them to promote supportive relationships with colleagues. Use of these skills is not exclusive to person/patient–nurse interactions. Try carrying out some of the activities within the skills chapters, changing the focus from the person/patient to other professionals. What do you know or think about other health-care professionals? Do you know what their job entails? Do you know what professional guidelines they have? Do you understand what their aim for person/patient care provision is? Developing more awareness of your own inner thoughts and feelings about the ways in which you can work alongside other professionals, valuing them and being valued yourself, will enhance your ability to develop a supportive inter-professional working environment. The skills identified in this book, of being attentive, responsive, encouraging, understanding, and challenging are not skills that can be switched on and off at will. Enactment of these skills on a daily basis in the work environment creates a sound basis for the development of a supportive environment.

There are recommendations in the use of these skills that are specific to colleague interactions. The content of supportive discussions between health-care colleagues needs to focus on specific *work-related* difficulties and the emotions they engender (Gray-Toft and Anderson 1983; Llewelyn and Payne 1995). These are related to the individual personalities of the professional, but are not personal problems *per se*. Reflective listening clarifies these difficulties and emotions, and promotes mutual understanding, but it alone is not sufficient in providing effective colleague support.

Challenging is needed in the case of colleague support (Richman 1988) because it offers new perspectives, reframes existing perspectives, spurs health care professionals on to improve their work, and helps to overcome obstacles to meeting goals. Challenging can only be effective in a general climate of trust and openness, and requires an ability to be assertive. Trust is promoted within teams when individual differences are tolerated and feedback is given directly and honestly. Conflict is not absent within this climate, but these conditions establish a context in which effective resolution of conflict can occur. A supportive work environment for health-care professionals is one in which each individual is:

- Acknowledged
- Validated
- Respected
- Listened to
- Accepted
- Understood
- Encouraged
- Challenged
- Offered feedback
- Appreciated
- Assisted.

A supportive environment is responsive to the individual's needs if, and when, colleague support is requested and received. Another member of the health-care team may indicate the need for support directly or indirectly, and his/her team members are in a prime position to respond to the cues indicating a need for support.

The following example, provided by a newly registered nurse in the field of learning disabilities, offers some insight into the benefits of responding to such cues: the terms 'supportive living environment' and 'tenants' are the terms currently used in learning-disabilities care because these people are not patients but a group who need some support to live normally within today's society.

I had been working for about six months, the whole time in a supported care environment. I was working one evening with another experienced nurse from a learning disability care background. I always liked it when I worked with Ruth because she knew what she was doing and helped me whenever I needed it.

This particular evening was busy but not really hectic. One of the tenants had become really upset while on an outing and attempted to jump in front of a moving car. As a result, all of the tenants on the outing returned to the supportive care environment early. I can't recall exactly what had upset her, but I was staying with her in her room, providing close one-to-one support.

Ruth was busy ensuring the other tenants were getting their dinner in the room next to me. Then the tenant I was with had a *grand mal* seizure. I had seen and even managed a few seizures prior to this, and although a bit scared, basically knew what to do. Everything was pretty much as it usually is during a seizure, but then something strange and frightening began to happen.

The seizure hadn't stopped, wouldn't stop, and seemed to go on for an interminable time. The tenant stopped breathing and began to turn blue. I began to panic inside, but kept my head while I opened her airway in the way I'd been instructed to do. I remember thinking to myself, 'CO_2 needs to build up in order to kick in the breathing response. That *is* what I learnt, isn't it?' I checked for a pulse. It was present.

After what felt like an eternity, the tenant began breathing spontaneously. It was funny because it was at this point that I began to panic openly. I shouted for Ruth and she was there in a flash, asking me what was happening. I quickly explained while we positioned the tenant and made her comfortable. Ruth stayed with the tenant and told me to go and call the doctor. In the end it all worked out. The tenant was OK but I ended up feeling terrible. Later, in the office, while Ruth and I were documenting the occurrence in the tenant's records, I suddenly blurted out, 'I handled that situation so badly. I was scared, panicked, and had to call you. I don't think I'll ever make a good nurse.'

Ruth looked at me and said, 'What do you mean?'

'Well, I couldn't manage alone. I called you', I replied.

She said, 'It seemed perfectly reasonable to me, you did everything correctly, and the whole thing was pretty frightening.' Then she turned toward me, looked me straight in the eye, and added, 'Anyway, who ever told you that you were Superwoman?'

I looked at her a bit sheepishly and said, 'Me?'

We both laughed, then had a chat, reflecting on the situation step-by-step, with Ruth reinforcing my clinical judgement and actions. She said had it been her in that room, she would have called out for me as well, especially if I was just next door. I mean, it's not like I abandoned the tenant and ran down the hall.

Ruth probably never realized just how much she helped that evening. Her comment about Superwoman was right on target. It challenged me to think about my expectations of myself. Her comment still echoes in my ears whenever I get caught up in those unreal expectations. I think every nurse should have a Ruth to remind her that she can't be Superwoman.

This story illustrates a caring, concerned and helpful response from an experienced nurse to a newly registered nurse. Ruth's reactions were based on an understanding of the situation and an awareness of this newly registered nurse's needs. She supported her by affirming her clinical actions, but challenged her at the same time to reconsider her expectations. This demonstrates support by offering an alternative perspective, a reappraisal of the situation. Ruth could have been supportive by just saying, 'You did the right thing, you handled the situation correctly, knew what to do and did it'. While this might have sufficed, she enhanced the support by using the situation to help the new graduate learn from it. The lesson stayed with this member of staff, probably throughout her career, and helped to ease some of her stress in future situations. The power of colleague support cannot be underestimated.

This example provides a sound rationale for the continued development of preceptorship role for nurses. The Nursing and Midwifery Council (2003) advocate that the support and guidance of an experienced practitioner is invaluable to newly registered, or returning-to-practice nurses. They advise that all newly registered nurses should have a period of support and guidance – this they refer to as a period of 'preceptorship', where a named person who is an experienced practitioner will advise and support the new member of staff for an agreed period of time.

CHAPTER SUMMARY

A necessary backdrop to supportive inter-professional working relationships and good communication is a working environment that acknowledges and validates each member of the team as a person, and is responsive to each individuals' reactions, feelings, anxieties, and confusions. Interpersonal skills training is unlikely to be successful unless there is active support for health-care professionals who employ these skills (Fielding and Llewelyn 1987). Health-care professionals cannot be expected to give of themselves without such support, from other working colleagues and the health-care organization that employs them, because work-related stress and disempowerment are addressed most effectively in the work environment.

REFERENCES

Annandale, E., Clark, J. and Allen, E. (1999). Interprofessional working: an ethnographic case study of emergency health care. *Journal of Interprofessional Care*, 13, 139–50.

Barnes, M. and Battersby, R. (2001). *Taking Over the Asylum: Empowerment and Mental Health*. UK: Palgrave.

Battersby, D., Hemmings, L., Kermode, S., Sutherland, S. and Cox, J. (1990). *Factors Influencing the Turnover and Retention of Registered Nurses in New South Wales Hospitals.* Sydney: New South Wales College of Nursing.

Benner, P. and Wrubel, J. (1989). *The Primacy of Caring: Stress and Coping in Health and Illness.* Menlo Park, CA: Addison-Wesley.

Bergagliotti, L. A. and Trygstad, L. N. (1987). Differences in stress and coping findings: a reflection of social realities or methodologies? *Nursing Research*, 36(3), 170–3.

Chiriboga, D. A., Jenkins, G. and Baily, J. (1983). Stress and coping among hospice nurses: test of an analytic model. *Nursing Research*, 32(5), 294–9.

Clothier, C., MacDonald, C. A. and Shaw, D. A. (1994) *The Allitt Inquiry: Independent Inquiry Relating to Deaths and Injuries on the Children's Ward at Grantham and Kesteven General Hospital During the Period February to April 1991.* London: HMSO.

Cronin-Stubbs, D. and Rooks, C. A. (1985). The stress, social support, and burnout of critical care nurses: the results of research. *Heart & Lung*, 14(1), 31–9.

Cross, D. G. and Kelly, J. G. (1983). Stress and coping strategies in hospitals: a comparison of ICU and ward nurses. *The Australian Nurses Journal*, 13(2), 43–6.

Davidson, B. (1997). The role of the psychiatric nurse. In P. J. Barker and B. Davidson (eds), *Psychiatric Nursing: The Ethical Goalposts.* London: Edward Arnold.

Decker, F. H. (1985). Socialization and interpersonal environment in nurses affective reactions to work. *Social Science and Medicine*, 20(5), 449–509.

DeFeo, D. (1987). The hunt for the really bad nurse. *American Journal of Nursing*, 87(2), 270.

Department of Health (1989). *Caring for People: Community Care in the Next Decade and Beyond.* London: HMSO.

Department of Health (1998). *A First Class Service: Quality in the New NHS.* London: HMSO.

Department of Health (2000). *The NHS Plan: A Plan for Investment, a Plan for Reform.* London: HMSO.

Department of Health (2001). *Your Guide to the NHS.* London: Department of Health, Crown Copyright.

Dunn, L. A., Rout, U., Carson, J. and Ritter, S. A. (1994). Occupational stress amongst care staff working in nursing homes: an empirical investigation. *Journal of Clinical Nursing*, 3, 177–83.

Fielding, R. G. and Llewelyn, S. P. (1987). Communication training in nursing may damage your health and enthusiasm: some warnings. *Journal of Advanced Nursing*, 12, 821–9.

Firth, H., McIntee, J., McKeown, P. and Britton, P. (1986). Interpersonal support amongst nurses. *Journal of Advanced Nursing*, 11, 273–82.

Forbes, E. J. and Fitzsimons, V. (1993). The key for holistic interdisciplinary collaboration. *Holistic Nursing Practice*, 7(4), 1–10.

Forrest, D. (1989). The experience of caring. *Journal of Advanced Nursing*, 14, 815–23.

Fry, S. (1988) The ethics of caring: can it survive nursing? *Nursing Outlook*, 36(1), 8.

Gentry, W. D. and Parkes, K. R. (1982). Psychological stress in intensive care unit and non-intensive care unit nursing: a review of the past decade. *Heart & Lung*, 11(1), 43–7.

Gray-Toft, P. A. and Anderson, J. G. (1981). Stress among hospital nursing staff: its causes and effects. *Social Science and Medicine*, 15A, 639–47.

Gray-Toft, P. A. and Anderson, J. G. (1983). A hospital staff support program: design and evaluation. *International Journal of Nursing Studies*, 20(3), 137–47.

Gray-Toft, P. A. and Anderson, J. G. (1985). Organizational stress in the hospital: development of a model for diagnosis and prediction. *Health Services Research*, 19(6), 753–74.

Hipwell, A. E., Tyler, P. A. and Wilson, C. M. (1989). Sources of stress and dissatisfaction among nurses in four hospital environments. *British Journal of Medical Psychology*, 62, 71–9.

Humphrey, J. H. (1988). *Stress in the Nursing Profession*. Springfield, IL: Charles C. Thomas.

Irvine, D. M. and Evans, M. G. (1996). Job satisfaction and turnover among nurses: integrating research findings across studies. *Nursing Research*, 44(4), 246–53.

Kavanagh, K. H. (1989). Nurses' networks: obstacles and challenge. *Archives of Psychiatric Nursing*, 3(4), 226–33.

Kushnir, T., Rabin, S. and Azulai, S. (1997). A descriptive study of stress management in a group of pediatric oncology nurses. *Cancer Nursing*, 20, 414–21.

LaRocco, J. M., House, J. S. and French, J. R. P. (1980). Social support, occupational stress, and health. *Journal of Health and Social Behaviour*, 21, 202–18.

Larson, D. G. (1987). Helper secrets. *Journal of Psychosocial Nursing*, 25(4), 20–6.

Lartin, J. M. (1988). Scapegoating: identifying and reversing the process. *Journal of Nursing Administration*, 18(9), 25–31.

Lazarus, R. S. and Folkman, S. (1984). *Stress, Appraisal and Coping*. New York: Springer.

Lee, V. and Henderson, M. C. (1996). Occupational stress and organizational commitment in nurse administrators. *Journal of Nursing Administration*, 26(5), 21–8.

Linder-Pelz, S. (1985). Occupational stressors and stress levels among Australian nurses: a review of research. *The Journal of Occupational Health and Safety – Australia and New Zealand*, 1(1), 9–15.

Llewelyn, S. and Payne, S. (1995). Caring: the costs to nurses and relatives. In A. Broome and S. Llewelyn (eds), *Health Psychology: Processes and Applications*, second edition (pp. 109–22). London: Chapman and Hall.

MacNeil, J. M. and Weisz, G. M. (1987). Critical care nursing stress: another look. *Heart & Lung*, 16(3), 274–7.

McMahon, R. (1990). Power and collegial relations among nurses on wards adopting primary nursing and hierarchical ward management structures. *Journal of Advanced Nursing*, 15, 232–9.

Mossholder, K. W., Bedeian, A. G. and Armenakis, A. A. (1982). Group process – work outcome relationships: a note on the moderating impact of self-esteem. *Academy of Management Journal*, 25(3), 575–85.

Ness, A. (1982). Stress: its effect on registered nurses and patient care. *The Australian Nurses Journal*, 12(1), 47–8.

Nichols, K. A., Springford, V. and Searle, J. (1981). An investigation of distress and discontent in various types of nursing. *Journal of Advanced Nursing*, 6, 311–18.

Nursing and Midwifery Council (2003) *Preceptorship*. London: NMC Publications.

Norbeck, J. S. (1985). Types and sources of social support for managing job stress in critical care nursing. *Nursing Research*, 34(4), 225–30.

Norbeck, J. S., Lindsey, A. M. and Carrieri, V. L. (1981). The development of an instrument to measure social support. *Nursing Research*, 30(5), 264–9.

Oskins, S. L. (1979). Identification of situational stressors and coping methods by intensive care nurses. *Heart & Lung*, 8(5), 953–60.

QAA (2001) *Benchmarking Academic and Practitioner Standards in Health Care Subjects*. Bristol: Quality Assurance Agency for Higher Education.

Reeves, S., Meyer, J., Glynn, M. and Bridges, J. (1999). Coordination of interprofessional health care teams in a general and emergency directorate. *Advanced Clinical Nursing*, 3, 49–59.

Richman, J. M. (1988). Social support groups. *Journal of Nursing Administration*, 18(2) 3–19

Ritchie, J. H., Dick, D. and Lingham, R. (1994). *Report of the Inquiry into the Care and Treatment of Christopher Clunis*. London: HMSO.

Roberts, S. J. (1983). Oppressed group behaviour: implications for nursing. *Advances in Nursing Science*, 5, 21–31.

Ryle, S. M. (1999). A concept analysis of empowerment: its relationship to mental health nursing. *Journal of Advanced Nursing*, 29, 600–7.

Salvage, J. (1988). Professionalisation – or struggle for survival? A consideration of current proposals for the reform of nursing in the UK. *Journal of Advanced Nursing*, 13, 515–19.

Salvage, J. (1990). The theory and practice of 'new nursing'. *Nursing Times*, 86, 4.

Salvage, J. (1992). The new nursing: empowering patients or empowering nurse? In J. Robinson, A. Gray and R. Elkan (eds), *Policy Issues in Nursing*. Buckingham: Open University Press.

Snape, J. and Cavanagh, S. J. (1993). Occupational stress in neurosurgical nursing. *Intensive and Critical Care Nursing*, 9(3), 162–70.

Styles, M. M. (1982). *On Nursing: Toward a New Endowment*. St Louis, MS: Mosby.

Tyler, P. A., Carroll, D. and Cunningham, S. E. (1991). Stress and well-being in nurses: a comparison of the public and private sectors. *International Journal of Nursing Studies*, 28, 125–30.

Weaver, D. (1990). Cost-effective use of professional resources: a pivotal time for nurse administrators. In N. Chaska (ed.), *The Nursing Profession: Turning Points*. St Louis, MS: Mosby.

West, M. and Rushton, R. (1986). The drop-out factor. *Nursing Times*, 82, 31 December, 29–31.

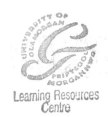